Nutrition and Diet Research Progress

Broccoli: Cultivation, Nutritional Properties and Effects on Health

NUTRITION AND DIET RESEARCH PROGRESS

Additional books in this series can be found on Nova's website under the Series tab.

Additional e-books in this series can be found on Nova's website under the e-book tab.

NUTRITION AND DIET RESEARCH PROGRESS

BROCCOLI: CULTIVATION, NUTRITIONAL PROPERTIES AND EFFECTS ON HEALTH

BERNHARD H. J. JUURLINK
EDITOR

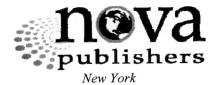

Copyright © 2016 by Nova Science Publishers, Inc.

All rights reserved. No part of this book may be reproduced, stored in a retrieval system or transmitted in any form or by any means: electronic, electrostatic, magnetic, tape, mechanical photocopying, recording or otherwise without the written permission of the Publisher.

We have partnered with Copyright Clearance Center to make it easy for you to obtain permissions to reuse content from this publication. Simply navigate to this publication's page on Nova's website and locate the "Get Permission" button below the title description. This button is linked directly to the title's permission page on copyright.com. Alternatively, you can visit copyright.com and search by title, ISBN, or ISSN.

For further questions about using the service on copyright.com, please contact:
Copyright Clearance Center
Phone: +1-(978) 750-8400   Fax: +1-(978) 750-4470   E-mail: info@copyright.com.

NOTICE TO THE READER

The Publisher has taken reasonable care in the preparation of this book, but makes no expressed or implied warranty of any kind and assumes no responsibility for any errors or omissions. No liability is assumed for incidental or consequential damages in connection with or arising out of information contained in this book. The Publisher shall not be liable for any special, consequential, or exemplary damages resulting, in whole or in part, from the readers' use of, or reliance upon, this material. Any parts of this book based on government reports are so indicated and copyright is claimed for those parts to the extent applicable to compilations of such works.

Independent verification should be sought for any data, advice or recommendations contained in this book. In addition, no responsibility is assumed by the publisher for any injury and/or damage to persons or property arising from any methods, products, instructions, ideas or otherwise contained in this publication.

This publication is designed to provide accurate and authoritative information with regard to the subject matter covered herein. It is sold with the clear understanding that the Publisher is not engaged in rendering legal or any other professional services. If legal or any other expert assistance is required, the services of a competent person should be sought. FROM A DECLARATION OF PARTICIPANTS JOINTLY ADOPTED BY A COMMITTEE OF THE AMERICAN BAR ASSOCIATION AND A COMMITTEE OF PUBLISHERS.

Additional color graphics may be available in the e-book version of this book.

Library of Congress Cataloging-in-Publication Data

ISBN: 978-1-63484-313-3

Library of Congress Control Number: 2015957368

Published by Nova Science Publishers, Inc. † New York

This book is dedicated to Professor Paul Talalay, the John Jacob Abel Distinguished Service Professor of Pharmacology at the Johns Hopkins University School of Medicine. His research, together with that of his students and colleagues, has made an enormous impact on the field of nutrigenomics and thereby giving a scientific basis to the Hippocratic dictum "Let food be your medicine and medicine your food."

Contents

Preface		ix
Chapter 1	Paul Talalay: The Catalyst *Teresa L. Johnson*	1
Chapter 2	Glucosinolates and their Distribution *Sabine Montaut and Patrick Rollin*	9
Chapter 3	Glucoraphanin and Other Glucosinolates in Heads of Broccoli Cultivars *Mark W. Farnham and Sandra E. Branham*	33
Chapter 4	The Xenobiotic Elimination System: An Overview *Jane Alcorn*	47
Chapter 5	Cellular Redox, Aging and Diet *Lida Sadeghinejad, Hossein Noyan and Bernhard H. J. Juurlink*	87
Chapter 6	The Nrf2 Signalling System *Bernhard H. J. Juurlink*	111
Chapter 7	Quercetin and Kaempferol Ameliorate Inflammation through NRF2 and Other Signaling Pathways *Sarah E. Galinn and Petra A. Tsuji*	121
Chapter 8	Radiomitigating Potential of Sulforaphane, a Constituent of Broccoli *Paban K. Agrawala and Omika Katoch*	145
Chapter 9	Broccoli Sprout Supplementation As a Novel Method for Preventing Perinatal Brain Injury *Jerome Y. Yager, Antoinette T. Nguyen, Jennifer Corrigan, Ashley M. A. Bahry, Ann-Marie Przyslupski and Edward A. Armstrong*	161

Contents

Chapter 10	The Multifaceted Role of Sulforaphane in Protection against UV Radiation-Mediated Skin Damage *Andrea L. Benedict, Elena V. Knatko, Rumen V. Kostov, Ying Zhang, Maureen Higgins, Sukirti Kalra, Jed W. Fahey, Sally H. Ibbotson, Charlotte M. Proby, Paul Talalay and Albena T. Dinkova-Kostova*	185
Chapter 11	Preclinical Studies on the Effect of Sulforaphane on Cardiovascular Disease and Fetal Determinants of Adult Health *Ali Banigesh and Bernhard H. J. Juurlink*	209
Chapter 12	Beneficial Effects of Broccoli Sprouts and Its Bioactive Compound Sulforaphane in Management of Type 2 Diabetes *Zahra Bahadoran and Parvin Mirmiran*	225
Chapter 13	Human Clinical Studies Involving Sulforaphane/Glucoraphanin *Bernhard H. J. Juurlink*	239
Chapter 14	Broccoli Cultivation in Warmer Climates *Karistsapol Nooprom*	251
Chapter 15	Broccoli: Agricultural Characteristics, Health Benefits and Post-Harvest Processing on Glucosinolate Content *Olga Nydia Campas-Baypoli, Ernesto Uriel Cantú-Soto and José Antonio Rivera-Jacobo*	263
Chapter 16	Broccoli: Nutritional Aspects, Health Benefits and Postharvest Conservation *José Guilherme Prado Martin, Natalia Dallocca Berno and Marta Helena Fillet Spoto*	283
Chapter 17	Innovative Industrial Cooking of Broccoli for Improving Health-Promoting Compounds *Ginés Benito Martínez–Hernández, Perla A. Gómez, Francisco Artés–Hernández and Francisco Artés*	299
Index		**335**

PREFACE

Hippocrates said: "Let food be your medicine and medicine your food." Until recently, this phrase has been essentially a mantra with little scientific support. We are now just beginning to understand how food and food constituents affect gene expression and thereby health. This is the area of research known as nutrigenomics. This book is about nutrigenomics, with a focus on some of the bioactive compounds found in broccoli. This book presents some scientific background to readers interested in nutrigenomics.

Many decades ago, Professor Paul Talalay together with his students and colleagues followed up on the observations of Lee Wattenberg that phytochemicals in our diet can decrease the probability of cancer formation. He and his colleagues were instrumental in discovering that many of these compounds were monofunctional inducers of phase 2 enzymes. They further played important roles in identifying the mechanisms whereby such compounds activate the transcription factor nuclear factor (erythroid-derived-2)-like 2 (Nrf2) resulting in the transcription of multiple genes, the protein products of most of these genes increase the endogenous capacity of cells to inactivate oxidants (including many carcinogens) or decrease the probability of producing strong oxidants. They also identified certain isothiocyanates (especially sulforaphane) metabolites of glucosinolates found in crucifers as potent activators of the Nrf2 signalling system. Paul Talalay and colleagues also identified the sprouts (germinated seeds) of certain cultivars of broccoli as being very rich sources of sulforaphane glucosinolate (glucoraphanin). This research has inspired other researchers such as Professor Richard Mithen of the UK Institute of Food Research to develop broccoli cultivars rich in sulforaphane glucosinolate. Furthermore, Professor Talalay and colleagues have chemically characterized a wide variety of phytochemicals that activate the Nrf2 signalling system. As pointed out in Chapter One, Professor Talalay's research has acted as a catalyst and has had major impacts on numerous laboratories around the world—including mine—in the area of nutrigenomics. This book is dedicated to Professor Paul Talalay to acknowledge his contribution to the field of nutrigenomics.

The organization of this volume is such that readers with only some background in phytochemicals and nutrition can get maximal benefit. The first chapter outlines some of the history of the ground-breaking nutrigenomic research by Professor Talalay and colleagues. Since major bioactive compounds found in broccoli are metabolites of glucosinolates, the next two chapters discuss glucosinolates in general (Chapter Two) and glucosinolate distribution in broccoli cultivars specifically (Chapter Three). Understanding xenobiotic metabolism is important in understanding how consumption of broccoli can affect metabolism. The reason behind this is that Nrf2 activators increase the expression of phase 2 enzymes involved in xenobiotic metabolism as well as phase 3 molecular transporters involved in the export of products of phase 2 enzyme actions, and inhibit the enzymatic activity of certain phase 1 enzymes. Xenobiotic metabolism is outlined in Chapter Four.

Oxidative stress and associated inflammation underlies many of the chronic diseases associated with aging; hence, Chapter Five outlines the role of oxidative stress on inflammation and aging, and sets the background on how Nrf2 activators can influence chronic disease. Many readers will have had little introduction to the Nrf2 signalling pathway and for them an introduction to Nrf2 signalling has been written in Chapter Six. Flavonoids, also found in broccoli, can influence the activation states of Nrf2 and influence other signaling pathways. They can also induce the expression of many phase 1 genes, whose protein products initiate xenobiotic metabolism. This is the rationale for basing Chapter Seven on flavonoids with a focus on quercetin and kaempferol, the dominant flavonoids found in broccoli.

Chapters Eight through Eleven of the book outline a number of preclinical studies examining the effects of sulforaphane on mitigating the effects of x-irradiation and UV irradiation, as well as mitigating prenatal brain injury. This is followed by Chapters Twelve and Thirteen, which review the human clinical trials that have been carried out with sulforaphane and/or glucoraphanin. Chapters Fourteen through Seventeen deal with agronomic aspects of broccoli cultivation, including post-harvest processing as well as how cooking affects the health-promoting phytochemicals found in broccoli.

I trust that this book will be most useful for the reader. I do end with a caveat: Not all broccoli cultivars are equal. Broccoli can contain a variety of glucosinolates, some glucosinolate species may yield goitrogenic metabolites (see Chapter Two). In general, goitrogenic glucosinolates are much lower in three-day-old broccoli sprouts than in mature plants, but there are exceptions. Three-day-old broccoli sprouts also typically have ten times the amount of glucosinolates/g tissue than mature broccoli. Broccoli sprout cultivars with high glucoraphanin content and low goitrogenic glucosinolates include Saga, Calabrese and the Hopkins cultivar trade-marked as 'BroccoSprouts.' Dr. Richard Mithen's research group has developed broccoli cultivar hybrids that have elevated glucoraphanin (two to three times that of standard hybrids) in the mature plant: these are marketed under the trade name 'Beneforté.' If one is to greatly increase one's consumption of broccoli, this should only consist of cultivars that are low in goitrogenic glucosinolates.

Finally, I thank Dr. Jed Fahey for suggestions on authors and chapters for this book.

Bernhard H. J. Juurlink, PhD
Professor emeritus, Department of Anatomy & Cell Biology
College of Medicine, University of Saskatchewan

In: Broccoli
Editor: Bernhard H. J. Juurlink

ISBN: 978-1-63484-313-3
© 2016 Nova Science Publishers, Inc.

Chapter 1

PAUL TALALAY: THE CATALYST

Teresa L. Johnson[*]
The Johns Hopkins University, Baltimore, MD, US

ABSTRACT

This chapter outlines the history of the groundbreaking chemopreventive research carried out by Dr. Paul Talalay and colleagues. This research has led to clinical trials examining the ability of Nrf2-activating compounds to ameliorate problems of oxidative stress, inflammation, and environmental pollutants. Such trials are anticipated to have a major impact in decreasing the burden of chronic diseases.

Keywords: broccoli, glucosinolate, isothiocyanate, sulforaphane, phase 2 enzymes

INTRODUCTION

The first era of nutrition research centered on the amelioration of deficiency-related diseases, providing robust, mechanistic insights into the physiological functions of macro- and micronutrients, and culminating in a series of evidence-based public health recommendations. In recent decades, however, a new era of nutrition research has emerged from data demonstrating specific molecular roles for non-nutrient, plant-derived dietary compounds that influence cellular signaling and gene expression, thereby providing protection against cellular injury and aging. The proposal of this concept, termed "chemoprotection," signaled a watershed event in nutritional research history, and provided a springboard for many arms of inquiry on bioactive plant-derived compounds. In particular, it led to the understanding of the molecular mechanisms that upregulate cellular cytoprotective proteins.

---

[*] Corresponding author: Teresa L. Johnson, The Johns Hopkins University, Baltimore, MD, US. E-mail:: tjohn143@jhu.edu, teresa@foodsynergies.net.

The impetus for these revolutionary ideas emerged in the mid 1960s, when University of Minnesota researcher Lee Wattenberg published a provocative paper in *Cancer Research* in which he described the beneficial effects of certain compounds on carcinogenesis, challenging earlier paradigms about cancer prevention, and raising the possibility that cancer could be thwarted [1]. The ensuing investigations demonstrated that phenolic antioxidants—in particular, the commonly used food preservatives butylated hydroxyanisole, butylated hydroxytoluene, and ethoxyquin—abrogated the carcinogenic effects of a diverse array of structurally unrelated compounds in animal models through enhancement of cells' capacity to increase their intrinsic chemoprotective potential [2].

Wattenberg's work (as well as others') suggested that chemical inhibition of carcinogenesis was achievable: The body's own protective mechanisms were accessible, and could be tapped—even enhanced—to reduce disease risk [3]. Although much of the scientific community understood that human cancers were caused by environmental, nutritional, and exogenous factors, many still considered cancer unavoidable, and the feasibility of its prevention far-fetched; nevertheless, Wattenberg's insights spurred a new emphasis on disease prevention.

A decade later, Paul Talalay, then director of the Department of Pharmacology at the Johns Hopkins University, turned his attention toward mediating the mutagenic effects of pharmaceutical agents, including several antischistosomal drugs. Inspired by (but skeptical about) Wattenberg's observations, Talalay and his colleagues expanded upon Wattenberg's work, focusing their investigations on other antioxidant compounds that might similarly boost cells' intrinsic defensive responses. Earlier investigators had noted that these cellular responses varied, were often non-sequential, and yielded different outcomes, not all of which were favorable—characteristic of the non-linear nature of xenobiotic detoxification, mediated by phase 1 and phase 2 drug-metabolizing enzymes, such as the cytochrome P-450 family of enzymes, or the glutathione S-transferases, respectively. Under Talalay's guidance, a multidisciplinary, collaborative approach soon yielded that considerable protection against chemical carcinogenesis could be achieved by induction of these enzymes responsible for carcinogen metabolism [4].

The child of Russian immigrants, Talalay was born in 1923, in Berlin, Germany. When Talalay was 10 years old, he and his family fled Nazi rule, landing first in France, then Belgium. The family eventually settled in London, England, where Talalay attended Bedford School, an all boys private school whose core values—integrity, responsibility, endeavor, and curiosity—would come to summarize his life and career. The years at Bedford also laid the groundwork for Talalay's future academic success, sparking a profound interest in science. Talalay is one of many illustrious "Old Bedfordians," notable alumni that include British politician Paddy Ashdown and Nobel Prize-winning chemist Archer Martin [5].

Talalay's fortuitous arrival in the United States came in July 1940, just two months prior to commencement of the London Blitz. He continued to pursue his scientific interests, earning his undergraduate degree in biophysics from Massachusetts Institute of Technology, and a medical degree from Yale University.

After serving two years as a general surgeon at Massachusetts General Hospital—a brief dalliance in clinical practice that profoundly influenced his research perspective—Talalay began working at the University of Chicago's Ben May Laboratory for Cancer Research. There he focused on the intersection of enzymology, steroid metabolism, and cancer treatment under the mentorship of the late Charles Huggins. In 1963, Talalay became professor and director of the Department of Pharmacology at the Johns Hopkins University. He stepped down from the directorship in 1974, and has remained at Johns Hopkins as the John Jacob Abel Distinguished Service Professor of Pharmacology and Molecular Sciences [3].

Talalay's extensive grounding in enzymology elucidated much of the work that was to come, and illuminated the critical physiological roles of the glutathione S-transferases, a family of phase 2 enzymes that drive glutathione conjugation via sulfhydryl groups to an array of endogenous and exogenous electrophilic compounds to facilitate their subsequent detoxification and elimination. Principally, glutathione conjugation serves as the inaugural event in the mercapturic acid pathway, and marshals a cascade of events critical in the protection of cellular macromolecules from electrophilic attack and oxidative stress, thus mediating the metabolic inactivation of proximate and ultimate carcinogens or mutagens [4].

Talalay and his colleagues noted that basal concentrations of hepatic and extrahepatic glutathione S-transferases typically are high, upregulate substantially when induced, and demonstrate an absolute requirement for glutathione [6]. Evidence mounted that other phase 2 antioxidant enzymes, including epoxide hydrolase, glucuronosyltransferases, heme oxygenase, and NADPH:quinone oxidoreductase 1 (NQO1), are similarly upregulated. NQO1, in particular, exhibits broad specificity, widespread distribution, and an ability to catalyze obligate two-electron quinone reduction [7]. As such, it demonstrates a significant local protective role in cells as it facilitates glucuronide and sulfate conjugation for subsequent conjugate elimination from the cell. Later work would reveal NQO1's "gatekeeping" roles, including its propensity to bind to and stabilize the tumor suppressor protein p53 against proteasomal degradation, serving a sentinel cytoprotective role [8].

By the early 1980s, Talalay and his colleagues provided evidence that the regulation of phase 1 and phase 2 enzymes was a function of a wide array of seemingly unrelated anticarcinogenic inducers, classified as either bifunctional or monofunctional inducers. The bifunctional inducers (e.g., 2,3,7,8-tetrachlorodibenzo-p-dioxin, polycyclic aromatic hydrocarbons, azo dyes, and naphthoflavone) promote the activities of both phase 1 and phase 2 enzymes, while monofunctional inducers (e.g., diphenols, thiocarbamates, isothiocyanates) stimulate only phase 2 enzymes. Whereas bifunctional inducers tend to be large planar aromatic molecules, monofunctional inducers share little structural concordance [9]. Since phase 1 enzymes promote activation of carcinogens to their more reactive forms, Talalay posited that monofunctional inducers are more promising candidates than bifunctional inducers as anticarcinogens [10].

Soon, three salient characteristics of chemoprotective enzyme inducers emerged: 1) the capacity for monofunctional rather than bifunctional induction; 2) the ability to raise phase 2 enzyme activity in multiple tissues; and 3) low toxicity (as evidenced by their widespread presence in foods or in living matter). This latter feature reduced the need for toxicity testing prior to clinical trials—a notable plus [11]. Quantitative assays already in use in Talalay's lab enabled the identification of a vast array of monofunctional inducers of cytoprotective proteins, including Michael reaction acceptors, diphenols, quinones, isothiocyanates, peroxides, vicinal dimercaptans, heavy metals, arsenicals, and others [12]. Typically, inducers exhibit electrophilicity, and thus serve as substrates for glutathione S-transferases. Increased intracellular glutathione levels accompany their induction, which enhances cellular protection [10].

Advances in cell culture techniques led to the development of a simple screening method for rapidly detecting and identifying anticarcinogenic components in human diets [13]. Evidence from epidemiological studies and animal feeding studies had indicated that high consumption of yellow and green vegetables, especially cruciferous vegetables, reduces cancer risk, suggesting vegetables were potential sources of inducer activity [14]. A systematic bioassay of several organically grown vegetables and fruits measured phase 2 enzyme induction, gauged inducer toxicity, and distinguished between monofunctional and bifunctional inducers. The breakthrough discovery came in the early 1990s when Talalay handed then-graduate student Hans Prochaska twenty dollars and sent him on a mission to Baltimore's Northeast Market to buy vegetables. When Prochaska returned to the lab, he began looking for substances in the vegetables that switched on the cells' protective mechanisms [3]. Of all the vegetables assayed, broccoli demonstrated particularly high phase 2-inducer activity. Sulforaphane, an isothiocyanate, was isolated and identified as the predominant chemical entity in broccoli responsible for phase 2 enzyme induction, exhibiting monofunctional inducer activity without phase 1 induction [15, 16].

The discovery that an isothiocyanate was responsible for the anticarcinogenic activity in broccoli generated considerable excitement and interest because it was a dietary component and readily available. Isothiocyanates and their glucosinolate precursors are present in many higher plants, especially among cruciferous vegetables [15]. Furthermore, the chemoprotective effects of isothiocyanates had been clearly demonstrated in rodents, likely due to isothiocyanates' capacity to induce phase 2 enzymes [15]. In addition, sulforaphane induces apoptosis, and inhibits cell-cycle progression, angiogenesis, and the activities of cytochrome P450s and histone deacetylases, collectively impeding tumor growth [16].

The results of the Talalay group's landmark five-year study, published in 1992 in *Proceedings of the National Academies of Science* (PNAS), hailed by the *New York Times* and *The Congressional Quarterly*, and declared one of the top 100 scientific discoveries of the 20th century by *Popular Mechanics,* was not viewed as a victory initially, and was in fact rejected by at least one notable publication before PNAS' acceptance [2, 3, 17, 18].

But the seminal paper produced a ripple effect that influenced dietary and, subsequently, agricultural practices worldwide. In 1991, the year before the study was published, per capita broccoli consumption in the United States averaged 5.29 pounds. In 2011, per capita consumption averaged 8.45 pounds, a 60% increase in two decades. More importantly, the study heralded a paradigm shift in cancer research: the disease once considered inevitable for many was, in fact, preventable, and dietary compounds—such as sulforaphane—could play a key role in the prevention equation.

Further investigation revealed, however, that sulforaphane was an artifact of isolation, and was in fact the degradation product of glucoraphanin, a glucosinolate—sulfur-rich precursor molecules characterized by a β-D-glucopyranose moiety, sulfur-linked to a β-thioglucoside-N-hydroxysulfate, and an amino acid-derived side chain [19]. Glucosinolates coexist with but are compartmentally segregated from plant myrosinases, endogenous β-thioglucosidase enzymes strategically sequestered throughout plants, whose sole known substrates are glucosinolates. Approximately 120 distinct glucosinolate structures have since been identified [20] – see also Chapters 2 and 3).

The trajectory of Talalay's research had changed course. The autumn of 1993 ushered in the inauguration of the Brassica Chemoprotection Laboratory at the Johns Hopkins School of Medicine, now the Lewis B. and Dorothy Cullman Chemoprotection Center, and a new era of discovery. Talalay's mission expanded, and the group now sought insights into the mechanisms by which plants develop self-protective chemical agents that can also afford animal cells protection against the damaging processes that lead to chronic disease.

Sulforaphane's isolation in particular facilitated identification of the elusive mechanisms by which antioxidant compounds prevent carcinogenesis. Specifically, tandem, coordinated phase 1 enzyme suppression inhibits ultimate carcinogen formation while phase 2 enzyme induction detoxifies residual electrophilic metabolites generated by phase 1 enzymes, thereby preventing DNA damage [21]. These highly inducible cytoprotective pathways, which typically function in "idle," escalate in the presence of sulforaphane.

There also came an understanding that many of the genes encoding cytoprotective proteins share common transcriptional regulation through the Keap1–Nrf2–ARE pathway, a key mediator of cytoprotective responses to oxidative and electrophilic stress. Keap1 (Kelch-like ECH-associated protein-1) presents transcription factor Nrf2 (nuclear factor-erythroid 2 p45-related factor-2) for ubiquitination and subsequent proteasomal degradation. Isothiocyanates such as sulforaphane react with highly reactive cysteine thiol groups on Keap1, eliminating the protein's ability to target Nrf2 for degradation. Consequently, Nrf2 amasses and then translocates to the nucleus where it binds to antioxidant response elements (AREs), specific DNA sequences in the upstream regulatory regions of cytoprotective genes.

This cascade of events sets in motion the coordinate transcription of a diverse group of cytoprotective proteins, altering the metabolism and elimination of environmental procarcinogens in humans, and affording protection against the damaging effects of environmental toxins by enhancing their detoxification. Sulforaphane is the most potent naturally occurring small molecule inducer of these cytoprotective proteins.

Talalay's group illuminated the relationship between inducer compounds' chemical structures and their potencies, and, together with the groups of Masayuki Yamamoto and Tom Kensler, identified the key players and events that mediate induction through the Keap1-Nrf2-ARE pathway, providing crucial insights into the molecular mechanisms by which phase 2 enzyme induction occurs. Yet, the impetus for induction remained an enigma. The mystery was solved when Albena Dinkova-Kostova, a young research associate and biochemist in Talalay's lab, noted that specific, highly reactive sulfhydryl groups located between the protein-binding domains of Keap1 likely serve as "cellular sensors" that recognize and interact with inducer compounds, thereby initiating phase 2 enzyme induction [22].

By the late 1990s, Talalay's work with sulforaphane was deeply rooted in basic science, and poised to move into clinical trials in humans. But the seasonal and practical aspects of broccoli acquisition had became problematic, so Talalay's team turned to production, which yielded the discovery that young broccoli sprouts contained substantially greater quantities of glucoraphanin than mature plants—a serendipitous event that enabled standardization for future investigations [19].

Production presented its own challenges, however. In a makeshift greenhouse comprised of steel growing racks, plastic tarps, and a portable electric space heater, Talalay colleagues Jed Fahey and Tom Kensler grew broccoli sprouts for a clinical trial to gauge sulforaphane bioavailability in humans. It was the winter of 2003 in rural China, and bitterly cold. The duo watered the sprouts every two hours, risking electrocution, freezing, and flooding.

In the end, they produced more than 200 kilograms of broccoli sprouts and one enormous batch of bitter-tasting broccoli sprout "tea." Future trials, which were among the first to "reduce-to-practice" the concept promulgated by Talalay so many years ago, relied on freeze-dried preparations developed in less spartan accommodations [23, 24].

The first trials were simple, proof-of-principle studies that provided both qualitative and quantitative evidence that sulforaphane-mediated enzyme induction, via broccoli-sprout infusion, was protective against cancer, and occurred in a dose dependent fashion [25]. Humans tolerate broccoli sprouts well, and nearly two decades of clinical trials involving broccoli sprouts and spanning a wide range of human disease states, including air pollution toxicity, asthma, autism, chronic obstructive pulmonary disease, radiation dermatitis, schizophrenia, and cancers of the bladder, breast, colon, lung, and prostate, among others, are complete or are currently underway. Nearly 25 years since the isolation and identification of sulforaphane, the research on broccoli, sulforaphane, and other plant-derived bioactive compounds remains robust and thriving. Current aims focus on refining the understanding of the mechanisms by which these compounds reduce chronic disease risk.

A diverse portfolio of activities has been ascribed to sulforaphane, most of which are related to its ability to upregulate cytoprotective proteins. However, in 2002, Jed Fahey heard of anecdotal evidence suggesting broccoli sprouts were effective in treating Helicobacter pylori infection, a gram-negative bacterium implicated in the etiology of peptic ulcers and gastric cancer. In the developing world, Helicobacter pylori infection rates exceed 90 percent and are associated with a significant cancer burden. Fahey discovered that sulforaphane is bactericidal for Helicobacter pylori and reduces gastric tumor formation in animal models. As such, Fahey's discovery speaks to the potentially immense public health applications for sulforaphane and other plant-derived bioactive compounds [24, 26, 27].

The Talalay group established (and continues to practice) a legacy of strong basic science applied against the backdrop of traditional medicine, anecdotal evidence, and epidemiological surveillance data, and successfully translated their findings to the clinic. The group's combined intellectual curiosity coupled with their scrupulous techniques likely stand unmatched in any setting.

In 2012, Talalay and colleagues Kensler and Fahey posited a new strategy to combat the escalating global burden of chronic disease: "green chemoprevention." In the near future, chronic disease treatment likely will exceed the healthcare delivery capabilities of many developing nations. However, a robust body of evidence demonstrates the "green" protective effects of isolated phytochemicals in many whole foods and their extracts. Insights into the mechanisms by which these phytochemicals exert their protective effects can be translated to native foods or potentially influence the introduction of other, culturally appropriate, protective foods.

Together, sulforaphane and broccoli sprouts serve as a model for green chemoprevention: Just as broccoli consumption increased in the wake of the overwhelming evidence supporting its chemoprotective effects, perhaps future identification of plant-derived foods with similarly chemoprotective systems that fit into the dietary practices of individual cultures might move populations toward consumption of those foods, especially in the developing world. In this way, green chemoprevention, the implementation of food-based, frugal, and culturally appropriate intervention strategies, will serve rich and poor alike [23, 24].

REFERENCES

[1] Wattenberg, L. W. Chemoprophylaxis of carcinogenesis: a review. *Cancer Res.* 1966;26(7):1520-6.

[2] Wattenberg, L. W. Inhibition of carcinogenic and toxic effects of polycyclic hydrocarbons by phenolic antioxidants and ethoxyquin. *J. Natl. Cancer Inst.* 1972;48(5):1425-30.

[3] Talalay, P. Paul Talalay, Interviewed by: Johnson, T. Baltimore 2015.

[4] Talalay, P. Mechanisms of induction of enzymes that protect against chemical carcinogenesis. *Adv. Enzyme Regul.* 1989;28:237-50.

[5] Our History: Bedford School; 2015 [cited 2015 10 April]. Available from: http://www.bedfordschool.org.uk/Our-History.

[6] Benson, A. M., Batzinger, R. P., Ou, S. Y., Bueding, E., Cha, Y. N., Talalay, P. Elevation of hepatic glutathione S-transferase activities and protection against mutagenic metabolites of benzo(a)pyrene by dietary antioxidants. *Cancer Res.* 1978;38(12):4486-95.

[7] Bueding, E., Batzinger, R. P., Cha, Y. N., Talalay, P., Molineaux, C. J. Protection from mutagenic effects of antischistosomal and other drugs. *Pharmacol. Rev.* 1978;30(4):547-54.

[8] Talalay, P., Benson, A. M. Elevation of quinone reductase activity by anticarcinogenic antioxidants. *Adv. Enzyme Regul.* 1982;20:287-300.

[9] Dinkova-Kostova, A. T., Talalay, P. NAD(P)H:quinone acceptor oxidoreductase 1 (NQO1), a multifunctional antioxidant enzyme and exceptionally versatile cytoprotector. *Arch. Biochem. Biophys.* 2010;501 (1):116-23.

[10] Prochaska, H. J., De Long, M. J., Talalay, P. On the mechanisms of induction of cancer-protective enzymes: a unifying proposal. *Proc. Natl. Acad. Sci. US.* 1985;82(23):8232-6.

[11] Talalay, P., De Long, M. J., Prochaska, H. J. Identification of a common chemical signal regulating the induction of enzymes that protect against chemical carcinogenesis. *Proc. Natl. Acad. Sci. US.* 1988;85(21):8261-5.

[12] Spencer, S. R., Wilczak, C. A., Talalay, P. Induction of glutathione transferases and NAD(P)H:quinone reductase by fumaric acid derivatives in rodent cells and tissues. *Cancer Res.* 1990;50(24):7871-5.

[13] Dinkova-Kostova, A. T., Fahey, J. W., Talalay, P. Chemical structures of inducers of nicotinamide quinone oxidoreductase 1 (NQO1). *Methods Enzymol.* 2004;382:423-48.

[14] De Long, M. J., Prochaska, H. J., Talalay, P. Induction of NAD(P)H: quinone reductase in murine hepatoma cells by phenolic antioxidants, azo dyes, and other chemoprotectors: a model system for the study of anticarcinogens. *Proc. Natl. Acad. Sci. US.* 1986;83(3):787-91.

[15] Prochaska, H. J., Santamaria, A. B., Talalay, P. Rapid detection of inducers of enzymes that protect against carcinogens. *Proc. Natl. Acad. Sci. US.* 1992;89(6):2394-8.

[16] Zhang, Y., Talalay, P., Cho, C. G., Posner, G. H. A major inducer of anticarcinogenic protective enzymes from broccoli: isolation and elucidation of structure. *Proc. Natl. Acad. Sci. US.* 1992;89(6):2399-403.

[17] Egner, P. A., Chen, J. G., Wang, J. B., Wu, Y., Sun, Y., Lu, J. H. et al. Bioavailability of Sulforaphane from two broccoli sprout beverages: results of a short-term, cross-over clinical trial in Qidong, China. *Cancer Prev. Res.* 2011;4(3):384-95.

[18] Angier, N. Potent Chemical To Fight Cancer Seen in Broccoli. *The New York Times.* 1992 March 15, 1992.

[19] Talalay, P. A fascination with enzymes: the journey not the arrival matters. *J. Biol. Chem.* 2005;280(32):28829-47.

[20] Fahey, J. W., Zhang, Y., Talalay, P. Broccoli sprouts: an exceptionally rich source of inducers of enzymes that protect against chemical carcinogens. *Proc. Natl. Acad. Sci. US.* 1997;94(19):10367-72.

[21] Fahey, J. W., Zalcmann, A. T., Talalay, P. The chemical diversity and distribution of glucosinolates and isothiocyanates among plants. *Phytochemistry.* 2001;56(1):5-51.

[22] Dinkova-Kostova, A. T., Holtzclaw, W. D., Cole, R. N., Itoh, K., Wakabayashi, N., Katoh, Y. et al. Direct evidence that sulfhydryl groups of Keap1 are the sensors regulating induction of phase 2 enzymes that protect against carcinogens and oxidants. *Proc. Natl. Acad. Sci. US.* 2002;99(18):11908-13.

[23] Kensler, T. W. Tom Kensler Interviewed by: Johnson, T. 2015.

[24] Fahey, J. W. Jed Fahey Interviewed by: Johnson, T. 2015.

[25] Zhang, Y., Talalay, P. Anticarcinogenic activities of organic isothiocyanates: chemistry and mechanisms. *Cancer Res.* 1994;54(7 Suppl.):1976s-81s.

[26] Fahey, J. W., Stephenson, K. K., Wallace, A. J. Dietary amelioration of Helicobacter infection. *Nutr. Res.* 2015;35(6):461-73.

[27] Fahey, J. W., Haristoy, X., Dolan, P. M., Kensler, T. W., Scholtus, I., Stephenson, K. K. et al. Sulforaphane inhibits extracellular, intracellular, and antibiotic-resistant strains of Helicobacter pylori and prevents benzo[a]pyrene-induced stomach tumors. *Proc. Natl. Acad. Sci. US.* 2002;99(11):7610-5.

[28] Shapiro, T. A., Fahey, J. W., Wade, K. L., Stephenson, K. K., Talalay, P. Human metabolism and excretion of cancer chemoprotective glucosinolates and isothiocyanates of cruciferous vegetables. *Cancer Epidemiol. Biomarkers Prev.* 1998;7(12):1091-100.

[29] Fahey, J. W., Kensler, T. W. Health span extension through green chemoprevention. *The virtual mentor: VM.* 2013;15(4):311-8.

[30] Fahey, J. W., Talalay, P., Kensler, T. W. Notes from the field: "green" chemoprevention as frugal medicine. *Cancer Prev. Res.* 2012;5(2):179-88.

In: Broccoli
Editor: Bernhard H. J. Juurlink

ISBN: 978-1-63484-313-3
© 2016 Nova Science Publishers, Inc.

Chapter 2

GLUCOSINOLATES AND THEIR DISTRIBUTION

Sabine Montaut[1,*] *and Patrick Rollin*[2,†]

[1]Laurentian University, Department of Chemistry & Biochemistry,
Biomolecular Sciences Programme, Sudbury, ON, Canada
[2] Université d'Orléans et CNRS, ICOA, UMR 7311, BP 6759,
F-45067 Orléans, France

ABSTRACT

Acting generally as bio-precursors of isothiocyanates (ITCs), glucosinolates (GLs) are important thiosaccharidic metabolites which occur in all plant families of the order Brassicales – namely in our daily vegetables. All known GLs (*ca* 130 characterized molecules) display a remarkable structural homogeneity invariably based on a β-D-glucopyrano unit and an O-sulfated anomeric *(Z)*-thiohydroximate function connected to a side chain which constitution, depending on plant species, is the sole structural variant. This chapter will focus on the distribution of GLs in the families of several plant orders (Brassicales, Malpighiales, Celastrales, Caryophyllales, and Gentianales), the mechanism of enzymatic degradation of GLs and the goitrogenic activity of this class of natural products and their enzymatic degradation products.

Keywords: Brassicales, secondary metabolites, thio-compounds, glucosinolates, myrosinase, isothiocyanates

INTRODUCTION

Sulfur-containing metabolites occur in several botanical classes and in particular crucifers, which belong to the Brassicale order. Brassicales encompass 17 families (Table 1)

---

[*] Corresponding Author address: Laurentian University, Department of Chemistry & Biochemistry, Biomolecular Sciences Programme, 935, Ramsey Lake Road Sudbury, ON P3E 2C6, Canada. Email: smontaut@laurentian.ca. Phone: +1 (705) 675-1151 ext: 2185.
[†] Email: patrick.rollin@univ-orleans.fr. Phone: +33 (0)238 417 370.

[1] of dicotyledonous angiosperms among which the Brassicaceae (synonymous of Cruciferae) are by far the most important, with more than 350 genera and 3,000 species [2, 3]. All plants in the order Brassicales (except plants from the family Koeberliniaceae) contain glucosinolates (GLs), thiosaccharidic secondary metabolites which display a remarkable structural homogeneity: a hydrophilic β-D-glucopyrano framework bearing a *O*-sulfated anomeric (*Z*)-thiohydroximate moiety connected to a hydrophobic aglycon side chain (Figure 1). GLs are therefore *S*-glucopyranosyl thioesters, although they have been currently called "thioglucosides." In the *ca* 130 known GLs, the aglycon chain is the sole structural variant, in which diversified aliphatic, arylaliphatic or indole-type arrangements can be found. Glucosinolates are found mainly in the order Brassicales but are also present in the orders Malpighiales, Celastrales, Caryophyllales, and Gentianales.

Table 1. The botanical order Brassicales

- Akaniaceae - Bataceae - Brassicaceae (*cabbages*) - Capparaceae (*capers*) - Caricaceae (*papaya*) - Cleomaceae - Emblingiaceae - Gyrostemonaceae	- Koeberliniaceae - Limnanthaceae - Moringaceae - Pentadiplandraceae - Resedaceae (*reseda*) - Salvadoraceae - Setchellanthaceae - Tovariaceae - Tropaeolaceae (*Indian cress*)

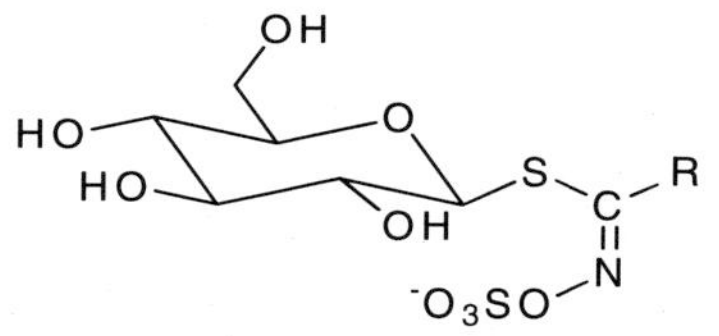

R = alkyl, alkenyl, arylalkyl, hydroxyalkenyl, indolylmethyl, thiofunctionalized

Figure 1. General structure of glucosinolates.

1. Glucosinolate Distribution in the Order BRASSICALES

a) General Considerations

Glucosinolates are biosynthesized from amino acids. They are divided into groups according to the amino acid precursor. Aliphatic GLs are biosynthesized from Ala, Leu, Ile, Val, and Met; arylaliphatic GLs from Phe and Tyr, and indole GLs from Trp. The biosynthesis follows a three-step process: 1) chain elongation of the amino acid (only Met and Phe), 2) formation of the core GL structure, and 3) secondary modifications of the amino acid side chain. Several enzymes and genes responsible of the biosynthesis of GLs have been identified. Reviews presenting the biosynthesis of GLs in details can be found in the literature [4, 5]. The modifications carried out during the biosynthesis of GLs are shown by the structural diversity of GLs (at least 130) which is reported in many reviews [2, 3, 6]. In the following subsections of this chapter we will give a brief overview of GLs in the families of the order Brassicales.

b) Akaniaceae Stapf

Bretschneidera sinensis Hemsl. (Akaniaceae) is the only known species of the genus *Bretschneidera*. A review of the scientific literature shows that 5,5-dimethyl-1,3-oxazolidine-2-thione can be isolated from *B. sinensis* leaves after a myrosinase hydrolysis of the plant extract, indicating the presence of 2-hydroxy-2-methylpropyl GL (**1**) (Figure 2). In addition, 3,4-dihydroxybenzyl GL (**2**) and other GLs in trace amounts were detected by GC-MS [7]. In 2010, benzyl (**3**), hydroxymethylpropyl, and hydroxybenzyl GLs were detected by LC-MS in leaves of a single herbarium specimen of *B. sinensis* collected from mainland China in 1919 [8]. Recently, the GL profile in several plant parts (leaf, branch, bark, root, and fruit) of *B. sinensis* from the People's Republic of China was established for the first time by HPLC. During this investigation, benzyl (**3**), 4-hydroxybenzyl (**4**), 2-hydroxy-2-methylpropyl (**1**), and 4-methoxybenzyl (**5**) GLs were identified. In addition, one new GL, 3-hydroxy-4-methoxybenzyl GL (**6**), was isolated in minor amount from the fruit. Furthermore, traces of 4-hydroxy-3-methoxyphenyl acetonitrile were detected by GC-MS analysis in the fruit, thus confirming the presence of the regioisomeric 4-hydroxy-3-methoxybenzyl GL (**7**) [9].

The GL profile of *B. sinensis* is close to that established for *Akania bidwillii* (R. Hogg) Mabb. (Akaniaceae), featuring benzyl (**3**), hydroxybenzyl, dihydroxybenzyl, and methoxybenzyl GLs [8].

c) Bataceae Mart. ex Perleb

A TLC analysis of myrosinase-degradation products obtained from an extract of *Batis maritima* L. (Bataceae) would suggest that the plant possesses indol-3-ylmethyl (**8**) and 4-hydroxyindol-3-ylmethyl (**9**) GLs [10]. Later, benzyl GL (**3**) has been reported in *B. maritima* [11]. More recently, the LC-MS analysis of an herbarium tissue of *B. maritima* showed the presence of benzyl (**3**) and indol-3-ylmethyl (**8**) GLs. However, the same analysis of *Batis argillicola* P. Royen sample failed to show the presence of any GL [8].

d) Brassicaceae Burnett

The most famous member of the family Brassicaceae is *Arabidopsis thaliana* L., which was the first plant to have its genome sequence completed [12]. 36 GLs have been identified in *A. thaliana*. The majority of GLs are chain-elongated compounds derived from Met [13, 14].

Some examples of edible and cultivated plants of the family Brassicaceae are rapeseed (*Brassica napus* L.), mustards (*Brassica juncea* (L.) Czern., *Brassica nigra* (L.) K. Koch, *Sinapis alba* L.), radishes (*Raphanus sativus* L.), cabbages (*Brassica oleracea*), rocket salad (*Eruca sativa* Mill.), rutabaga (*Brassica napobrassica* Mill.), turnip (*Brassica rapa* var. *rapa*

L.), horseradish (*Armoracia rusticana* P. Gaertn., B. Mey. & Scherb.), and broccoli (*Brassica oleracea* L. var. *italica*). In general, sulfur-containing, branched-aliphatic, olefinic, aryl and indole GLs are reported in *Brassica* sp. [2]. 3-Methylsulfinylpropyl (**10**), 2-hydroxy-3-butenyl (**11**), 4-methylsulfinylbutyl (**12**) (major), 5-methylsulfinylpentyl (**13**), 3-butenyl (**14**), 4-pentenyl (**15**), 4-hydroxyindol-3-ylmethyl (**9**), indol-3-ylmethyl (**8**), 2-phenylethyl (**16**), 4-methoxyindol-3-ylmethyl (**17**), and 1-methoxyindol-3-ylmethyl (**18**) GLs have been quantified in freshly harvested broccoli inflorescences [15, 16] and in different cultivars in inflorescences at various development stages [17].

Some GLs can be specific to certain genera. As an example, 4-methylsulfanyl-3-butenyl GL (**19**) is found only in five genera of the Brassicaceae family: *Brassica*, *Bunias*, *Matthiola*, *Raphanus*, and *Rapistrum* [18]. Information regarding the GL profile of a particular plant from the family Brassicaceae can be found in some research articles and reviews [2, 3, 19-21].

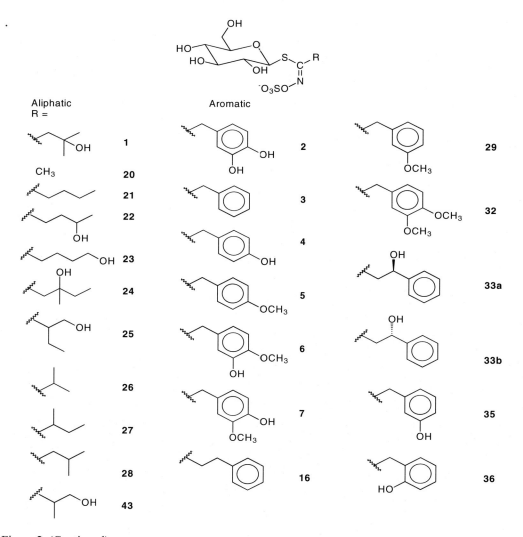

Figure 2. (Continued).

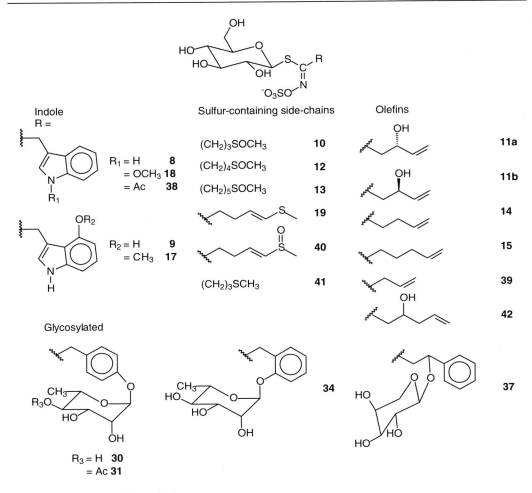

Figure 2. Examples of glucosinolate structures.

e) Capparaceae Juss.

The most known member of the family Capparaceae is the edible caper (*Capparis spinosa* L.). Methyl GL (**20**), the structurally simplest GL, seems to be widely present in many genera (*Atamisquea, Boscia, Cadaba, Capparis, Crataeva, Dhofaria, Dipterygium, Forchhammeria, Gynadropsis, Maerua, Puccionia, Ritchiea, Steriphoma,* and *Thylachium*) of the family Capparaceae [8, 21-26]. However, methyl GL (**20**) is not present in all *Atamisquea* sp., *Capparis* sp., and *Steriphoma* sp. [8, 27]. Furthermore, indole GLs can be found in *C. spinosa* and *Maerua triphylla* A. Rich. [8, 28]. Benzyl (**3**), butyl (**21**), 3-hydroxybutyl (**22**), 4-hydroxybutyl (**23**), 3-butenyl (**14**), and 2-hydroxy-3-butenyl (**11**) GLs have also been identified in *C. flexuosa* [24, 27]. *Boscia longifolia* Hadj-Moust. has high level of hydroxymethylbutyl GL and *Capparis tomentosa* Lam. has a high level of hydroxyethyl GL. Oxoalkyl GLs are found in *Capparis scabrida* Kunth. whereas methylsulfonylalkyl (nonyl to undecyl) GLs are the major GLs found in *Steriphoma elliptica* Sreng, *Steriphoma paradoxum*

(Jacq.) Endl., and *Steriphoma peruvianum* Spruce. In addition, several major and unknown GLs need to be characterized in some *Capparis* sp., *Atamisquea emarginata* Miers ex Hook. and Arn., and *Morisonia americana* L. [8]. For the detailed GL profiles of other specific plants of the family Capparaceae the reader is advised to refer to the review by Fahey *et al.* and to the references cited therein [2].

f) Caricaceae Dumort.

The most known member of the family Caricaceae is the edible tropical fruit, papaya (*Carica papaya* L.). Benzyl GL (**3**) seems to be the only GL identified throughout the family Caricaceae (genera *Jarilla*, *Carica* and *Cycliomorpha*) [2, 20, 29]. The presence of indol-3-ylmethyl GL (**8**) was tentatively suggested in papaya seeds however other investigations have failed to detect this GL [30].

g) Cleomaceae Bercht. & J. Presl

Cleome sp. (Cleomaceae) appear to biosynthetize methyl (**20**) and 2-hydroxy-2-methylbutyl (**24**) GLs [8, 23, 31, 32]. Furthermore, it was estimated via a thiocyanate ion measurement that the seeds of certain *Cleome* sp. produce 4-hydroxybenzyl GL (**4**) [20]. Indol-3-ylmethyl (**8**) and 1-methoxyindol-3-ylmethyl (**18**) GLs can be found in some *Cleome* sp. [32, 33]. 1-Ethyl-2-hydroxyethyl (**25**) and 2-hydroxy-2-methylpropyl (**1**) GLs are expected in *Cleome diandra* Burch thanks to the identification by GC of oxazolidinethiones produced by myrosinase degradation [20].

Polinisia sp (Cleomaceae) and *Wislizenia* sp. (Cleomaceae) seeds seem to both produce 4-hydroxybenzyl GL (**4**) (thiocyanate ion measurement). Additionally, *Polinisia* sp. seeds produce 2-hydroxy-2-methylbutyl GL (**24**) [20].

h) Emblingiaceae J. Agardh

Emblingia is a monospecific plant genus containing the species *Emblingia calceoliflora* F. Muell (Emblingiaceae). Hydroxy and hydroxymethoxybenzyl GLs were detected by LC-MS in a leaf tissue sampled from a single herbarium specimen of *E. calceoliflora* collected *ca.*1850 in Australia [8].

i) Gyrostemonaceae A. Juss.

2-Propyl, 2-butyl, and 2-methylpropyl isothiocyanates (ITCs) have been detected by GC in seeds and leaves of *Tersonia cyathifolia* (Fenzl) J. W. Green (syn. *Tersonia brevipes* Moq) (Gyrostemonaceae) after a myrosinase hydrolysis of the plant extract, indicating the presence of 1-methylethyl (**26**), 1-methylpropyl (**27**), and 2-methylpropyl (**28**) GLs [34]. In addition, (+)-*sec*-butyl ITC and benzyl cyanide have been identified in the essential oil from leaves of the Australian *Codonocarpus cotinifolius* (Desf.) F. Muell. (syn. *C. cotinifolia* (Desf.) F. Muell.) (Gyrostemonaceae) [35]. This study shows that 1-methylpropyl (**27**) and benzyl (**3**) GLs are present in the plant. Later, *sec*-butyl ITC and 5-ethyl-5-methyloxazolidine-2-thione were identified by GC after myrosinase hydrolysis of the plant's seed extract indicating the presence of 1-methylpropyl (**27**) and 2-hydroxy-2-methylbutyl (**24**) GLs [20]. Furthermore, it was estimated in the same study via thiocyanate ion measurement that the seeds of this plant produce 4-hydroxybenzyl GL (**4**) [20]. A C-5 hydroxyalkyl GL not entirely characterized was detected in *C. cotinifolius*, *Codonocarpus pyramidalis* (F. Muell.) F. Muell., and *T. cyathifolia* seeds. It was hypothesized on the basis of LC-MS analysis and literature data that it could be either 1-methyl-3-hydroxybutyl, 2-hydroxy-2-methylbutyl, or 2-hydroxypentyl GL [21].

Finally, the LC-MS analysis of *Gyrostemon sheathii* W. Fitzg. (Gyrostemonaceae) herbarium tissue showed that the plant contains hydroxy-methyl-propyl, methyl-ethyl, methyl-propyl, *n*-pentyl (likely to be methylbutyl), *n*-hexyl (likely to be methylpentyl), and indolyl-3-ylmethyl (**8**) GLs [8].

j) Koeberliniaceae Engl.

To our knowledge, no GL has been detected in plants of the family Koeberliniaceae [2, 3, 8, 36].

k) Limnanthaceae R. Br.

The oil obtained from steam-distilled seeds of *Limnanthes douglasii* R. Br. (Limnanthaceae) contains *m*-methoxybenzyl ITC indicating that *m*-methoxybenzyl GL (**29**) exists in the seeds [37]. The presence of this GL in the seeds of the plant was confirmed by LC-MS analysis [21]. Furthermore, the *m*-methoxybenzyl ITC has also been tentatively detected as a thiourea derivative by TLC in *Limnanthes alba* Benth., *Limnanthes alba* var. *versicolor* (Greene) C. T. Mason, *L. douglasii*, *Limnanthes douglasii* var. *nivea* C. T. Mason (two samples), *L. douglasii* var. *rosea* (Benth.) C. T. Mason (two samples), *Limnanthes floccosa* Howell, *Limnanthes gracilis* Howell, and *Limnanthes montana* Jepson [38]. In addition, an unidentified thiourea different from the *m*-methoxybenzyl thiourea was detected in one sample of *L. douglasii* var. *nivea* and in *Limnanthes bakeri* J. T. Howell. These results definitely need confirmations. Later, *m*-methoxybenzyl ITC and 5,5-dimethyl-1,3-oxazolidine-2-thione were obtained after steam distillation of *Limnanthes alba* Benth. var. *alba* seed indicating that this plant also contains *m*-methoxybenzyl (**29**) and 2-hydroxy-2-methylpropyl (**1**) GLs [39]. Finally, an HPLC analysis confirmed the presence of benzyl (**3**), methoxybenzyl and dimethoxybenzyl GLs in seeds of *Limnanthes* (species not specified) [8].

l) Moringaceae Martinov

Benzyl ITC was isolated from *Moringa oleifera* Lam. (syn. *Moringa pterygosperma* C. F. Gaertner) (Moringaceae). This indicates that the plant has benzyl GL (**3**) [40]. The presence of this GL was confirmed by HPLC analysis of the seed of *M. oleifera* [8]. In an other investigation, 1-methylethyl and 1-methylpropyl ITCs were identified by GC after myrosinase hydrolysis of the seed extract indicating the presence of 1-methylethyl (**26**) and 1-methylpropyl (**27**) GLs [20]. Furthermore, it was estimated in the same study via thiocyanate ion measurement that the seeds of this plant produced 4-hydroxybenzyl GL (**4**) [20]. Later a LC-MS analysis has shown that *M. oleifera* contained benzyl GL (**3**) (root), 4-(α-L-rhamnosyloxy)benzyl GL (**30**), (seed roots, bark, and leaves), and three monoacetyl isomers (leaves), the structures of which were not established [41]. It was shown in the same investigation that *Moringa stenopetala* L. contained also benzyl GL (**3**) (root), 4-(α-L-rhamnosyloxy)benzyl GL (**30**) (seeds, roots, leaves), and the same three monoacetyl regioisomers (leaves) observed in *M. oleifera* [41].

Myrosinase-treated seed extract of *Moringa peregrina* (Forssk.) Fiori. (Moringaceae) generated 2-propyl, 2-butyl, 2-methylpropyl, 4-(α-L-rhamnosyloxy)benzyl and 4-(4'-*O*-acetyl-α-L-rhamnosyloxy)benzyl ITCs, and 5,5-dimethyl-1,3-oxazolidine-2-thione. The presence of these enzymatic degradation products means that the seeds contain 1-methylethyl (**26**), 1-methylpropyl (**27**), 2-methylpropyl (**28**), 4-(α-L-rhamnosyloxy)benzyl (**30**) and 4-(4'-*O*-acetyl-α-L-rhamnosyloxy)benzyl (**31**), and 2-hydroxy-2-methylpropyl (**1**) GLs [42].

m) Pentadiplandraceae Hutch. & Daziel

The plant family Pentadiplandraceae possesses only one genus, *Pentadiplandra*, which contains a single species, *Pentadiplandra brazzeana* Baillon. Recently, the GLs present in root, seed, and leaf extracts of the plant *P. brazzeana* were characterized and quantified by us according to the HPLC analysis of desulfo-GLs. Benzyl (**3**), 3-methoxybenzyl (**29**), and 4-methoxybenzyl (**5**) GLs were shown to be present in the root extract, whereas the seed mainly contained 4-methoxybenzyl GL (**5**). 3,4-dimethoxybenzyl GL (**32**), indol-3-ylmethyl GL (**8**), and traces of benzyl GL (**3**) were detected in the leaf extract [43].

n) Resedaceae Martinov

2-Hydroxy-2-phenylethyl (**33**) and 4-hydroxybenzyl (**4**) GLs were deduced from the GC-MS analysis of myrosinase degradation product and a thiocyanate ion measurement in the seeds of *Caylusea abyssinica* (Fresen.) Fisch. & C. A. Mey. (Resedaceae) [20]. However, 2-phenylethyl (**16**), 2-(*R*)-hydroxy-2-phenylethyl (**33a**), and 2-(*S*)-hydroxy-2-phenylethyl (**33b**) GLs were identified in the seeds by LC-MS [21].

Seeds of *Reseda alba* L (Resedaceae) contain 2-hydroxy-2-methylpropyl GL (**1**) [44, 45] whereas a thiocyanate ion measurement demonstrated that the seeds of this plant produce 4-hydroxybenzyl GL (**4**) [20]. The presence of indol-3-ylmethyl GL (**8**) was established in etiolated seedlings [33]. 2-Hydroxy-2-methylpropyl GL (**1**) was also isolated in *R. alba* inflorescences [46]. The presence of 2-phenylethyl GL (**16**) in the roots of *R. alba* was deduced on the basis of paper chromatography of 2-phenylethyl ITC [47].

The presence of indol-3-ylmethyl GL (**8**) was reported in *Reseda lutea* L. (Resedaceae) [33]. It was also found that 8-week-old plants of *R. lutea* generate benzyl ITC after autolysis which indicates that the plants contains benzyl GL (**3**) [19]. Benzyl ITC was also detected in the roots [47]. Later, 2-(α-L-rhamnopyranosyloxy)benzyl GL (**34**) was identified by LC-MS in the seed of *R. lutea* [8, 21].

2-(*S*)-hydroxy-2-phenylethyl (**33b**), 2-phenylethyl (**16**), and indol-3-ylmethyl (**8**) GLs were identified in *Reseda luteola* L. (Resedaceae) [19, 33, 46-49]. In addition, 2-phenylethyl (**16**) and 2-hydroxy-2-phenylethyl (**33**) GLs were identified as their respective ITC aglycones in *R. luteola* tissue cultures [50]. 2-Hydroxyphenylethyl, indol-3-ylmethyl (**8**), and 2-hydroxy-2-methylpropyl GL or 1-ethyl-2-hydroxyethyl GL (insufficient data to distinguish between these two possibilities) were detected on the leaf surface of *R. luteola* by LC-MS [32]. More recently, 2-(*S*)-hydroxy-2-phenylethyl (**33b**), 2-(*R*)-hydroxy-2-phenylethyl (**33a**) and indol-3-ylmethyl (**8**) GLs were identified by LC-MS in the seed of *R. luteola* [21].

The green parts of *Reseda media* Lag. (Resedaceae) contain benzyl (**3**), 2-phenylethyl (**16**), *m*-hydroxybenzyl (**35**) (major) GLs and traces of indol-3-ylmethyl GL (**8**). Other unidentified GLs were also detected in trace amounts [51].

Reseda phyteuma L. and *Reseda crystallina* Webb. (Resedaceae) were both reported to contain indol-3-ylmethyl GL (**8**) whereas *Reseda complicata* Bory (Resedaceae) had indol-3-ylmethyl (**8**) and 1-methoxyindol-3-ylmethyl (**18**) GLs [33]. Furthermore, 2-(α-L-rhamnopyranosyloxy)benzyl GL (**34**) was identified by LC-MS in *R. phyteuma* [8].

The occurrence of methyl GL (**20**) was reported in seeds of *Reseda odorata* L. (Resedaceae) but never confirmed in other studies [52]. The presence of indol-3-ylmethyl GL (**8**) was reported in *R. odorata* [33]. Moreover, 2-(α-L-rhamnopyranosyloxy)benzyl GL (**34**) is the major GL in green parts of *R. odorata* L. but is also present in roots, stems and leaves. Chromatographic evidence indicates that another GL, present in low concentration, does not seem to be the indole derivative but rather *o*-hydroxybenzyl GL (**36**) [8, 46]. In addition, 2-(*S*)-hydroxy-2-phenylethyl (**33b**), 2-(*R*)-hydroxy-2-phenylethyl (**33a**) and indol-3-ylmethyl (**8**) GLs were identified by LC-MS in seeds of *R. odorata* [21].

2-(α-L-Rhamnopyranosyloxy)benzyl GL (**34**) was identified by LC-MS in *R. stricta* Pers. (Resedaceae) [8].

Reseda suffruticosa Loefl. (Resedaceae) herbarium tissue contains 2-phenylethyl GL (**16**) and GLs synthesized from Leu, Ile, Val [8].

Finally, 2-(α-L-arabinopyranosyloxy)-2-phenylethyl (**37**), 2-hydroxy-2-phenylethyl (**33**), and 2-phenylethyl (**16**) GLs have been identified in green parts of *Sesamoides canescens* (L.) Kuntze var. *canescens* (Resedaceae) and *Sesamoides pygmaea* (Scheele) Kuntze (Resedaceae). Two other GLs in minor amounts have been detected but their structure was not elucidated [53].

o) Salvadoraceae Lindl.

Benzyl ITC was found in the volatile produced by steam distillation of the seeds of *Salvadora oleoides* Decne. (Salvadoraceae) [54]. It was reported that the seeds of *Salvadora persica* L. (Salvadoraceae) produced also benzyl ITC upon myrosinase hydrolysis indicating that the plant possesses benzyl GL (**3**) [20]. Later, benzyl ITC was found to be the major constituent of the root essential oil of *S. persica* [55]. These studies indicate that *S. oleoides* and *S. persica* seeds contain benzyl GL (**3**).

An LC-MS analysis has shown that *Azima tetracantha* Lam (Salvadoraceae) contains indol-3-ylmethyl GL (**8**) (seed, root, young leaves, and stem-thorns), *N*-methoxyindol-3-ylmethyl GL (**18**) (seed, root, young leaves, old leaves, and stem-thorns), and provisionally *N*-hydroxyindol-3-ylmethyl GL (root, young leaves, old leaves, and stem-thorns) [21, 56].

More recently, indole GLs were noted to be the major GLs of dried herbarium tissue of *A. tetracantha*, *S. persica*, *Dobera loranthifolia* (Warb) Harms (Salvadoraceae), and *Dobera glabra* (Forssk) Juss. ex Poir. (Salvadoraceae), along with benzyl and hydroxybenzyl GL in *S. persica* [8].

p) Setchellanthaceae Iltis

The family Setchellanthaceae contains only one species, *Setchellanthus caeruleus* Brandegee, a shrub found in Mexico. The only LC-MS analysis of three samples of herbarium tissue of *S. caeruleus* showed the presence of hydroxy-methylpropyl, methylethyl, methylpropyl and hydroxybenzyl GLs [8].

q) Tovariaceae Pax

In *Tovaria pendula* Ruiz and Pavón, methylethyl (**26**), benzyl (**3**), indol-3-ylmethyl (**8**), 4-hydroxyindol-3-ylmethyl (**9**), 4-methoxyindol-3-ylmethyl (**17**), 1-methoxyindol-3-ylmethyl (**18**), and *N*-acetylindol-3-ylmethyl (**38**) GLs were identified [8, 33, 57, 58].

r) Tropaeolaceae Juss. ex DC.

Benzyl GL (**3**) seems to be present in all *Tropaeolum* species [21, 50, 59]. The most known member of the family Tropaeolaceae is the edible and ornamental garden nasturtium (*Tropaeolum majus* L.). In addition to benzyl GL (**3**), *T. majus* seeds and leaf surface have 4-methoxybenzyl GL (**5**) [20, 32, 52, 59, 60]. Traces of indol-3-ylmethyl GL (**8**) have been detected on the leaf surface and in the seeds of the plant [21, 32]. 2-Propenyl GL (**39**) was detected in the flowers of *T. majus* [61].

In *Tropaeolum peregrinum* L. seeds, isopropyl and *sec*-butyl ITCs were detected after myrosinase hydrolysis of the plant extract [52]. Those results indicate that the seeds contain the 1-methylethyl (**26**) and 1-methylpropyl (**27**) GLs. In another investigation on the seeds, methoxybenzyl ITC and 5,5-dimethyloxazolidinethione were released upon myrosinase hydrolysis which would indicate that the seeds have methoxybenzyl GL and 2-hydroxy-2-methylpropyl GL (**1**) [20]. The presence of benzyl GL (**3**) (major) in the seeds was confirmed by HPLC and an unknown GL was also detected [21].

Seeds of the Andean isaño (*Tropaeolum tuberosum* Ruíz & Pav.) were reported to produce benzyl, 2-propyl and 2-butyl ITCs upon enzymatic hydrolysis of the extract. This led to think that benzyl (**3**), 1-methylethyl (**26**) and 1-methylpropyl (**27**) GLs are present in the plant species [59]. In another study, seeds, tubers and flowers of *T. tuberosum* (syn *T. tuberosum* subsp. *tuberosum*) produced only 4-methoxybenzyl ITC upon myrosinase hydrolysis from the parent GL. Futhermore, only 4-methoxybenzyl GL (**5**) was detected by

HPLC in *T. tuberosum* tubers [62]. On the contrary, *T. tuberosum* subsp. *silvestre* produced benzyl, 2-propyl and 2-butyl ITCs, thus confirming the presence of benzyl (**3**), 1-methylethyl (**26**) and 1-methylpropyl (**27**) GLs [63].

Seeds of *Tropaeolum boliviense* Loes., *Tropaeolum longiflorum* Killip, and *Tropaeolum seemannii* Buch. produced benzyl, 2-propyl, and 2-butyl ITCs, upon myrosinase hydrolysis, confirming the presence of benzyl (**3**), 1-methylethyl (**26**), and 1-methylpropyl (**27**) GLs [59]. In the same study, seeds of *Tropeaolum hjertingii* Sparre and *Tropaeolum minus* L. were shown to produce only benzyl ITC upon myrosinase hydrolysis, confirming the presence of only benzyl GL (**3**) in the seeds [59].

Finally, it has been established that benzyl (**3**), 4-methoxybenzyl (**5**), 1-methylethyl (**26**), 1-methylpropyl (**27**) and 2-methylpropyl (**28**) GLs are present in the seeds of *Tropaeolum cochabambae* Buch [59].

2. GLUCOSINOLATE DISTRIBUTION IN THE ORDERS MALPIGHIALES, CELASTRALES, CARYOPHYLLALES, AND GENTIANALES

The occurrence of GLs in some of the following plant orders are questionable and would need further confirmations.

Glucosinolates have been identified in the families Putranjivaceae (*Drypetes* genus), Violaceae (*Rinorea* genus), Euphorbiaceae (genera *Croton*, *Euphorbia*, and *Phyllanthus*), all belonging to the order Malpighiales. Benzyl GL (**3**) is expected in *Drypetes gossweileri* S. Moore because of the identification of benzyl ITC in the essential oil of the bark of this plant [64, 65]. The same GL is also expected in *Rinorea subintegrifolia* O. Ktze [65]. In another investigation, 3-methylsulfinylpropyl (**10**) and 2-propenyl (**39**) GLs were identified by HPLC in the seeds of *Croton liglium* L., 4-methylsulfinyl-3-butenyl (**40**) and 3-methylsulfanylpropyl (**41**) GLs in the herbs of *Euphorbia humifusa* Willd., and 2-propenyl (**39**) in the roots of *Phyllanthus emblica* L. [61].

In the order Celastrales, the family Hippocrateaceae is expected to contain GLs. Benzyl, 4-methoxybenzyl, and dimethoxybenzyl ITCs have been detected in the essential oil of the root of *Hippocratea welwitschii* Oliv. (Hippocrateaceae) indicating that the parent GLs would exist in the plant [66].

GLs have also been claimed in the family Phytolaccaceae (order Caryophyllales). It was shown by that the seeds of *Phytolacca dioica* L. (Phytolaccaceae) produced benzyl and *m*-hydroxybenzyl ITCs upon myrosinase hydrolysis indicating that the plant possesses benzyl (**3**) and *m*-hydroxybenzyl (**35**) GLs [20]. Moreover, researchers claimed to have detected 4-methylsulfinylbutyl GL (**12**) by HPLC in the seeds of *Phytolacca acinosa* Roxb. (Phytolaccaceae) [61].

Finally, a low total GL content measured by spectrophotometry in plants (*Knoxia valerianoides* Thorel et Pitard and *Gardenia jasminoides* Ellis) of the family Rubiaceae (order Gentianales) is claimed without specifying the GL(s) [61]. Other investigations are needed to confirm the presence of GL(s) in this family.

3. MECHANISMS OF ENZYMATIC DEGRADATION OF GLUCOSINOLATES

a) Isothiocyanates

Without exception, GL-containing plants also contain myrosinase (thioglucoside glucohydrolase EC 3.2.3.147), the only enzyme able to break an anomeric carbon-sulfur bond and therefore to catalyze the hydrolytic cleavage of the glucosidic C-S bond of GLs [67, 68]. Over the years, many research efforts have been put into clarifying this unique enzyme-substrate relationship and the mechanistic versatility of myrosinase. Being located in different cell sites, GLs and myrosinase cohabit in the cells of all Brassicaceae species. In fact the term "myrosinase" stands for a group of glycoproteins containing various thiol groups, disulfide and salt bridges. Depending on the source, they can assume multiple forms with different molecular weights (135-480 kD), a different number of subunits (2-12) and a high content of carbohydrate (up to 22.5%), mostly hexoses [69, 70]. The main myrosinase isoform isolated from ripe seeds of *Sinapis alba* - a typical source for myrosinase - consists of two identical subunits with a molecular weight of 71.7 kD [71, 72], containing 499 residues and stabilized by a Zn^{2+} ion bound on a 2-fold axis, with tetrahedral coordination. This isoenzyme has three disulfide bridges per sub-unit and 21 carbohydrate residues distributed in 10 glycosylation sites on the surface.

The myrosinase-catalyzed hydrolysis of GLs generally releases a sulfate anion and D-glucose and produces unstable aglycones, which can follow various transformation processes depending on the reaction conditions. The detached aglycones generally undergo a fast Lossen-type rearrangement to deliver a variety of strongly electrophilic ITCs and/or closely related bio-active thio-compounds (Figure 3).

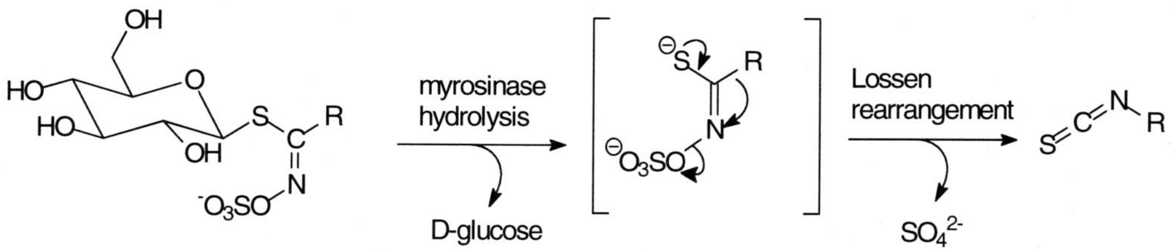

Figure 3. Myrosinase-assisted hydrolytic cleavage of glucosinolates to deliver isothiocyanates.

b) Nitriles and Epithionitriles

However, apart from the delivery of ITCs, the catabolism of GLs is likely to follow less common pathways [73]. A collection of related thio-compounds can also form, depending mainly on the chemical structure of the aglycon chain and the experimental conditions. Neutral pH values generally favour the production of ITCs (Figure 3), whereas acidic conditions and/or the presence or a reducing agent (ferrous ion, cysteine) favour the formation of nitriles, with concomitant extrusion of elemental sulfur [74, 75] (Figure 4).

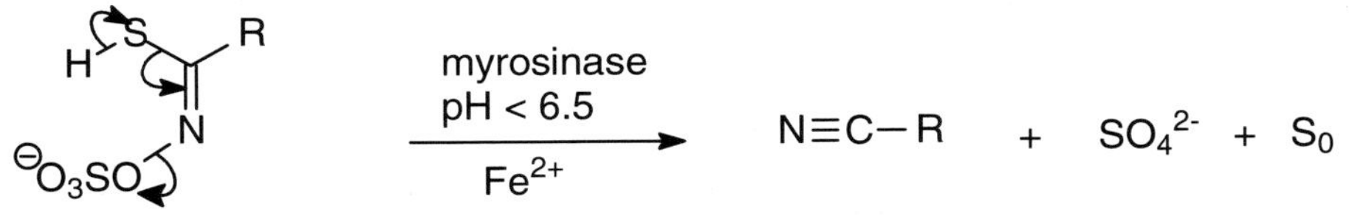

Figure 4. Formation of nitriles from GLs.

In the presence of an epithiospecifier protein (ESP) [76-78], the myrosinase-catalyzed hydrolysis of alkenyl GLs bearing a terminal vinyl group can also produce epithionitriles [79] (Figure 5).

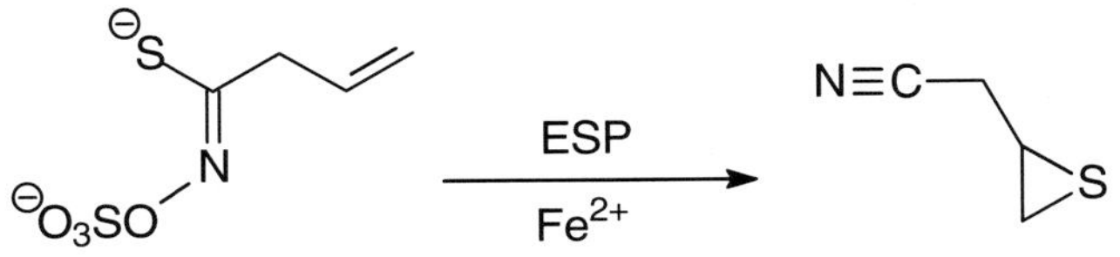

Figure 5. Formation of epithionitriles from GLs.

c) Goitrin and Oxazolidinethiones

In the case of GLs bearing in the aglycon a β-positioned hydroxyl group *viz.* 2-(R)-hydroxy-3-butenyl GL (**11b**, progoitrin), 2-(S)-hydroxy-3-butenyl GL (**11a**, *epi*-progoitrin), 2-(R)-hydroxy-2-phenylethyl GL (**33a**, glucobarbarin), 2-hydroxy-4-pentenyl GL (**42**, gluconapoleiferin), 2-hydroxy-2-methylbutyl GL (**24**, glucocleomin), 2-hydroxy-2-methylpropyl GL (**1**, glucoconringiin), and 2-hydroxy-1-methylethyl GL (**43**, glucosysimbrin), the ITCs produced cannot be isolated because they undergo a fast cyclization process to afford 1,3-oxazolidine-2-thiones [80-82] (Figure 6).

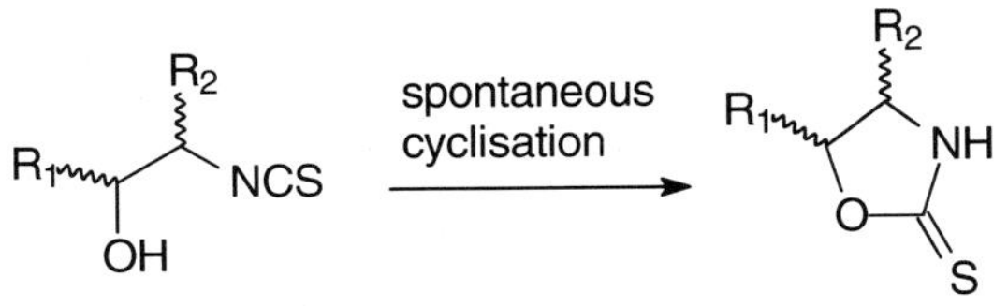

Figure 6. Formation of 1,3-oxazolidine-2-thiones from GLs.

d) Thiocyanates

Under the influence of an isomerizing co-factor (thiocyanate-forming protein), thiocyanates can also be produced in some limited cases [83, 84] (Figure 7).

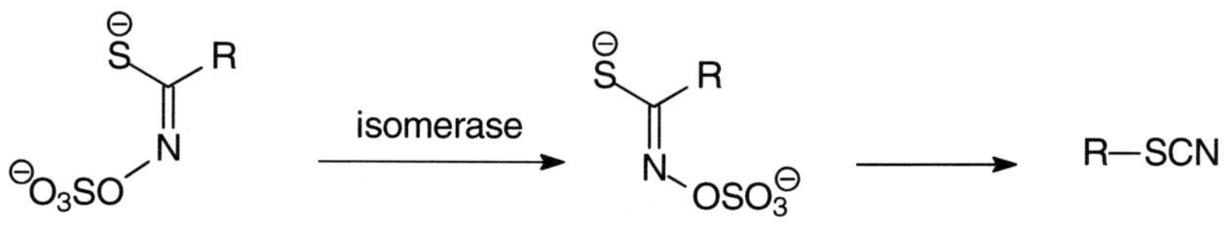

Figure 7. Formation of thiocyanates from GLs.

4. GOITROGENICITY ON ANIMALS AND HUMANS

a) Consumption of Crucifers by Humans and Animals

Goiter refers to the abnormal enlargement of the thyroid gland. One of the causes of such disorder can be ingestion of goitrogens in the diet and this can be managed by elimination of the goitrogen or by adding sufficient thyroxine to shut off thyroid-stimulating hormone activity. There are reports of endemic goiter, the origin of which is suggested to be caused by eating cruciferous plants [85]. However, it has not been proved that eating such plants causes goiter in humans. Most human goiters (hypothyroid) may be due to iodine deficiency [86]. The only goiters related to GLs are those associated with hypothyroidism.

GLs and their myrosinase-degradation products (ITCs, oxazolidine-2-thiones, nitriles and thiocyanate ion) can exhibit goitrogenic or antithyroid activity on humans and animals. Despite high iodide supplementation, a GL load (19 mmol kg^{-1} diet of rapeseed meals) decreased the growth rate, the feed intake, the iodine store of the thyroid and serum concentration of thyroid hormone and resulted in goiter formation in pigs. In the case of diets with less than 6 mmol kg^{-1}, iodine prevented antithyroid effects. Iodine administration prevents the effects of a low GL intake only, by overcoming the depressed thyroxine released of the thyroid, resulting in regression of goiter [87].

Thyroid peroxidase oxidizes iodide ions to form iodine atoms for addition onto Tyr residues on thyroglobulin for the production of thyroxine (T4) or triiodothyronine (T3), the thyroid hormones. *In vitro*, the activity of thyroid peroxidase is reduced by raw cauliflower and cabbage. The activity is almost the same as that of raw extracts. The activity is more reduced with boiled extracts. In the presence of extra iodide ions, the recovery in thyroid peroxidase activity was maximum with raw extract, moderate for boiled extract and remained almost unchanged for cooked extract of plants. Regarding mustard, turnip and radish, the maximum inhibition of thyroid peroxidase activity was found with boiled extracts, followed by cooked extracts, and raw extracts. Extra iodide had reversed the anti-thyroid peroxidase activity of raw extracts of radish or mustard, but the recovery after boiled and cooked extracts was less than for the raw extracts [88].

b) Goitrin and Other Oxazolidinethiones

The antithyroid factor of rutabaga root was proved to be L-5-vinyl-1,3-oxazolidine-2-thione (commonly called goitrin). This compound was also isolated from other *Brassica* species seeds such as turnip, cabbage, kale, rape, and quantified in Brussels sprouts and kohlrabi. It was found to have antithyroid activity equal to that of thiouracil in normal human subjects. In rats, goitrin is one-fifth as active as thiouracil and similar in activity to oxazolidine-2-thione and 5,5-dimethyloxazolidine-2-thione [89]. In another study, (±)-5-vinyl-1,3-oxazolidine-2-thione fed to chicks at 0.15% of the ration provoked depression of growth rate, hyperplasia, and hypertrophy of the thyroid. The uptake of I^{131} by the thyroid was depressed during the initial feeding. However, after a longer feeding of 25 days, the thyroid function returned to normality. It was concluded that the chicken eventually reached physiological equilibrium at an increased ratio of thyroid to body weight [90]. Other investigations confirmed that goitrin can cause enlargement of thyroid in chicks [91, 92]. First, it was concluded that the incorporation of blood I^{131} by the thyroid gland was not inhibited, but the slow release of I^{131} and the depressed thyroid hormone in blood, some steps of thyroid hormone synthesis and furthermore secretion of thyroid hormone into blood or deiodination of some of iodo-amino acids in thyroid gland are inhibited by goitrin [91]. Later, the results indicated that thyroid hormone synthesis is not so much suppressed to the degree expected from the enlargement of thyroid gland when goitrin is administered orally to chicks [92]. Moreover, the depression in metabolism of thyroid hormone induced by administration of goitrin to chicks may be restored in a relatively short time after withdrawal of goitrin, despite hypertrophy of thyroid gland which persists for relatively longer time [93].

In rats fed with a low-iodine diet, propylthiouracil was found to be 150 times as potent as goitrin after oral administration but only 40 times as potent after parenteral administration [94]. Furthermore, in humans, a significant decrease of radioiodine uptake was observed following a single dose of 50 mg of goitrin in 6 subjects, and of 25 mg of goitrin in 13 subjects, whereas a dose of 2 × 10 mg of goitrin was without effect in 18 subjects [95]. This product is released by myrosinase degradation of 2-(R)-hydroxy-3-butenyl GL (**11b**).

Mild hyperplastic goiter occurred in rats fed meal containing 0.23% of (R)-goitrin [96]. Rats fed with rapeseed isolate composed largely of butenyl ITC and butenyl cyanide showed depressed live-weight gain and intake and, although thyroid weight was unaffected, tracer studies with I^{125} suggested that biosynthesis of thyroid hormones was affected by the feeding [97].

5,5-Dimethyloxazolidine-2-thione was found to be approximately one-fifth as active as thiouracil in rats. This oxazolidine-2-thione is found in the seeds of *Conringia orientalis* (L.) Dumort. (Brassicaceae) [86].

5-Phenyloxazolidine-2-thione, which can be obtained from the myrosinase degradation of 2-hydroxy-2-phenylethyl GL (**33**), was shown to possess antithyroid activity when given parenterally to rats whereas it was ineffective when given orally [94]. It was also found to possess approximately 50% the antithyroid activity of goitrin in both man and rats [86].

c) Thiocyanate Ion and Isothiocyanates

At pH 7, when plant cells are broken, indole GLs (**8, 18**) can be cleaved by myrosinase into glucose, sulfate, indolyl alcohols, 3,3'-bis-indolylmethane (or substituted) and thiocyanate ion (SCN⁻) [98]. Upon enzymatic hydrolysis, 4-hydroxybenzyl GL (**4**) can give 4-hydroxybenzyl ITC which undergoes further degradation to 4-hydroxybenzyl alcohol and SCN⁻ [99]. The thiocyanate ion (SCN⁻) can block uptake of iodide by the thyroid gland through competitive inhibition of the iodide transport mechanism.

It was shown that the treatment of hypertension by the administration of SCN⁻ can provoke enlargement of the thyroid gland in some patients [100]. In rats, it was observed that SCN⁻ inhibits preferential concentration of iodide by thyroid tissue. It causes also the discharge of iodide from the thyroid as well as prevents its uptake. In the experimental conditions, SCN⁻ had a partial inhibitory effect on thyroid iodide concentration 5 hours after injection [101]. In pigs, SCN⁻ induced clinical hypothyroidism in the absence of supplemental iodine [87].

Methyl ITC, myrosinase-degradation product of methyl GL (**20**), had no effect on the thyroid and its function in rats [102]. However, allyl ITC depressed iodine uptake in rat thyroids. In addition, the administration of allyl ITC to rats for 60 days, in doses corresponding approximately to the total content of mustard oils in cabbage, caused thyroid changes similar to those observed after cabbage feeding [103]. Feeding rats with a combination of SCN⁻, goitrin and allyl ITC produced a greater alteration in thyroid function and increase in thyroid size than did administration of any one of them individually. The results led to think that the goitrogenicity of cabbage and other cruciferous plants may be explained by the combined action of the SCN⁻, goitrin and allyl ITC contained therein [104]. 3-Methylsulfonylpropyl ITC (also called cheirolin) displayed antithyroid effect in an acute test in rats. It was shown to be more active that *n*-propyl ITC [105].

d) Intact Glucosinolates

2-(*R*)-Hydroxy-3-butenyl GL (**11b**) was found to induce antithyroid activity after being administered to humans and rats [86, 106]. Thyroid hyperplasia occurred in rats fed meal containing 2-(*S*)-hydroxy-3-butenyl GL (**11a**) plus active thioglucosidase enzyme(s) [96].

CONCLUSION

The objective of this chapter was not to present a comprehensive review of the GLs found in the plant kingdom but rather a general overview to introduce their structural diversity. It is worth noting that some GLs are specific to certain plant families, genera and sometimes species. Many early investigations have used indirect methods to characterize the structure of GLs by determining the structure of myrosinase-degradation products. Nowadays, the structures are established thanks to the isolation of intact GLs. Next, the structures are established using spectroscopic methods (NMR and mass spectrometry). The discovery of new GL structures is still relevant because the GL profiles of certain plants are partially known and some structures are not completely ascertained. Some underinvestigated species, genera, and families (especially endemic plants) need to be explored. Moreover, researchers will have to direct their efforts towards the identification of minor GLs.

Benign goiter may be accentuated by eating excessive amounts of *Brassica* vegetables in geographic areas where iodide content is low in soil and water. Humans will use iodized salt in their diet or ingest iodide supplements to reduce or prevent goiter. Nowadays, goiter does not seem to be a public health concern for humans in affluent countries where the diet is diversified. Finally, a double zero rapeseed (low erucic acid and low total GL content) has been developed and this rapeseed meal can be safely used to feed animals.

REFERENCES

[1] APG III. An update of the angiosperm phylogeny group classification for the orders and families of flowering plants: APGIII. (2009). *Bot. J. Linn. Soc.* 161, 105–121.

[2] Fahey, J. W., Zalcmann A. T., Talalay, P., (2001). The chemical diversity and distribution of glucosinolates and isothiocyanates among plants. *Phytochemistry* 56, 5–51.

[3] Agerbirk, N., Olsen, C. E., (2012). Glucosinolate structures in evolution. *Phytochemistry* 77, 16-45.

[4] Sønderby, I. E., Geu-Flores, F., Halkier, B. A., (2010). Biosynthesis of glucosinolates – gene discovery and beyond. *Trends Plant Sci.* 15, 283-290.

[5] Grubb, C. D., Abel, S., (2006). Glucosinolate metabolism and its control. *Trends Plant Sci.* 11, 89-100.

[6] Clarke, D. B., (2010). Glucosinolates, structures and analysis in food. *Anal. Methods* 2, 310-325.

[7] Boufford, D. E., Kjær, A., Madsen, J. Ø., Skrydstrup, T., (1989). Glucosinolates in Bretschneideraceae. *Biochem. Syst. Ecol.* 17, 375-379.

[8] Mithen, R., Bennett, R., Marquez, J., (2010). Glucosinolate biochemical diversity and innovation in the Brassicales. *Phytochemistry* 71, 2074-2086.

[9] Montaut, S., Zhang, W.-D., Nuzillard, J.-M., De Nicola, G. R., Rollin P., (2015). Glucosinolate diversity in *Bretschneidera sinensis* of Chinese origin. *J. Nat. Prod.* 78, 2001-2006.

[10] Schraudolf, H., Schmidt, B., Weberling, F., (1971). Das Vorkommen von "Myrosinase" als Hinweis auf die systematische Stellung der Batidaceae. *Experientia* 27, 1090-1091.

[11] Mabry, T. J., (1976) Pigment dichotomy and DNA-RNA hybridization data for centrospermous families. *Plant. Syst. Evol.* 126, 79-94.

[12] The Arabidopsis Genome Initiative, (2000). Analysis of the genome sequence of the flowering plant *Arabidopsis thaliana*. *Nature* 408, 796-815.

[13] Kliebenstein, D. J., Kroymann, J., Brown, P., Figuth, A., Pedersen, D., Gershenzon, J., Mitchell-Olds, T., (2001). Genetic control of natural variation in *Arabidopsis* glucosinolate accumulation. *Plant Physiol.* 126, 811-825.

[14] Reichelt, M., Brown, P. D., Schneider, B., Oldham, N. J., Stauber, E., Tokuhisa, J., Kliebenstein, D. J., Mitchell-Olds, T., Gershenzon, J., (2002). Benzoic acid glucosinolate esters and other glucosinolates from *Arabidopsis thaliana*. *Phytochemistry* 59, 663-671.

[15] Vallejo, F., Tomás-Barberán, F., García-Viguera, C., (2003). Health-promoting compounds in broccoli as influenced by refrigerated transport and retail sale period. *J. Agric. Food Chem.* 51, 3029-3034.

[16] Borrowski, J., Szajdek, A., Borrowska, E. J., Ciska, E., Zieliński, H., (2008). Content of selected bioactive components and antioxidant properties of broccoli (*Brassica oleracea* L.). *Eur. Food Res. Technol.* 226, 459-465.

[17] Vallejo, F., García-Viguera, C., Tomás-Barberán, F., (2003). Changes in broccoli (*Brassica oleracea* L. var. *italica*) health-promoting compounds with inflorescence development. *J. Agric. Food Chem.* 51, 3776-3782.

[18] Montaut, S., Barillari, J., Iori, R., Rollin, P., (2010). Glucoraphasatin: chemistry, occurrence, and biological properties. *Phytochemistry*, 71, 6-12.

[19] Cole, R. A., (1976). Isothiocyanates, nitriles and thiocyanates as products of autolysis of glucosinolates in *Cruciferae*. *Phytochemistry* 15, 759-762.

[20] Daxenbichler, M. E., Spencer, G. F., Carlson, D. G., Rose, G. B., Brinker, A. M., Powell, R. G., (1991). Glucosinolate composition of seeds from 297 species of wild plants. *Phytochemistry* 30, 2623-2638.

[21] Bennett, R. N., Mellon, F. A., Kroon, P. A., (2004). Screening crucifer seeds as sources of specific intact glucosinolates using ion-pair high-performance liquid chromatography negative ion electrospray mass spectrometry. *J. Agric. Food Chem.* 52, 428-438.

[22] Ahmed, Z. F., Rizk, A. M., Hammouda, F. M., Seif El-Nasr, M. M., (1972). Naturally occurring glucosinolates with special reference to those of family Capparidaceae. *Planta Med.* 21, 35-60.

[23] Kjær, A., Thomsen, H., (1963). Isothiocyanate-producing glucosides in species of Capparidaceae. *Phytochemistry* 2, 39-32.

[24] Gmelin, R., Kjær, A., (1970). Glucosinolates in some new world species of Capparidaceae. *Phytochemistry* 9, 601-602.

[25] Hedge, I. C., Kjær, A., Malver, O., (1980). *Dipterygium* – *Cruciferae* or *Capparaceae*? *Notes Roy. Bot. Gard. Edinburgh* 38, 247-250.

[26] Lüning, B., Kers, L. E., Seffers, P., (1992). Methyl glucosinolate confirmed in *Puccionia* and *Dhofaria* (Capparidaceae). *Biochem. Syst. Ecol.* 20, 394.

[27] Kjær, A., Schuster, A., (1971). Glucosinolates in *Capparis flexuosa* of Jamaican origin. *Phytochemistry* 10, 3155-3160.

[28] Schraudolf, H., (1989). Indole glucosinolates of *Capparis spinosa*. *Phytochemistry* 28, 259-260.

[29] Gmelin, R., Kjær, A., (1970). Glucosinolates in the Caricaceae. *Phytochemistry* 9, 591-593.

[30] Williams, D. J., Pun, S., Chaliha, M., Scheelings, P., O'Hare, T., (2013). An unusual combination in papaya (*Carica papaya*): The good (glucosinolates) and the bad (cyanogenic glycosides). *J. Food Comp. Anal.* 29, 82-86.

[31] Kjær, A., Gmelin, R., Larsen, I., (1955). Isothiocyanates XIII. Methyl isothiocyanate, a new naturally occurring mustard oil, present as glucoside (glucocapparin) in Capparidaceae. *Acta Chem. Scand.* 9, 857-858.

[32] Griffiths, D. W., Deighton, N., Birch, A. N. E., Patrian, B., Baur, R., Städler, E., (2001). Identification of glucosinolates on the leaf surface of plants from the Cruciferae and other closely related species. *Phytochemistry* 57, 693-700.

[33] Schraudolf, H., (1965). Zur Verbreitung von Glucobrassicin und Neoglucobrassicin in höheren Pflanzen. *Experientia* 21, 520-522.

[34] Kjær, A., Malver, O., (1979). Glucosinolates in *Tersonia brevipes* (Gyrostemonaceae). *Phytochemistry* 18, 1565.

[35] Bottomley, W., White, D. E., (1950). The chemistry of Western Australian plants. II. The essential oil of *Codonocarpus cotinifolius* (Desf.). *Roy. Australian Chem. Inst. J. Proc.* 17, 31-32.

[36] Rodman, J. E., Soltis, P. S., Soltis, D. E., Sytsma, K. J., Karol, K. G., (1998). Parallel evolution of glucosinolate biosynthesis inferred from congruent nuclear and plastid gene phylogenies. *Am. J. Bot.* 85, 997-1006.

[37] Ettlinger, M., Lundeen, A., (1956). The mustard oil of *Limnanthes douglasii* seed, *m*-methoxybenzyl isothiocyanate. *J. Am. Chem. Soc.* 78, 1952-1954.

[38] Miller, R. W., Daxenbichler, M. E., Earle, F. R., (1964). Search for new industrial oils. VIII. The genus *Limnanthes*. *J. Am. Oil Chem. Soc.* 41, 167-169.

[39] Daxenbichler, M. E., VanEtten, C. H., (1974). 5,5-Dimethyloxazolidine-2-thione formation from glucosinolate in *Limnanthes alba* Benth. seed. *J. Am. Oil Chem. Soc.* 51, 449-450.

[40] Kurup, P. A., Narasimha Rao, P. L., (1954). Antibiotic principle from *Moringa pterygosperma*. Part II. Chemical nature of pterygospermin. *Ind. J. Med. Res.* 42, 85-95.

[41] Bennett, R. N., Mellon, F. A., Foidl, N., Pratt, J. H., Dupont, M. S., Perkins, L., Kroon, P. A., (2003). Profiling glucosinolates and phenolics in vegetative and reproductive tissues of the multi-purpose trees *Moringa oleifera* L. (horseradish tree) and *Moringa stenopetala* L. *J. Agric. Food Chem.* 51, 3546-3553.

[42] Kjær, A., Malver, O., El-Menshawi, B., Reisch, J., (1979). Isothiocyanates in myrosinase-treated seed extracts of *Moringa peregrina*. *Phytochemistry* 18, 1485-1487.

[43] De Nicola, G. R., Nyegue, M., Montaut, S., Iori, R., Menut, C., Tatibouët, A., Rollin, P., Ndoyé, C., Amvam Zollo, P.-H., (2012). Profile and quantification of glucosinolates in *Pentadiplandra brazzeana* Baill. *Phytochemistry*, 73, 51-56.

[44] Gmelin, R., Kjær, A., (1970). 2-Hydroxy-2-methylpropyl glucosinolate in *Reseda alba*. *Phytochemistry* 9, 599-600.

[45] Kiddle, G., Bennett, R. N., Botting, N. P., Davidson, N. E., Robertson, A. A. B., Wallsgrove, R. M., (2001). High-performance liquid chromatographic separation of natural and synthetic desulfoglucosinolates and their chemical validation by UV, NMR and chemical ionisation-MS methods. *Phytochem. Anal.* 12, 226-242.

[46] Olsen, O., Sørensen, H., (1979). Isolation of glucosinolates and the identification of *O*-(α-L-rhamnopyranosyloxy)benzylglucosinolate from *Reseda odorata*. *Phytochemistry* 18, 1547-1552.

[47] Delaveau, P., (1957). Sur la multiplicité des hétérosides à sénévol et leur relation avec la physiologie et la taxinomie des Crucifères. *Bull. Soc. Bot. Fr.* 104, 148-152.

[48] Kjær, A., Gmelin, R., (1958). *Iso*thiocyanates XXXIII. An *iso*thiocyanate glucoside (glucobarbarin) of *Reseda luteola* L. *Acta Chem. Scand.* 12, 1693-1694.

[49] Underhill, E., Kirkland, D. F., (1972). L-2-Amino-4-phenylbutyric acid and 2-phenylethylglucosinolate, precursors of 2-hydroxy-2-phenylethylglucosinolate. *Phytochemistry* 11, 1973-1979.

[50] Kirkland, D. F., Matsuo, M., Underhill, E. W., (1971). Detection of glucosinolates and myrosinase in plant tissue cultures. *Lloydia* 34, 195-198.

[51] Olsen, O., Sørensen, H., (1980). Glucosinolates and amines in *Reseda media*. *Phytochemistry* 19, 1783-1787.

[52] Kjær, A., Conti, J., Larsen, I., (1953). Isothiocyanates IV. Systematic investigation of the occurrence and chemical nature of volatile isothiocyanates in seeds of various plants. *Acta Chem. Scand.* 7, 1276-1283.

[53] Olsen, O., Rasmussen, K. W., Sørensen, H., (1981). Glucosinolates in *Sesamoides canescens* and *S. pygmaea*: 2-(α-L-arabinopyranosyloxy)-2-phenylethylglucosinolate. *Phytochemistry* 20, 1857-1981.

[54] Patel, C., Narayana Iyer, S., Sudborough, J. J., Watson, H. E., (1926). The fat from '*Salvadora oleoides*': khakan fat. *J. Indian Inst. Sci.* 9A, 117-132.

[55] Bader, A., Flamini, G., Cioni, P. L., Morelli, I., (2002). The composition of the root oil of *Salvadora persica* L. *J. Essent. Oil Res.* 14, 128-129.

[56] Bennett, R. N., Mellon, F. A., Rosa, E. A. S., Perkins L., Kroon, P. A., (2004). Profiling glucosinolates, flavonoids, alkaloids, and other secondary metabolites in tissues of *Azima tetracantha* L. (Salvadoraceae). *J. Agric. Food Chem.* 52, 5856-5862.

[57] Schraudolf, H., Bäuerle, R., (1986). ¹N-acetyl-3-indolylmethyl-glucosinolate in seedlings of *Tovaria pendula* Ruiz et Pav. *Z. Naturforsch.* 41c, 526-528.

[58] Christensen, B. W., Kjær, A., Øgaard Madsen, J., Olsen, C. E., Olsen O., Sørensen, H., (1982). Mass-spectrometric characteristics of some per-trimethylsilylated desulfoglucosinolates. *Tetrahedron* 38, 353-357.

[59] Kjær, A., Ogaard-Madsen, J., Maeda, Y., (1978). Seed volatiles within the family Tropaeolaceae. *Phytochemistry* 17, 1285-1287.

[60] Gadamer, J., (1899). Das ätherische Oel von *Tropaeolum majus*. *Arch. Pharm.* 237, 111-120.

[61] Hu, Y., Linag, H., Yuan, Q., Hong, Y., (2010). Determination of glucosinolates in 19 Chinese medicinal plants with spectrophotometry and high-pressure liquid chromatography. *Nat. Prod. Res.* 24, 1195-1205.

[62] Ramallo, R., Wathelet, J.-P., Le Boulengé, E., Torres, E., Marlier, M., Ledent, J.-F., Guidi, A., Larondelle, Y., (2004). Glucosinolates in isaño (*Tropaeolum tuberosum*) tubers: qualitative and quantitative content and changes after maturity. *J. Sci. Food Agric.* 84, 701-706.

[63] Johns, T., Towers, G. H. N., (1981). Isothiocyanates and thioureas in enzyme hydrolysates of *Tropaeolum tuberosum*. *Phytochemistry* 20, 2687-2689.

[64] Eyele Mvé-Mba, C., Menut, C., Bessière, J. M., Lamaty, G., Nzé Ekekang, L., Denamganai J., (1997). Aromatic plants of tropical Central Africa. XXIX. Benzyl isothiocyanate as major constituent of bark essential oil of *Drypetes gossweileri* S. Moore. *J. Essent. Oil Res.*, 9, 367-370.

[65] Agnaniet, H., Mounzeo, H., Menut, C., Bessière, J.-M., Criton, M., (2003). The essential oils of *Rinorea subintegrifolia* O. Ktze and *Drypetes gossweileri* S. Moore occurring in Gabon. *Flavour Frag. J.* 18, 207-210.

[66] Iwu, M. W., Unaeze, N. C., Okunji, C. O., Corley, D. G., Sanson, D. R., Tempesta, M. S. (1991). Antibacterial aromatic isothiocyanates from the essential oil of *Hippocratea welwitschii* roots. *Int. J. Pharmacognosy* 29, 154-158.

[67] Burmeister, W. P., Cottaz, S., Driguez, H., Iori, R., Palmieri, S., Henrissat, B., (1997). The crystal structure of *Sinapis alba* myrosinase and a covalent glycosyl-enzyme

intermediate provide insights into the substrate recognition and active site machinery of an *S*-glycosidase. *Structure* 5, 663-675.

[68] Burmeister, W. P., Cottaz, S., Rollin, P., Vasella, A., Henrissat, B., (2000). High resolution X-ray crystallography shows that ascorbate is a cofactor for myrosinase and substitutes for the function of the catalytic base. *J. Biol. Chem.* 275, 39385-39393.

[69] Björkman, R., (1976). Properties and function of plant myrosinases. In *The Biology and Chemistry of the Cruciferae*; Vaughan, J. G., MacLeod, A. J., Jones, B. M. G., Eds.; Academic Press: London; pp.191-205.

[70] Bones, A. M. and Rossiter, J. T., (1996). The myrosinase-glucosinolate system, its organization and biochemistry. *Physiol. Plant.* 97, 194-208.

[71] Björkman, R., Janson, J.-C., (1972). Studies on myrosinases. I. Purification and characterization of a myrosinase from white mustard seed (*Sinapis alba* L.). *Biochim. Biophys. Acta* 276, 508-518.

[72] Pessina, A., Thomas, R. M., Palmieri, S., Luisi, P. L., (1990). An improved method for the purification of myrosinase and its physicochemical characterization. *Arch. Biochem. Biophys.* 280, 383-315.

[73] Benn, M., (1977). Glucosinolates. *Pure Appl. Chem.* 49, 197-210.

[74] Daxenbichler, M. E., VanEtten, C. H., Spencer, G. F., (1977). Glucosinolates and derived products in cruciferous vegetables. Identification of organic nitriles from cabbage. *J. Agric. Food Chem.* 25, 121-124.

[75] Uda, Y., Kurata, T., Arakawa, N., (1986). Effects of thiol compounds on the formation of nitriles from glucosinolates. *Agric. Biol. Chem.* 50, 2741-2746.

[76] Tookey, H. L., (1973). Crambe thioglucoside glucohydrolase (EC 3.2.3.1.). Separation of a protein required for epithiobutane formation. *Can. J. Biochem.* 51, 1654-1660.

[77] Bernardi R., Negri A., Ronchi S., Palmieri S., (2000). Isolation of the epithiospecifier protein from oil-rape (*Brassica napus* ssp. *oleifera*) seed and its characterization. *FEBS Lett.* 467, 296-298.

[78] Foo, H. L., Gronning, L. M., Goodenough, L., Bones, A. M., Danielsen, B.-E., Whiting, D. A., Rossiter, J. T., (2000). Purification and characterization of epithiospecifier protein from *Brassica napus*: enzymic intramolecular sulphur addition within alkenyl thiohydroximates derived from alkenyl glucosinolate hydrolysis. *FEBS Lett.* 468, 243-246.

[79] Bones, A. M., Rossiter, J. T., (2006). The enzymatic and chemically induced decomposition of glucosinolates. *Phytochemistry* 67, 1053-1067.

[80] VanEtten, C. H., Daxenbichler, M. E., Peters, J. E., Tookey, H. L., (1966). Variation in enzymatic degradation products from the major thioglucosides in *Crambe abyssinica* and *Brassica napus* seed meals. *J. Agric. Food Chem.* 14, 426-430.

[81] Leoni, O., Bernardi, R., Gueyrard, D., Rollin, P., Palmieri, S., (1999). Chemo-enzymatic preparation from renewable resources of enantiopure 1,3-oxazolidine-2-thiones. *Tetrahedron: Asymmetry* 10, 4775-4780.

[82] Galletti, S., Bernardi, R., Leoni, O., Rollin, P., Palmieri, S., (2001). Preparation and biological activity of four epiprogoitrin myrosinase-derived products. *J. Agric. Food Chem.* 49, 471-476.

[83] Hasapis, X., MacLeod, A. J., (1982). Benzyl glucosinolate degradation in heat-treated *Lepidium sativum* seeds and detection of a thiocyanate-forming factor. *Phytochemistry* 21, 1009-1013.

[84] Burow, M., Bergner, A., Gershenzon, J., Wittstock, U., (2007). Glucosinolate hydrolysis in *Lepidium sativum* – identification of the thiocyanate-forming protein. *Plant Mol. Biol.* 63, 49-61.

[85] Clements, F. W., Wishart, J. W., (1956). A thyroid-blocking agent in the etiology of endemic goiter. *Metab. Clin. Exp.* 5, 623-639.

[86] Greer, M. A., (1962). II. Thyroid hormones. The natural occurrence of goitrogenic agents. *Recent Prog. Horm. Res.* 18, 187-219.

[87] Schöne, F., Groppel, B., Hennig, A., Jahreis, G., (1997). Rapeseed meals, methimazole, thiocyanate and iodine affect growth and thyroid. Investigations into glucosinolate tolerance in the pig. *J. Sci. Food Agric.* 74, 69-80.

[88] Chandra, A. K., Mukhopadhyay, S., Lahari, D., Tripathy, S., (2004). Goitrogenic content of Indian cyanogenic plant foods & their *in vivo* anti-thyroid activity. *Indian J. Med. Res.* 119, 180-185.

[89] Astwood, E. B., Monte, A. G., Ettlinger, M. A., (1949). L-5-vinyl-2-thiooxazolidone, an antithyroid compound from yellow turnip and from *Brassica* seeds. *J. Biol. Chem.* 181, 121-130.

[90] Clandinin, D. R., Bayly, L., Caballero, A., (1966). Effects of (±)-5-vinyl-2-oxazolidinethione, a goitrogen in rapeseed meal, on the rate of growth and thyroid function of chicks. *Poult. Sci.* 45, 833-838.

[91] Matsumoto, T., Itoh, H., Akiba, Y., (1968). Goitrogenic effects of (-)-5-vinyl-2-oxazolidinethione, a goitrogen in rapeseed, in growing chicks. *Poult. Sci.* 47, 1323-1330.

[92] Akiba, Y., Matsumoto, T., (1976). Antithyroid activity of goitrin in chicks. *Poult. Sci.* 55, 716-719.

[93] Akiba, Y., Matsumoto, T., (1973). Thyroid function of chicks after withdrawal of (-)-5-vinyl-2-oxazolidinethione, a goitrogen in rapeseed. *Poult. Sci.* 52, 562-567.

[94] Faiman, C., Ryan, R. J., Eichel, H. J., (1967). Effect of goitrin analogues and related compounds on the rat thyroid gland. *Endocrinology* 81, 88-92.

[95] Langer, P., Michajlovskij, N., Sedlák, J., Kutka, M., (1971). Studies on the antithyroid activity of naturally occuring L-5-vinyl-2-thiooxazolidone in man. *Endokrinologie* 57, 225-229.

[96] VanEtten, C. H., Gagne, W. E., Robbins, D. J., Booth, A. N., Daxenbichler, M. E., Wolff, I. A., (1969). Biological evaluation of crambe seed meals and derived products by rat feeding. *Cereal Chem.* 46, 145-155.

[97] Lo, M.-T., Bell, J. M., (1972). Effects of various dietary glucosinolates on growth, feed intake, and thyroid function of rats. *Can. J. Anim. Sci.* 52, 295-302.

[98] Gmelin, R., Virtanen, A. I., (1962). Neoglucobrassicin, ein zweiter SCN⁻-Precursor vom Indoltyp in *Brassica*-Arten. *Acta Chem. Scand.* 16, 1378-1384.

[99] Kawakishi, S., Namiki, M., Wanatabe, H., Muramatsu, K., (1967). Studies on the decomposition of sinalbin Part II. The decomposition products of sinalbin and their degradation pathways. *Agric. Biol. Chem.* 31, 823-830.

[100] Barker H., (1936). The blood cyanates in the treatment of hypertension. *J. Am. Med. Assoc.* 106, 762-767.

[101] Vanderlaan, J. E., Vanderlaan, W. P., (1947). The iodide concentration mechanism of the rat thyroid and its inhibition by thiocyanate. *Endocrinology* 40, 403-416.

[102] Astwood, E. B., Bissell, A., Hughes, A. M., (1945). Further studies on the chemical nature of compounds which inhibit the function of the thyroid gland. *Endocrinology* 37, 456-481.

[103] Langer, P., Štolc, V., (1965). Goitrogenic activity of allyl isothiocyanate a widespread natural mustard oil. *Endocrinology* 76, 151-155.

[104] Langer, P., (1966). Antithyroid action in rats of small doses of some naturally occurring compounds. *Endocrinology* 79, 1117-1122.

[105] Bachelard, H. S., McQuillan, M. T., Trikojus, V. M., (1963). Studies on endemic goitre III. An investigation of the antithyroid activities of isothiocyanates and derivatives with observations of fractions of milk from goitrous areas. *Aust. J. Biol. Sci.* 16, 177-191.

[106] Greer, M. A., Deeney, J. M., (1959). Antithyroid activity elicited by the ingestion of pure progoitrin, a naturally occurring thioglycoside of the turnip family. *J. Clin. Invest.* 38, 1465-1474.

In: Broccoli
Editor: Bernhard H. J. Juurlink

ISBN: 978-1-63484-313-3
© 2016 Nova Science Publishers, Inc.

Chapter 3

GLUCORAPHANIN AND OTHER GLUCOSINOLATES IN HEADS OF BROCCOLI CULTIVARS

Mark W. Farnham[*] *and Sandra E. Branham*

U.S. Department of Agriculture, Agricultural Research Service,
U.S. Vegetable Laboratory, Charleston, SC, US

ABSTRACT

Broccoli (*Brassica oleracea* L. var. *italica*) emerged as an increasingly popular vegetable of North American consumers during the second half of the 20th Century, with per capita consumption increasing nearly eight fold during this period. Likewise, production and consumption of broccoli has also increased in Europe and Asia in recent decades. The discovery in 1992 that broccoli heads contain sulforaphane, an isothiocyanate breakdown product thant induces anticarcinogenic protective enzymes in mammalian cells, has stimulated consumer recognition of broccoli as a health-promoting vegetable and likely stimulated increased consumption of this vegetable through present day. This chapter summarizes the results of studies that have examined the concentrations of glucosinolates in broccoli heads harvested from known cultivars grown in field studies. Based on those results, we present best estimates of the concentrations of specific compounds like glucoraphanin, glucoiberin, and glucobrassicin that could be expected in broccoli heads purchased by consumers. The importance of genotype as a factor influencing glucosinolate levels is also considered based on results of studies that have examined this. Breeding approaches aimed at enhancing levels of glucoraphanin and progress toward that goal are also presented. Lastly, broccoli seed, which has been shown to contain high levels of glucoraphanin and also glucoiberin, is examined as a potential valuable source for delivery of these glucosinolates.

Keywords: *Brassica oleracea* L. var. *italica*, sulforaphane, glucoiberin, progoitrin, glucobrassicin, neo-glucobrassicin, methoxyglucobrassicin, chemoprotection

---

[*] USDA-ARS-U.S. Vegetable Laboratory, 2700 Savannah Hwy., Charleston, SC 29414 USA. Email: Mark.Farnham@ars.usda.gov.

INTRODUCTION

The 41st President of the United States, George H. W. Bush, declared in the spring of 1990 that "I do not like broccoli, and I haven't liked it since I was a little kid and my mother made me eat it. And I'm president of the United States, and I'm not going to eat any more broccoli!" [1]. It is unlikely that President Bush (born in 1924) actually saw broccoli on his plate very often in his youth. Broccoli (*Brassica oleracea* L. var. *italica*) was a minor garden vegetable in North America at that time, cultivated primarily by Italians who brought it with them when they emigrated from Europe around the beginning of the 20th Century. Broccoli remained a minor crop in the U.S. until the mid-1960s when per capita consumption was estimated at only about one pound per person per year (Figures 1; 2). At the time of President Bush's above declaration, consumption had increased to about five pounds per person per year (Figure 1). There is no evidence that Bush's lack of appreciation for broccoli had any lasting effect on the consumption of this vegetable in the U.S.

President William Jefferson Clinton put broccoli back on the White House menu following his election in 1992. However, a more important event for broccoli occurring in that same year was the reported discovery by Zhang et al. [3] at the John Hopkins University School of Medicine that sulforaphane, an isothiocyanate breakdown product isolated from broccoli heads, was a major inducer of anticarcinogenic protective enzymes in mammalian cells. In this landmark study for broccoli, the Hopkins researchers led by Paul Talalay showed that extracts from the hybrid cultivar 'Saga' readily induced quinone reductase activity in Hepa 1c1c7 murine hepatoma cells. They also demonstrated that sulforaphane, as well as its sulfide and sulfone analogues, all induced quinone reductase and glutathione transferase activities in several mouse tissues, and suggested that the induction of such detoxifying enzymes might be related to anticarcinogenic activity by broccoli. The publication of these findings brought a media spotlight on broccoli as a health-promoting vegetable and led to numerous studies focused on sulforaphane, its precursor glucosinolate glucoraphanin, as well as other glucosinolates found in broccoli. This collective body of research has likely been a factor influencing even greater per capita consumption of broccoli through the late 1990s and into the new millennium (Figure 1).

Hybrid cultivars of broccoli were introduced to vegetable producers in the 1960s as an alternative to improved open-pollinated cultivars (like 'Waltham 29') that had been grown since the introduction of the crop to North America. Within a decade of their introduction, hybrid cultivars were adopted by producers due to a more vigorous and uniform growth habit, and higher quality harvested heads that were more compact and durable than heads harvested from the open-pollinated cultivars (Figure 2). The durable head produced by hybrids was more resistant to wilting and amenable to cold storage and long distance transport, allowing it to be shipped across the states, west to east. Ultimately, it made its way into more and more grocery stores and onto dinner tables throughout the country. We have postulated previously that the gradual increase in broccoli consumption that began in the 1960s and 70s is closely associated with the introduction and adoption of hybrid cultivars [4]. Today, broccoli has become one of the most economically important vegetable crops produced in the U.S. with a farm gate value estimated at about $700 M [2]. Its popularity is also increasing throughout the world with increased consumption now occurring throughout Europe and also in China.

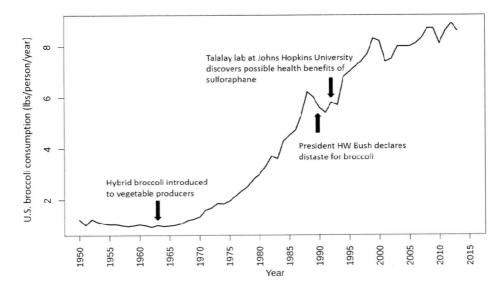

Figure 1. U.S. per capita broccoli consumption (1950–2013) with relevant historical events highlighted.

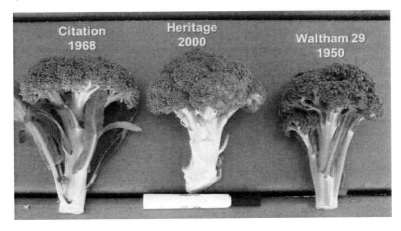

Figure 2. Broccoli heads representative of cultivar development in different decades (all harvested from a single field study). 'Waltham 29' is an open-pollinated cultivar, while both 'Citation' and 'Heritage' are hybrid cultivars. The marker was included in the photograph as a size reference and it measures 16 cm in length.

GLUCOSINOLATE PROFILES AND CONCENTRATIONS IN HEADS OF BROCCOLI CULTIVARS

Studies Prior to 1992

Glucosinolates have been well studied as constituents of the Brassicaceae family of plants [5], and a relatively large body of research has focused on the glucosinolates as chemicals that may have evolved as defense compounds against plant predators, especially insects [6]. Most of the studies examining inter-relationships between host glucosinolates and insect predators have focused on various Brassica species other than *B. oleracea*, or they focused on specific *B. oleracea* crops other than broccoli. This topic has been widely reviewed previously, and since broccoli was not considered in the studies reviewed [6, 7, 8], no results from this line of research are discussed herein.

Table 1. Mean concentrations and ranges of three aliphatic glucosinolates [glucoraphanin (GR), glucoiberin (GI) and progoitrin (PG)] and of three indole glucosinolates [glucobrassicin (GB), neo-glucobrassicin (NGB), and 4-methoxy-glucobrassicin (MGB)] frequently measured in broccoli cultivars and reported in referenced studies since 1987

	Aliphatic Glucosinolates			Indole Glucosinolates		
Reference [# hybrids]	GR	PG	GI	GB	NGB	MGB
Baik et al. (13) [10]	0.85-6.45 (3.69)[b]	0.17-1.65 (0.56)	nm[c]	0.23-3.27 (1.53)	0.00-3.46 (1.03)	0.00-0.28 (0.08)
Brown et al. (14)[5]	2.40-18.40 (9.54)	0.30-1.51 (0.75)	nm	nm	nm	nm
Carlson et al. (10) [6][a]	2.98-8.83 (6.39)	0.00-0.37 (0.07)	0.14-1.12 (0.48)	4.22-7.17 (5.94)	nm	nm
Charron et al. (15) [8]	0.41-15.35 (7.89)	0.00-2.14 (0.97)	0.00-1.02 (0.46)	0.10-5.49 (2.59)	0.01-6.76 (2.50)	0.00-0.24 (0.12)
Farnham et al. (16) [5][a]	2.74-13.46 (10.44)	nm	nm	1.10-2.74 (1.98)	0.14-1.36 (0.74)	nm
Faulkner et al. (17) [3]	0.80-11.10 (5.77)	nm	0.10-1.00 (0.50)	nm	nm	nm
Hansen et al. (18) [5]	15.20-38.40 (24.94)	0.80-16.10 (6.10)	0.00-7.80 (1.90)	10.70-33.40 (18.80)	2.60-19.90 (13.58)	0.70-2.00 (1.24)
Kim & Juvik (19) [3]	2.10-4.20 (2.90)	nm	nm	2.50-10.0 (5.27)	3.20-9.00 (6.37)	nm
Kushad et al. (20) [20]	1.50-21.70 (8.32)	0.00-2.60 (0.71)	nm	0.10-2.80 (0.99)	nm	nm
Lewis & Fenwick (9) [17][a]	1.78-6.17 (4.00)	0.00-2.37 (0.58)	0.42-1.46 (0.95)	1.74-7.96 (4.24)	1.94-10.26 (6.08)	0.23-0.84 (0.55)
Rosa & Rodrigues (21) [9]	6.00-15.05 (9.48)	0.10-5.40 (1.57)	nm	4.00-9.25 (6.51)	0.90-6.95 (3.50)	1.45-3.00 (2.21)
Sarikamis et al. (22) [3]	5.00-10.60 (7.00)	nm	0.40-3.60 (1.57)	3.10-5.90 (4.27)	0.50-0.70 (0.60)	1.60-2.40 (2.03)
Schonhof et al. (23) [4][a]	1.50-7.76 (4.18)	0.15-2.65 (0.84)	0.06-0.89 (0.51)	1.55-2.70 (2.06)	0.18-1.33 (0.65)	0.09-0.28 (0.20)
Reference [# hybrids]	GR	PG	GI	GB	NGB	MGB
Vallejo et al. (24) [6]	1.30-4.30 (2.85)	nm	nm	1.60-12.60 (4.40)	0.10-0.70 (0.33)	nm
Wang et al. (25) [5]	1.57-5.95 (3.52)	1.77-6.07 (3.20)	0.01-0.17 (0.08)	1.84-8.83 (5.28)	0.24-4.25 (1.87)	0.43-1.24 (0.79)

[a]Original values reported in fresh weight and converted to dry weight for comparison using a 1:10 ratio.
[b]Values in the table are in the form of: min-max (mean); units = µmol/g dry weight.
[c]nm = not measured or reported.

Two studies prior to 1992 examined glucosinolate profiles and their concentrations in broccoli cultivars. Lewis and Fenwick [9] compared glucosinolate concentrations in harvested heads from 24 different broccoli cultivars (grown in 1985), most of which were hybrids available in the mid-1980s. Although these authors measured glucosinolate concentrations on a fresh tissue basis, all fresh weight reported values discussed in this chapter have been converted to a dry weight (dw) basis (e.g., µmol/g dw), since this has been the most widely reported measure and also to allow ease in comparing results from different studies. Lewis and Fenwick [9] found that more than 90% of the total glucosinolate content of broccoli heads could be attributed to the aliphatic glucosinolate, glucoraphanin, and two indole glucosinolates, glucobrassicin and neo-glucobrassicin (Table 1). They observed similar mean ranges (from more than 1.00 to 10.00 µmol/g dw or less) in the concentrations of these three glucosinolates among cultivars they examined. In the same year that Lewis and Fenwick reported their findings, Carlson et al. [10] reported observations of glucosinolates in broccoli heads from six cultivars that were actually grown and sampled in 1975. Most of their sampled cultivars were early hybrids (e.g., 'Green Comet' and 'Green Duke'), which were developed in the late 1960s or early 1970s. They identified glucoraphanin and glucobrassicin as the most predominant glucosinolates in broccoli heads (Table 1), observing relatively similar ranges as Lewis and Fenwick [9]. Carlson et al. [10] and Lewis and Fenwick [9] were interested in glucosinolates as nutritional or possibly anti-nutritional components, but they were unaware of the importance of glucoraphanin as the precursor of the isothiocyanate sulforaphane. However, they were the first authors to identify glucoraphanin as one of the most prevalent glucosinolates in the increasingly popular broccoli crop.

Studies after 1992

Following the first report on sulforaphane by Zhang et al. [3] and subsequent papers about this compound that followed (e.g., [11, 12]), researchers increasingly turned their attention to the intact glucosinolate glucoraphanin, the immediate precursor to sulforaphane. Although sulforaphane is the biologically active compound of greatest import in broccoli, glucoraphanin is relatively easy to assay with established methods, is relatively stable when samples are handled appropriately (i.e., rapidly frozen and subsequently lyophilized), and researchers assumed that a measure of intact glucoraphanin would indirectly indicate the potential of a given broccoli sample to induce a beneficial effect when consumed. Thus, numerous studies were undertaken, starting in the late 1990s up until recent years, in which investigators were trying to ascertain expected levels of glucoraphanin and other glucosinolates in a collection of cultivars (mostly hybrids) grown in various field environments. Of fifteen total studies examined (including the two 1987 studies described above), three studies evaluated 3 or 4 hybrids, eight evaluated 5 to 9 hybrids, and three evaluated 10 or more hybrids [9, 10, 13-25]. In general, there is little overlap between studies in regard to the specific hybrids that were tested. A few hybrids (e.g., Marathon) are included in a number of studies, but most investigators examined a unique set of hybrid cultivars, most of which were being grown commercially at the time their respective studies were undertaken. We have examined data from these studies (summarized in Table 1) to provide a synopsis of what is generally known about glucosinolate levels in heads harvested from broccoli cultivars.

Glucoraphanin was the primary focus of study in research papers examined and all of them detected and reported levels of this glucosinolate in broccoli heads. More than half of the studies reported concentrations of two other aliphatic glucosinolates, progoitrin and glucoiberin. Thirteen of 15 studies reported concentrations of the most prevalent indole glucosinolate glucobrassicin, and more than half of them also reported levels of neoglucobrassicin and 4-methoxyglucobrassicin, two additional indole glucosinolates. The above six glucosinolates appear to be the most consistent and abundant ones found in broccoli hybrids (Table 1).

The original ranges in mean concentrations of glucoraphanin in broccoli heads that were measured and reported by Carlson et al. [10] and Lewis and Fenwick [9] were repeated by most researchers who evaluated this trait subsequently (Table 1). Virtually all broccoli cultivars evaluated contain at least a small concentration of glucoraphanin; none were reported to contain zero in the 15 studies examined. Seven out of those 15 studies reported high concentration means below 10 µmol/g dw, and seven reported high concentration means between 10 and 22 µmol/g dw (Table 1). Hansen et al. [18] reported a range in head glucoraphanin concentrations from 15.2 to 38.4 µmol/g dw. Those concentrations are much greater than concentrations cited by all other researchers, and interestingly, the authors evaluated some hybrids (e.g., Shogun and Premium Crop) examined by others. We conclude that these concentrations are not the norm and that Hansen et al. [18] may have overestimated glucoraphanin. In general, mean concentrations of glucoraphanin in conventional broccoli are most likely to range from 2 to 12 µmol/g dw or somewhat higher, and levels of glucoraphanin in such heads should not be expected to exceed 15 µmol/g dw.

Glucoiberin breaks down to the isothiocyanate iberin, and this compound has some biological activity similar to sulforaphane, albeit less potent [11]. Of the eight studies that reported concentrations of glucoiberin, six observed concentration ranges from zero or near zero to 1.5 µmol/g dw or less (Table 1). Sarikamis et al. [22] reported a high concentration of 3.60 µmol/g dw in one hybrid, and Hansen et al. [18] reported a high of 7.80 µmol/g dw in another. Clearly, glucoiberin concentrations in harvested broccoli heads are lower than those of glucoraphanin (e.g., possibly one tenth of the glucoraphanin level), and glucoiberin can be undetectable in some hybrids. The aliphatic glucosinolate progoitrin is more often considered an anti-nutrient (e.g., causing goitrogenic effects in some individuals) and it does not have a potential benefit similar to glucoraphanin or glucoiberin. Ten of 15 examined studies reported measuring progoitrin, and seven of these had ranges from zero or near zero to 2.65 µmol/g dw or less. The remaining three studies reported high concentrations of 5.40, 6.07, and 16.10 µmol/g dw in heads from different hybrid broccoli cultivars. As in other comparisons, Hansen et al. [18] observed much higher maximum concentrations than any other researchers. In general, mean concentrations of progoitrin in broccoli heads can be expected to be 2.0 µmol/g dw or less and to occur at higher concentrations than for glucoiberin; however, progoitrin is not likely to approach the higher levels (e.g., 10-15 µmol/g dw) observed for glucoraphanin.

Glucobrassicin and neo-glucobrassicin are the most abundant indole glucosinolates found in heads of broccoli cultivars. Both of these glucosinolates can break down to unstable glucosinolates that readily breakdown further to various other compounds including indole-3-carbinol (I3C). I3C is a biologically active compound that may combat cancer cells in mammalian systems by interfering with cell division processes [26, 27, 28]. Although I3C may have a significant chemoprotective effect when consumed, the potential effects of this compound are much less studied than those of sulforaphane. Thirteen out of 15 examined studies measured glucobrassicin in broccoli with low cultivar means ranging from less than 1 to approximately 4 µmol/g dw, and high cultivar means about 3 to more than 12 µmol/g dw (Table 1). Very similar low and high means have also been reported for neo-glucobrassicin (Table 1). As with nearly all other glucosinolates, much higher means of these indole glucosinolates were observed by Hansen et al. [18]. Eight out of 15 studies we looked at also reported levels of 4-methoxy-glucobrassicin. Cultivar means for this glucosinolate were much lower than for the other two indoles, with maximum values typically below 3 µmol/g dw. Several of the studies examined herein reported concentrations of glucobrassicin and neo-glucobrassicin in cultivar heads that were very similar to concentrations of glucoraphanin in those same materials. Interest in the indole glucosinolates has never approached that shown for glucoraphanin, but they may play a significant role in imparting any health-promoting impact conveyed due to the consumption of broccoli.

There are nine additional glucosinolates that have been identified at low concentrations in certain hybrids with a limited number of the studies. Mean head concentrations of sinigrin among hybrids studied [9, 10, 14, 17, 20, 23, 25] ranged from 0 to 0.80 µmol/g dw. Epiprogoitrin concentrations [13, 25] ranged from 0 to 0.65 µmol/g dw, 4-hydroxyglucobrassicin concentrations [9, 13, 16, 22, 23, 24, 25] ranged from 0 to 0.97 µmol/g dw, glucoerucin [10, 25] ranged from 0.01 to 0.56 µmol/g dw, glucoalyssin [13, 18, 25] ranged from 0 to 0.40 µmol/g dw, and gluconapoleiferin [10, 13, 23] ranged from 0 to 1.45 µmol/g dw (Table 1). Most studies in which investigators were able to measure gluconapin head concentrations among hybrids reported similar cultivar means and a range of about 0-1.62 µmol/g dw looking across most studies [10, 13, 15, 17, 18, 23, 25]. However, Kim and Juvik [19] reported up to 4.13 µmol/g dw. These same authors also found a higher mean concentration (2.27 µmol/g dw) of gluconasturtiin, than reported in five other studies [10, 13, 18, 20, 25] that assayed levels of this glucosinolate and found ranges around 0 to 1.15 µmol/g dw. Of the two studies that attempted to measure glucoiberverin, the first found from 2.7 to 4.9 µmol/g dw [17], while the second could not detect any in the broccoli hybrids examined [23].

INFLUENCE OF GENOTYPE VERSUS ENVIRONMENT ON EXPRESSION OF GLUCORAPHANIN AND OTHER GLUCOSINOLATES

Effects of Cultural Practices on Glucosinolates

A few studies have examined the possibility that glucosinolates in broccoli heads might be enhanced by cultural practices like sulfur fertilization. Most of these studies [29, 30, 31] tend to show that increased applications of sulfur are often associated with increased concentrations of glucosinolates in general (and sometimes glucoraphanin specifically). However, these studies also typically conclude that individual cultivars respond differently to varying sulfur fertility [29], and more than one study has found that the effects of sulfur fertilization can be largely influenced by nitrogen nutrition [31, 32].

Although increasing sulfur fertilization sometimes increases glucosinolate concentration in broccoli heads, applications of selenium tend to decrease glucosinolate concentrations [19, 33]. This is believed to occur due to the fact that selenium (taken up as SeO$_4$: selenate) replaces sulfur and interferes with normal glucosinolate metabolism [34]. In different studies, Shelp et al. [35, 36] examined the effects of boron nutrtition on the concentrations of glucosinolates in harvested broccoli heads. They found that boron nutrition had little or no effect on concentrations of most glucosinolates, but they consistently observed significant differences in glucosinolate concentrations between the two hybrids included in their studies.

Another approach to enhancing glucosinolates involves the exogenous application of compounds (e.g., methyl jasmonate) that may result in an upregulation in the production of glucosinolates, effectively increasing concentrations. In one such study, Kim and Juvik [19] demonstrated that the application of methyl jasmonate significantly increased concentrations of aromatic and indole glucosinolates in heads of broccoli cultivars, but did not increase concentrations of aliphatic glucosinolates like glucoraphanin. Ku et al. [37] attempted to standardize application methods to bring about maximum glucosinolate concentrations. At this time, we are unaware of any concerted efforts to use methyl jasmonate as a means to increase the health-promoting potential of broccoli.

Importance of Genotype versus Environment

Several researchers have tried to determine if different broccoli culivars might perform differently in different growing seasons, especially in spring versus fall environments, which present very different temperature conditions when heads are maturing [21, 29, 38]. With spring broccoli crops grown in temperate regions, seedlings begin the growing season under cool conditions, but finish it as temperatures are increasingly warmer. On the contrary, fall crops begin with seedings at very warm temperatures in late summer, but they reach maturity when conditions are cooling and becoming optimal for the crop in the late fall. These studies are not particularly informative because they typically report that cultivar and season effects are highly significant, as well as are all related two-way and three-way interaction effects. The significant interactions make it especially difficult to generalize about any seasonal factors, because one often observes a paricular hybrid exhibiting higher concentrations in spring compared to fall, while another exhibits higher concentrations in fall over spring. Additionally, when cultivars are tested in more than one spring environment or more than one fall environment [21, 38], head glucosinolate concentrations for a given cultivar often differ between the two fall tests or between the two spring tests.

Brown et al. [14] and Farnham et al. [16] tried to measure the relative effects of genotype versus environment in multi-environment tests using a limited number of conventional hybrid cultivars and inbred breeding lines. Brown et al. [14] observed significant differences in genetic variability for aliphatic glucosinolates, including glucoraphanin, but not for indole glucosinolates. For example, they found that 54% of variability in glucoraphanin concentrations and 71% of variability in progoitrin concentrations could be attributed to genetic variation. Their observations indicated that variation observed for indole glucosinolates is largely attributable to other, nongenetic factors. Farnham et al. [16] reported similar findings as Brown et al. [14] in that they observed highly significant genotype effects for levels of glucoraphanin in broccoli heads, while environment and genotype by environment effects were found to be much less significant. On the contrary, they could not detect any genotypic effects on head concentrations of three indole glucosinolates including glucobrassicin, neo-glucobrassicin, or hydroxy-glucobrassicin. All variation for these indole compounds was attributed to environmental effects.

Abercrombie et al. [39] undertook a diallel breeding study to determine whether general combining ability or specific combining ability were most important when making new hybrids using inbreds that express known levels of glucoraphanin. In one fall test, glucoraphanin concentration of broccoli heads ranged from 0.83 to 6.00 µmol/g dw, and in a spring environment, from 0.26 to 7.82 µmol/g dw. Significant general combining ability was observed for glucoraphanin concentration in both years. Conversely, no significant specific combining ability was observed in either year. Based on these results, Abercrombie et al. [39] concluded that a given inbred will combine with others to make hybrids with relatively predictable levels of head glucoraphanin and that this should allow identification of inbreds that typically contribute high glucoraphanin levels when hybridized with others. This last study and those described above by Brown et al. [14] and Farnham et al. [16] provide information that can and is being applied to conventional breeding efforts aimed at enhancing glucosinolate (and especially glucoraphanin) concentrations in broccoli heads. These efforts attempt to exploit existing genetic variation within conventional broccoli germplasm to breed for higher concentrations of specific glucosinolates, and they help to verify the important role that genotype plays in the expressed levels of glucoraphanin.

Faulkner et al. [17] embarked on a unique effort to transfer relatively high levels of aliphatic glucosinolates from a relatively wild, but related species (*Brassica villosa* L.) to broccoli (*B. oleracea*). This effort was undertaken over the last couple decades and it followed a strategic plan laid out by a group led by Richard Mithen [22, 40]. This effort ultimately resulted in the development of the commercial hybrid 'Beneforte' which is currently marketed by the Monsanto Vegetable Seeds Co. Results of Traka et al. [41] compiled from multi-year trials indicate that 'Beneforte' and related hybrids consistently exhibit higher (e.g., up to 2.5 times more) glucoraphanin and glucoiberin concentrations in their heads than do several standard commercial hybrids. For instance, glucoraphanin levels for 'Beneforte' were reported to be 20-25 µmol/g dw of head, while other conventional hybrids had levels around 10 µmol/g dw head. 'Beneforte' and others very similar to it contain an introgressed *B. villosa* chromosome segment associated with the elevated levels of glucoraphanin and glucoiberin. This is a significant development for broccoli; however, the high aliphatic glucosinolate concentrations reported for 'Beneforte' by Traka et al. [41] have not been verified by different researchers other than those who developed it. Seed of 'Beneforte' does not appear to be available on the open market, and may only be grown by specific vegetable growers producing broccoli under contract. In total, work to develop 'Beneforte' and other studies described in this section show that genotype is critical in the expression of glucoraphanin and glucoiberin levels in broccoli heads, and that it is possible to manipulate genotype and alter glucosinolate concentration in a deliberative fashion.

And What about Those Broccoli Seeds and Sprouts?

In 1997, Talalay's group made another interesting discovery that broccoli seedling sprouts contain glucoraphanin at concentrations nearly ten times greater than occur in vegetable heads [42]. This discovery brought considerable attention to broccoli seedling sprouts as a potential vehicle for delivering glucoraphanin and sulforaphane, and it also paved the way for a tremendous amount of research aimed at using broccoli sprouts to impart a health enhancing or disease prevention benefit. The existing research covering this specific topic goes far beyond the scope of this chapter and must be explored elsewhere; however, it is useful to examine studies since that the 1997 discovery wherein researchers examined levels of glucoraphanin in seed and the influence that cultivar or genotype might have on this trait. Several studies quickly showed that high levels of glucoraphanin in sprouts are simply a reflection of high levels of glucoraphanin deposition in broccoli seed. For example, West et al. [43] showed that different hybrid and open-pollinated cultivars exhibit significantly different levels of glucoraphanin and other glucosinolates in seed. They observed a range in glucoraphanin concentration from 5 to 104 µmol/g fw of dry seed. Rangkadilok et al. [44] observed a wider range in glucoraphanin concentrations from 44 to 275 µmol/g fw of dry seed of different broccoli genotypes (inbreds and hybrids). Additionally, Velasco et al. [45] examined glucoraphanin in seed of broccoli accessions from a germplasm seed bank and found significant differences among entries, observing a range in concentration from 48 to 140 µmol/g fw of dry seed. None of these studies looked at seed lots for the same genotype produced in different environments, and none of the researchers generated their own seed used in the research.

Farnham et al. [46] examined different glucoraphanin and glucoiberin levels in seed lots produced from the same self-compatible inbred lines (genotypes) in different years and in different greenhouse and outdoor cage environments. They observed a range in glucoraphanin concentration from 6 to 91 µmol/g fw of dry seed among the inbreds and showed that genotype plays a much more important role than environment in the ultimate expression of glucoraphanin concentration in seed. Farnham et al. [46] also observed a range of glucoiberin concentrations from 0 to almost 40 µmol/g fw of dry seed among inbreds and also concluded that genotype was critical in expressed levels of this glucosinolate. These authors were the first to look at seed lots they generated from self-compatible inbred lines. They pointed out that hybrid cultivar (e.g., Marathon) seed would not be a good source of seed for sprouting simply because it is too expensive to produce, and open-pollinated cultivar (e.g., DeCicco) seed would not be a good source because glucosinolate concentration is too variable and inconsistent. Their work [46, 47] demonstrated that seed from inbred lines (grown as cultivars) would prove to be the best source of cheap, uniform seed containing consistent levels of glucoraphanin, making it ideal for producing seedling sprouts. As a result of their work a high-glucoraphanin inbred expressing levels of glucoraphanin consistently greater than 60 µmol/g fw of dry seed was released under the name 'Hopkins' [48].

CONCLUSION

Numerous studies have looked at the glucosinolates present in broccoli heads, and the reported concentrations of glucosinolates from those collective works provide a good picture of what is expected to be found in broccoli produce purchased by consumers. Six different glucosinolates account for the majority of these compounds in broccoli. Three of the most prevalent are aliphatic glucosinolates including glucoraphanin, progoitrin, and glucoiberin. The other three prominent compounds are all indole glucosinolates, and these are glucobrassicin, neo-glucobrassicin, and 4-methoxy-glucobrassicin. Glucoraphanin is the most abundant aliphatic glucosinolate and it is expected to occur at concentrations of 2-12 µmol/g dw, and probably never higher than 15 µmol/g dw, in heads of conventional hybrid cultivars. Glucobrassicin is the most abundant indole glucosinolate, and it is likely to be found at concentrations in the same range as is glucoraphanin. Several studies support the finding that genotype is the critical factor influencing levels of glucoraphanin and glucoiberin concentrations in broccoli heads. However, concentrations of indole glucosinolates in heads do not appear to be under similar genetic control. Researchers have shown that it is possible to select for increased concentrations of glucoraphanin in broccoli heads as well as in broccoli seed. It is feasible that new cultivars available in the marketplace will be advertised as "high glucoraphanin" broccoli that is able to confer a health-promoting effect. Such marketing may help to bring added attention to a popular vegetable that grew dramatically in popularity during the latter half of the 20th Century and that is increasingly consumed in North America as well as in the rest of the world through the present day.

REFERENCES

[1] Dowd, M. (1990). 'I'm president, so no more broccoli! [Newspaper article]. Retrieved from http://www.nytimes.com/1990/03/23/us/i-m-president-so-no-more-broccoli.html. Accessed on Aug. 25, 2015.

[2] National Agricultural Statistics Service, U.S. Department of Agriculture. (1950-2013). Agricultural Statistics Annual. [database]. Retrieved from http://www.nass.usda.gov/ Publications/Ag_Statistics/ index.asp. Accessed on Aug. 25, 2015.

[3] Zhang, Y., Talalay, P., Cho, C. G., & Posner, G. H. (1992). A major inducer of anticarcinogenic protective enzymes from broccoli: isolation and elucidation of structure. *Proceedings of the National Academy of Sciences of the United States of America, 89*(6), 2399–2403.

[4] Farnham, M. W., Keinath, A. P., & Grusak, M. A. (2011). Mineral Concentration of Broccoli Florets in Relation to Year of Cultivar Release. *Crop Science, 51*(6), 2721.

[5] Fahey, J. W., Zalcmann, A T., & Talalay, P. (2001). The chemical diversity and distribution of glucosinolates and isothiocyanates amoung plants. *Phytochemistry, 56*, 5–51.

[6] Hopkins, R. J., van Dam, N. M., & van Loon, J. J. (2009). Role of glucosinolates in insect-plant relationships and multitrophic interactions. *Annual Review of Entomology, 54*, 57–83.

[7] Chew, F. (1988). Biological effects of glucosinolates. *In Biologically Active Natural Products*, ed. H. G. Cutler, Washington, DC: ACS, pp. 155-181.

[8] Louda, S., & Mole, S. (1991). Glucosinolates: chemistry and ecology. *In Herbivores: Their Interactions with Secondary Plant Metabolites*, ed. B. M. Rosenthal GA, New York: Academic, pp. 123-164.

[9] Lewis, J., & Fenwick, G. R. (1987). Glucosinolate content of brassica vegetables: Analysis of twenty-four cultivars of calabrese (green sprouting broccoli, *Brassica oleracea* L. var. botrytis subvar. cymosa Lam.). *Food Chemistry, 25*(4), 259–268.

[10] Carlson, D. G., Daxenbichler, M. E., & Vanetten, C. H. (1987). Glucosinolates in Crucifer Vegetables : Broccoli, Brussels Sprouts, Cauliflower, Collards, Kale, Mustard Greens, and Kohlrabi. *J. Amer. Soc. Hort. Sci, 112*(1), 173–178.

[11] Zhang, Y., Kensler, T. W., Cho, C. G., Posner, G. H., & Talalay, P. (1994). Anticarcinogenic activities of sulforaphane and structurally related synthetic norbornyl isothiocyanates. *Proceedings of the National Academy of Sciences of the United States of America, 91*(8), 3147–3150.

[12] Talalay, P., Fahey, J. W., Holtzclaw, W. D., Prestera, T., & Zhang, Y. (1995). Chemoprotection against cancer by Phase 2 enzyme induction. *Toxicology Letters, 82-83*, 173–179.

[13] Baik, H., Juvik, J., Jeffery, E., Wallig, M., Kushad, M., & Klein, B. (2003). Relating glucosinolate content and flavor of broccoli cultivars. *Journal of Food Science, 68*(3), 1043–1050.

[14] Brown, A. F., Yousef, G. G., Jeffery, E. H., Klein, B. P., Wallig, M. A., Kushad, M. M., & Juvik, J. A. (2002). Glucosinolate Profiles in Broccoli: Variation in Levels and Implications in Breeding for Cancer Chemoprotection. *J. Amer. Soc. Hort. Sci., 127(5)*, 807–813.

[15] Charron, C. S., Sams, C. E., & Canaday, C. H. (2002). Impact of Glucosinolate Content in Broccoli (*Brassica oleracea* (Italica Group)) on Growth of Pseudomonas marginalis, a Causal Agent of Bacterial Soft Rot. *Plant Disease, 86*(8), 629–632.

[16] Farnham, M. W., Wilson, P. E., Stephenson, K. K., & Fahey, J. W. (2004). Genetic and environmental effects on glucosinolate content and chemoprotective potency of broccoli. *Plant Breeding, 123*, 60–65.

[17] Faulkner, K., Mithen, R., & Williamson, G. (1998). Selective increase of the potential anticarcinogen 4-methylsulphinylbutyl glucosinolate in broccoli. *Carcinogenesis, 19*(4), 605–609.

[18] Hansen, M., Laustsen, A., Olsen, C., Poll, L., & Sorensen, H. (1997). Chemical and sensory quality of broccoli (*Brassica oleracea* L. var *Italica*). *Journal of Food Quality, 20*, 441–459.

[19] Kim, H. S., & Juvik, J. A. (2011). Effect of Selenium Fertilization and Methyl Jasmonate Treatment on Glucosinolate Accumulation in Broccoli Florets. *J. Amer. Soc. Hort. Sci., 136*(4), 239–246.

[20] Kushad, M. M., Brown, A. F., Kurilich, A. C., Juvik, J. A., Klein, B. P., Wallig, M. A., & Jeffery, E. H. (1999). Variation of glucosinolates in vegetable crops of Brassica oleracea. *J. Ag. and Food Chemistry, 47*(4), 1541–8.

[21] Rosa, E. A. S., & Rodrigues, A. S. (2001). Total and individual glucosinolate content in 11 broccoli cultivars grown in early and late seasons. *HortScience, 36*(1), 56–59.

[22] Sarikamis, G., Marquez, J., Maccormack, R., Bennett, R. N., Roberts, J., & Mithen, R. (2006). High glucosinolate broccoli: a delivery system for sulforaphane. *Molecular Breeding, 18*(3), 219–228.

[23] Schonhof, I., Krumbein, A., & Brückner, B. (2004). Genotypic effects on glucosinolates and sensory properties of broccoli and cauliflower. *Nahrung - Food, 48*(1), 25–33.

[24] Vallejo, F., Toms-Barbern, F. A., & Garca-Viguera, C. (2002). Potential bioactive compounds in health promotion from broccoli cultivars grown in Spain. *J. Sci. Food and Agriculture, 82*(11), 1293–1297.

[25] Wang, J., Gu, H., Yu, H., Zhao, Z., Sheng, X., & Zhang, X. (2012). Genotypic variation of glucosinolates in broccoli (*Brassica oleracea* var. *italica*) florets from China. *Food Chemistry, 133*(3), 735–741.

[26] 26) Aggarwal, B. B., & Ichikawa, H. (2005). Molecular targets and anticancer potential of indole-3-carbinol and its derivatives. *Cell Cycle, 4*(9), 1201–1215.

[27] Chinni, S. R., Li, Y., Upadhyay, S., Koppolu, P. K., & Sarkar, F. H. (2001). Indole-3-carbinol (I3C) induced cell growth inhibition, G1 cell cycle arrest and apoptosis in prostate cancer cells. *Oncogene, 20*(23), 2927–2936.

[28] Sarkar, F. H., & Li, Y. (2004). Indole-3-Carbinol and Prostate Cancer. *The Journal of Nutrition, Supplement*, 3493S–3498S.

[29] Vallejo, F., Tomás-Barberán, F. A., Gonzalez Benavente-García, A., & García-Viguera, C. (2003). Total and individual glucosinolate contents in inflorescences of eight broccoli cultivars grown under various climatic and fertilisation conditions. *J. Sci. Food and Agriculture, 83*(4), 307–313.

[30] Jones, R. B., Imsic, M., Franz, P., Hale, G., & Tomkins, R. B. (2007). High nitrogen during growth reduced glucoraphanin and flavonol content in broccoli (*Brassica oleracea* var. *italica*) heads. *Australian Journal of Experimental Agriculture, 47*(12), 1498–1505.

[31] Schonhof, I., Blankenburg, D., Müller, S., & Krumbein, A. (2007). Sulfur and nitrogen supply influence growth, product appearance, and glucosinolate concentration of broccoli. *Journal of Plant Nutrition and Soil Science, 170*(1), 65–72.

[32] Omirou, M. D., Papadopoulou, K. K., Papastylianou, I., Constantinou, M., Karpouzas, D. G., Asimakopoulos, I., & Ehaliotis, C. (2009). Impact of nitrogen and sulfur fertilization on the composition of glucosinolates in relation to sulfur assimilation in different plant organs of broccoli. *J. Ag. and Food Chemistry, 57*(20), 9408–9417.

[33] Robbins, R. J., Keck, A., Banuelos, G., & Finley, J. W. (2005). Cultivation conditions and selenium fertilization alter the phenolic profile, glucosinolate, and sulforaphane content of broccoli. *Journal of Medicinal Food, 8*(2), 204–214.

[34] Charron C. S., Kopsell D. A., Randall W. M. and Sams C. E. (2001) Sodium selenate fertilisation increases selenium accumulation and decreases glucosinolate concentration in rapid-cycling Brassica oleracea. *J Sci Food Agric 81*, 962–966.

[35] Shelp, B. J., Shattuck, V. I., McLellan, D & Liu, L. (1992). Boron nutrition and the composition of glucosinolates and soluble nitrogen compoiunds in two broccoli (Brassica olerace var. italica) culivars. *Can. Journal Plant Science, 72*, 889–899.

[36] Shelp, B. J., Liu, L., & McLellan, D. (1993). Glucosinolate concentrantration of broccoli (*Brassica oleracea* var. *italica*) grown under various boron treatments at three Ontario sites. *Can Journal Plant Science, 73*, 885–888.

[37] Ku, K. M, E. H. Jeffery, & J. A. Juvik (2014) Optimization of methyl jasmonate application to broccoli florets to enhance health-promoting phytochemical content. *J. Sci. Food Agric., 94*(10), 2090-2096.

[38] Charron, C. S., Saxton, A. M., & Sams, C. E. (2005). Relationship of climate and genotype to seasonal variation in the glucosinolate-myrosinase system. I. Glucosinolate content in ten cultivars of *Brassica oleracea* grown in fall and spring seasons. *J. Sci. Food and Agriculture, 85*(4), 671–681.

[39] Abercrombie, J. M., M. W. Farnham, & J. W. Rushing. (2005) Genetic combining ability of glucoraphanin level and other horticultural traits of broccoli. *Euphytica 143*, 145-151.

[40] Mithen, R., Faulkner, K., Magrath, R., Rose, P., Williamson, G., & Marquez, J. (2003). Development of isothiocyanate-enriched broccoli, and its enhanced ability to induce phase 2 detoxification enzymes in mammalian cells. *Theor. Appl. Genetics 106*(4), 727–734.

[41] Traka, M. H., Saha, S., Huseby, S., Kpriva, S., Walley, P. G., Barker, G. C., Moore, J., Mero, G., van den Bosch, F., Constant, H., Kelly, L., Schepers, H., Boddupalli, S., & Mithen, R. F. (2013) Genetic regulation of glucoraphanin accumulation in Beneforte broccoli. *New Phytologist 198,* 1085-1095.

[42] Fahey, J. W., Zhang, Y., & Talalay, P. (1997). Broccoli sprouts: an exceptionally rich source of inducers of enzymes that protect against chemical carcinogens. *Proceedings of the National Academy of Sciences of the United States of America, 94*(19), 10367–10372.

[43] West, L. G., Meyer, K. A., Balch, B. A., Rossi, F. J., Schultz, M. R., & Haas, G. W. (2004). Glucoraphanin and 4-Hydroxyglucobrassicin Contents in Seeds of 59 Cultivars of Broccoli, Raab, Kohlrabi, Radish, Cauliflower, Brussels Sprouts, Kale, and Cabbage. *J. Ag. and Food Chemistry, 52*(4), 916–926.

[44] Rangkadilok, N., Nicolas, M. E., Bennett, R. N., Premier, R. R., Eagling, D. R., & Taylor, P. W. J. (2002). Determination of sinigrin and glucoraphanin in Brassica species using a simple extraction method combined with ion-pair HPLC analysis. *Scientia Horticulturae, 96*(1-4), 27–41.

[45] Velasco, L., & Becker, H. C. (2000). Variability for seed glucosinolates in a germplasm collection of the genus Brassica. *Genetic Resources and Crop Evolution, 47*(3), 231–238.

[46] Farnham, M. W., Stephenson, K. K., & Fahey, J. W. (2005). Glucoraphanin level in broccoli seed is largely determined by genotype. *HortScience, 40*(1), 50–53.

[47] Farnham, M. W. and Harrison, H. F. (2003), Using self-compatible inbreds of broccoli as seed producers. *Hort Science 38*, 85-87.

[48] U.S. Government as represented by the Secretary of Agriculture and Caudill Seed and Warehouse Company, Inc. Plant Variety Protection Certificate 200700022. "Hopkins" broccoli. Issued June 22, 2010.

In: Broccoli
Editor: Bernhard H. J. Juurlink

ISBN: 978-1-63484-313-3
© 2016 Nova Science Publishers, Inc.

Chapter 4

THE XENOBIOTIC ELIMINATION SYSTEM: AN OVERVIEW

*Jane Alcorn**

College of Pharmacy and Nutrition, University of Saskatchewan, Saskatoon, SK, Canada

ABSTRACT

The chapter presents an overview of the xenobiotic elimination system from the perspective of an oral xenobiotic exposure. It notes the interrelationship of the three elimination organs, liver, kidney, and intestine, and their respective roles in limiting systemic exposures. The polarized epithelia of each elimination organ are highlighted as these are the 'workhorses' of xenobiotic elimination and express the transporters and enzymes that ultimately cause xenobiotic removal from the body. Emphasis is placed on the four phases of xenobiotic elimination, phase 0 transporter-mediated xenobiotic uptake into the polarized epithelia, phase I and phase II xenobiotic metabolism within the polarized epithelia, and phase III transporter-mediated xenobiotic efflux from the polarized epithelium. Hence, the chapter provides a general summary of the solute carrier transporters of phase 0 elimination, the cytochrome P450 enzymes of phase I metabolism, the conjugating enzymes of phase II metabolism, and the ATP binding cassette transporters of phase III elimination. Finally, it offers an overview of the genetic, environmental, and host factors influencing the activity of these individual elimination mechanisms, as well as the transcriptional factors that regulate and coordinate their expression. An extensive interplay between the various xenobiotic elimination mechanisms requires that the xenobiotic is positioned within an integrated xenobiotic elimination system to truly understand xenobiotic exposure outcomes.

INTRODUCTION

Our daily lives expose us to a vast array of chemically disparate natural and synthetic foreign substances collectively referred to as xenobiotics. To prevent or eradicate any

---

* E-mail: jane.alcorn@usask.ca.

pharmacodynamic or toxicodynamic sequelae from such exposures, the human body must conscript its xenobiotic elimination mechanisms to limit xenobiotic entrance into the body and cause its removal from the body. The xenobiotic elimination system is composed of highly versatile cellular and system wide mechanisms whose interplay ultimately defines the outcome of a xenobiotic exposure. Simple knowledge of the involvement of an individual elimination pathway is not sufficient to fully understand the fate of a xenobiotic subsequent to its exposure. This chapter will first offer a framework of the xenobiotic elimination system that integrates the major organs and key mechanisms of elimination conceptualizing the sequential and simultaneous processes involved in xenobiotic elimination. This will be done from the perspective of an oral exposure since this route represents the most significant source of xenobiotics. This chapter then proceeds to a succinct overview of the individual xenobiotic elimination pathways and the mechanisms that regulate and coordinate their expression. The chapter's conceptual framework is designed to remind the reader that the overall fate of a xenobiotic exposure goes well beyond an individual elimination pathway. The reader is challenged to maintain perspective on the xenobiotic within the whole integrated xenobiotic elimination system.

THE XENOBIOTIC ELIMINATION SYSTEM DETERMINES SYSTEMIC EXPOSURE

Every interface with the external environment exposes our bodies to a multitude of xenobiotics. Although these chemicals can mediate local interactions at these interfaces, our principal concern is systemic exposure, the ability of a xenobiotic to gain entrance into the blood circulatory system and cause whole body exposure. Systemic exposure considers the total time course and magnitude of xenobiotic concentrations in the body and a xenobiotic may cause toxicity and possibly death with systemic persistence and/or accumulation. To avoid such undesirable outcomes, the xenobiotic elimination system functions to limit the magnitude and time course of systemic xenobiotic concentrations. Bear in mind, this same system also contributes to homeostatic control of endobiotics [1]. As a consequence, the xenobiotic elimination system requires significant versatility to manage this plethora of chemically divergent endobiotics and xenobiotics and confronts important challenges in its role to maintain tight control over endobiotic systemic levels while limiting xenobiotic systemic exposures.

The gastrointestinal tract represents one of the most significant interfaces with the external environment [2]. Following an oral exposure, the body employs a number of barrier mechanisms to limit xenobiotic bioavailability, or that fraction of the oral exposure dose that enters the systemic blood circulation as an unmodified xenobiotic. A xenobiotic's oral bioavailability depends upon its absorption properties and presystemic elimination processes. Absorption refers to its ability to remain intact within the gastrointestinal lumen and permeate the gastrointestinal mucosal membrane, while presystemic elimination refers to processes that eliminate the xenobiotic before it reaches the systemic blood supply. For any xenobiotic that evades these barrier mechanisms, systemic elimination, determined principally by renal and hepatic mechanisms, also functions to limit systemic exposure to the xenobiotic. When xenobiotics present at the gastrointestinal interface, then, systemic exposure can be significantly limited either at the time of oral absorption and presystemic elimination and/or by the efficiency of the systemic elimination mechanisms (Figure 1).

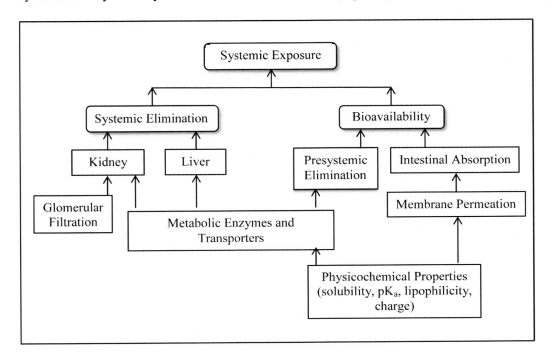

Figure 1. Xenobiotic systemic exposure following an oral exposure depends upon the factors influencing oral bioavailability and systemic elimination. Presystemic elimination and absorption processes determine oral bioavailability. Presystemic elimination depends upon hepatic and intestinal metabolic enzymes and transporters that function to prevent the xenobiotic from becoming available to the systemic circulation. Once in the systemic circulation, systemic exposure is influenced by the elimination mechanisms of the major systemic elimination organs, the kidney and liver.

XENOBIOTIC ELIMINATION: AN INTEGRATED SYSTEM

Xenobiotic elimination involves a significant number of competing and/or collaborating processes such that elimination must be viewed from the context of the whole integrated system. This integrated system is composed of a hierarchy of distinct organizational units whose spatiotemporal relationships and sum of events within this dynamic hierarchal architecture determine the ultimate fate of a xenobiotic exposure (Figure 2) [3]. At the pinnacle of this hierarchal system is the whole physiological system. A blood circulatory system interconnects each major elimination organ, the gastrointestinal tract, liver, and kidney, with a parallel blood supply such that xenobiotics are delivered simultaneously to each elimination organ by the systemic circulation. The elimination organs are further subdivided into repeating functional units, the villi of the intestine, the acini of the liver, and the nephrons of the kidney. Each of the functional units is composed of polarized epithelia, which contain the individual xenobiotic metabolizing enzymes and transporters that contribute to xenobiotic elimination. Lower levels of arrangement must also include the genes and the protein machinery responsible for functional enzyme and transporter expression and regulation. For most xenobiotics, the organization of the xenobiotic elimination system in this manner effectively limits their overall systemic exposure.

Each elimination organ contributes variably to the systemic elimination of a xenobiotic, while the gastrointestinal tract and the liver can further contribute to presystemic elimination. Only unbound xenobiotic can be made available to the elimination processes and its rate of delivery to the elimination organs by the organ blood flow can, in some cases, be a limiting factor in the extent of elimination by that organ. Following an oral route of exposure, though, a xenobiotic passes through key elimination organs in series, the gastrointestinal tract, the portal blood supply, and then the liver, before it gains entrance into the systemic circulation. In this case, elimination mechanisms act sequentially such that only a fraction of the total external exposure dose of a xenobiotic reaches the systemic circulation. This sequential elimination of xenobiotics is referred to as presystemic elimination, which often is the major contributor to reduced xenobiotic bioavailability (bioavailability being defined as the fraction of the xenobiotic exposure dose that becomes available as an unmodified xenobiotic to the systemic circulation) [4]. Once in the systemic circulation the various elimination organs may act simultaneously to effect removal of the xenobiotic and its metabolites from the body.

Each organ of elimination has a substantive capacity for xenobiotic elimination. Their parenchymal masses are largely composed of repeating functional units, the hepatic acinus, the renal nephron, and the gastrointestinal tract villus-crypt structure (Figure 2). The hepatic acinus consists of single layers of hepatocytes (the polarized epithelia) that exist between sinusoids such that hepatocytes are extensively in contact with the blood supply. Hepatocytes also have direct contact with bile canaliculi, which connect to the gall bladder and subsequently the intestine. The renal nephron consists of the glomerulus, the filtration component of the nephron, and the tubules, which contain the glomerular filtrate and are lined with the renal tubule polarized epithelium. A significant vasculature surrounds the tubular system (peri-tubular capillaries) which positions the systemic blood supply near the polarized epithelium of the renal tubules. This allows for the tubules to further function in the excretion of various xenobiotics from the systemic circulation. The intestinal mucosa consists of villus and crypt structures lined with the enterocytic polarized epithelium. Villi, luminal projections of the intestinal wall, provide a remarkably large surface area for absorption of xenobiotics from the intestinal lumen.

The anatomical nature of the functional units results in a zonal differentiation of function with respect to xenobiotic elimination capacity. The hepatic acinus is delineated into three zones along the longitudinal axis between the portal triad (zone 1) and the central vein (zone 3) (intermediate hepatocytes representing zone 2). Differences in the expression of individual elimination pathways exist between and within the hepatic zones [5, 6]. Given the liver's relative size, the functional unit mass, and extent of expression of the xenobiotic metabolizing enzymes and transporters within the acini, the liver contributes considerably to overall xenobiotic presystemic and systemic elimination.

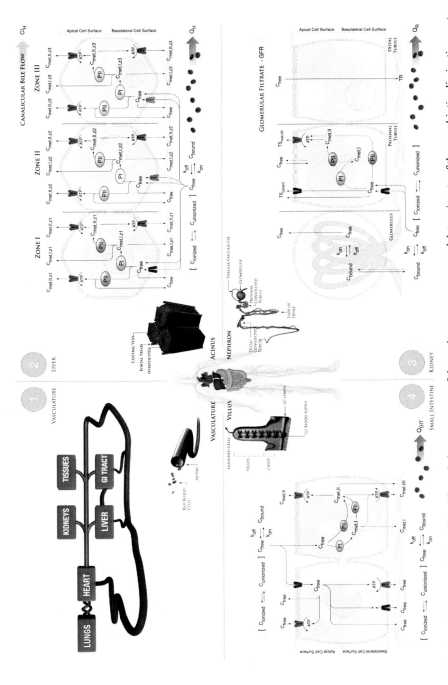

Figure 2. A schematic representation of the hierarchal arrangement of the various components and determinants of the xenobiotic elimination system. The physiological system represents the highest level. Descent through the hierarchy follows the path from the individual xenobiotic elimination organ (liver, kidney, gastrointestinal tract), their functional units (hepatic acinus, renal nephron, intestinal villus-crypt), the polarized epithelia of the functional units, and the individual elimination pathways (i.e., phase I and phase II enzymes, phase 0 uptake and phase 3 efflux transporters, glomerulus). The blood circulatory system (left upper quadrant) interconnects the major elimination organs by parallel blood supplies. A xenobiotic absorbed from the gastrointestinal is delivered sequentially to the liver via the portal circulation before its entry into the systemic circulation. The gastrointestinal tract (lower left quadrant) may contribute

significantly to presystemic elimination. The villus-crypt creates a large surface area for xenobiotic absorption (by passive diffusion and/or carrier-mediated processes) and mucosal blood flow (Q_M) maintains a gradient for absorption. Xenobiotic phase I and II metabolizing enzymes and phase 0 and III uptake and efflux transporters are expressed in the mature villus enterocyte. The kinetic processes of drug ionization, binding within the GIT lumen, and enterocyte uptake and/or efflux processes precede metabolism. The rate of transport and metabolism is dependent on the concentration of unbound xenobiotic (C_{free}). For the hepatic elimination system (upper right quadrant), a xenobiotic is delivered to the acinus by the portal venous circulation and hepatic artery, respectively, at a rate defined by hepatic blood flow (Q_H). Only the unbound xenobiotic (C_{free}) undergoes passive diffusion or carrier-mediated uptake into the hepatocyte. Intracellular free concentrations will determine the rate of metabolism by phase I (PI) and/or phase II (PII) enzymes to a drug metabolite (C_{met}) as well as carrier-mediated efflux (phase 3, PIII). The metabolites undergo passive diffusion or phase 3 efflux at the basolateral membrane into the systemic circulation or can be sequentially metabolized by PII enzymes before its removal from the hepatocyte by efflux transporters in the basolateral or canalicular membranes. At the canalicular membrane xenobiotic or xenobiotic metabolite is excreted into the bile. Renal blood flow (Q_R) determines rate of xenobiotic delivery to the kidney (lower right quadrant). Unbound xenobiotic is removed from the systemic blood supply by glomerular filtration or by nephron tubule elimination mechanisms. Filtered xenobiotic may undergo tubular reabsorption (TR) and return to the systemic blood circulation. Xenobiotic elimination by the proximal renal tubule polarized epithelium depends on plasma protein binding and transporter-mediated uptake at the basolateral membrane. Once within the epithelial barrier competing processes of PI (usually very limited) or PII enzyme-mediated metabolism and intracellular binding will determine the free concentration available for transporter-mediated excretion into the glomerular filtrate. The quantitative and qualitative contribution of the individual xenobiotic metabolizing enzymes and transporters may change with location in the functional unit (i.e., intestine-colon axis, hepatic acinus zones 1, 2, and 3; proximal-distal tubule axis of renal nephron) (*Graphic courtesy of Dr. Sam Gilchrist, Ph.D.* (http://www.seabass.smugmug.com)).

The kidney divides aspects of xenobiotic elimination into different spatial zones within the functional unit, the nephron. As a consequence, xenobiotic elimination by the kidney nephron involves three distinct processes, glomerular filtration, renal tubule reabsorption, and renal tubule excretion or metabolism. All xenobiotics not bound to plasma proteins are filtered at the glomerulus, while proximal tubule epithelial cells are principally responsible for the majority of xenobiotic excretion and renal metabolism as well as reabsorption of filtered lipophilic xenobiotics. The proximal tubule epithelium's contribution to xenobiotic metabolism is rather limited relative to the other elimination organs [7, 8]. However, the proximal tubule exhibits extensive heterogeneity in excretory capacity due to the wide expression of diverse xenobiotic transporters [9]. These transporters are vital to the elimination of some xenobiotics and xenobiotic metabolites.

Finally, the gastrointestinal tract exhibits a functional differentiation both along the crypt-villus axis and duodenal-colonic axis [10]. Enzymes and transporters are expressed in gradient patterns from proximal to distal portions of the gastrointestinal tract and from villus tip to crypt region [11]. The villus shows an increasing pattern of differentiation from crypt to villus tip and the individual xenobiotic elimination pathways (i.e., the enzymes and transporters) are principally found in the mature epithelial cells at the tips of the villi [2, 12-14]. Such expression gradients within the functional units of the elimination organs suggest the relative ratio of the xenobiotic metabolizing enzymes and transporters will significantly impact the nature of presystemic elimination and will be variably responsive to shifts in the proportions of the various enzymes and transporters. The position of the gastrointestinal tract in the xenobiotic elimination system indicates its very important role in presystemic elimination.

The next sublevel in the hierarchal arrangement of the xenobiotic elimination system are the polarized epithelia, a layer of tightly knit epithelial cells that line luminal or external compartments to create a selective physical and functional barrier to control entrance of xenobiotics into the functional units and to maintain organ homeostasis [15]. Hepatocytes, renal tubule cells, and enterocytes compose the polarized epithelium, which is arranged such that the basolateral side of the polarized epithelium faces a blood supply and the apical side faces a lumen, either the bile canaliculi, renal tubule lumen, or gastrointestinal lumen, respectively. The kidney glomerulus is also lined with a leaky polarized epithelium, the vascular endothelium.

The polarized epithelia have important barrier mechanisms to limit xenobiotic access. First, the lipoidal epithelial plasma membranes function as semipermeable barriers limiting permeation by passive diffusion to unbound, uncharged lipid soluble solutes. Water soluble and charged xenobiotics and endobiotics require membrane protein carriers (transporters) and channels to gain access to or removal from the cell. For both passive diffusion and carrier-mediated transport xenobiotic physicochemical characteristics such as molecular weight, acid/base character and pK_a, and lipophilicity influence the rate and mechanism of transport across the membrane [15]. Second, tight junctions between the epithelial cells preclude paracellular (i.e., between cells) movement and most xenobiotics cross the barrier via transcellular transport mechanisms. The tight junctions also create distinct apical and basolateral membrane surfaces. The polarized nature of these epithelia ensures directionality of transcellular drug movement (i.e., vectorial transport) at the epithelial barrier by passive and/or transporter-mediated processes [16]. Finally, the polarized epithelia contain xenobiotic metabolizing enzymes that function to biotransform xenobiotics usually to more polar and inactive metabolites before they can gain access to the systemic circulation. Each barrier mechanism has a key function in the three organs of elimination but each has variable importance as determined by the location of the elimination organ in the overall physiological system.

The polarized epithelia represent the 'workhorses' of xenobiotic elimination. Their plasma membranes and tight junction structures represent an important first barrier to xenobiotic exposure. However, the plethora of membrane transporters and xenobiotic metabolizing enzymes expressed within the polarized epithelia are significantly responsible for limiting systemic exposure to a xenobiotic. The arrangement of the elimination organs and the distribution of xenobiotic transporters and enzymes within the polarized epithelia divide xenobiotic elimination into four phases and it is the complex interplay between the phases that critically defines the nature of xenobiotic elimination in the intact physiological system [17]. The transporters and enzymes also represent the adaptable barrier mechanisms, as these proteins are highly responsive to environmental influences and alterations in whole body and organ homeostasis. Such adaptability depends upon post-transcriptional mechanisms and transcriptional regulation controlled by highly interrelated nuclear receptor pathways and other regulatory factors, the final level of the hierarchal system. These mechanisms sense the external environment to respond quickly to regulate xenobiotic transporters and enzymes in a coordinated fashion to ensure maintenance of whole body homeostasis while limiting xenobiotic systemic exposures [18, 19].

THE FOUR PHASES OF XENOBIOTIC ELIMINATION

Our growing understanding of the role of plasma membrane transporters in xenobiotic absorption and disposition required a redefinition of the phases of xenobiotic metabolism, phase I and phase II, first articulated by Williams in the 1950's [20, 21]. Since xenobiotic metabolizing enzymes are expressed in the cytosol and certain cellular organelles of the polarized epithelia, access to these enzymes requires the xenobiotic to permeate across the cell membrane and undergo intracellular transport to the active site of the xenobiotic metabolizing enzymes. Historically, passive diffusion was believed to be the principal process in the permeation of xenobiotics and their polar metabolites. Today, a clear role exists for the importance of transporters in cellular membrane permeability for both hydrophilic and lipophilic xenobiotics [20, 22, 23]. For many xenobiotics transporters are important determinants of their intracellular concentrations, presystemic and systemic elimination, and pharmacological or toxicological outcome [24-27]. As an important factor in cellular uptake and efflux, then, changes in transporter activity alone may affect the overall rate and pattern of xenobiotic metabolism without concomitant changes in xenobiotic metabolizing enzyme expression. Often, the xenobiotic transporters and metabolizing enzymes work in cooperation, a so-called transporter-enzyme interplay, to limit xenobiotic systemic exposure (Figure 3) [28, 29]. The relative interplay of membrane transporters and xenobiotic metabolizing enzymes becomes a critical consideration in defining the overall rate and pattern of elimination for xenobiotics in general.

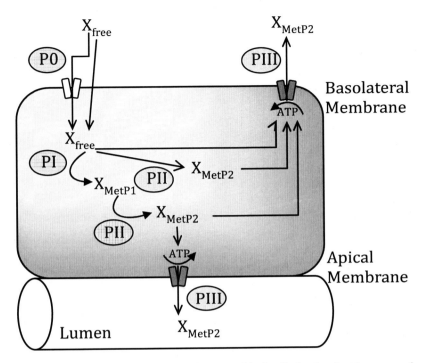

Figure 3. The four phases of xenobiotic elimination. Xenobiotic elimination involves a number of competing and sequential steps at the polarized epithelia of the elimination organs. Uptake into the polarized epithelium may involve passive diffusion of the unbound xenobiotic (X_{free}) or require a phase 0 (P0) uptake transporter (white double bars). Phase III (PIII) efflux transporters (grey double bars) may actively efflux the xenobiotic (X_{free}) back across the apical membrane to limit overall xenobiotic uptake into the polarized epithelium. In the intracellular environment of the polarized epithelial cell, xenobiotics may undergo phase I (P1) or phase II (PII) metabolism to form more polar inactive metabolites (X_{MetPI}, X_{MetPII}). Sometimes metabolism results in bioactivation, the production of a reactive intermediate or active metabolite. Phase I (X_{MetPI}) metabolites may undergo sequential phase II metabolism (PII). The unmetabolized xenobiotic and its phase I and phase II metabolites may require a phase III efflux transporter (PIII) to effect its removal from either the basolateral membrane into the systemic blood supply or apical membrane into a luminal space. Once in the blood circulation the unmetabolized xenobiotic and its metabolites undergo a similar process in the epithelia of other elimination organs until they are permanently removed from the body via the feces and/or urine.

Today xenobiotic elimination consists of four phases to acknowledge the role of transporters in presystemic and systemic elimination. Phase 0 constitutes the uptake transporters at the enterocytic apical and hepatocellular basolateral polarized epithelial membranes, which influence oral bioavailability, as well as transporters at the renal tubular basolateral membrane, which facilitate xenobiotic uptake from the systemic circulation into the renal epithelium for excretion. Phase 0 usually has limited relevance for the lipid soluble xenobiotic that undergoes passive diffusion, although increasing evidence suggests phase 0 transporters have a significant role in the uptake of water soluble and some lipophilic xenobiotics [22, 30, 31]. Phase III involves the efflux transporters expressed in the hepatocellular polarized epithelium (apical and basolateral) and luminal apical epithelium of the intestine and renal tubule system to cause xenobiotic and metabolite removal from the cell or to prevent their entrance into the polarized epithelium (Figure 3). These transporters can impact the availability of xenobiotics to the phase I and phase II xenobiotic metabolizing enzymes. Phase I involves enzymes that mediate oxidation, reduction, and hydrolysis reactions while phase II enzymes mediate conjugation reactions. The phase I and phase II processes usually produce metabolites with enhanced aqueous solubility [32]. Removal of the polar metabolite (or parent xenobiotic) from the polarized epithelial cell often requires an efflux transporter, so-called phase III elimination. Hence, these four phases of xenobiotic elimination often occur sequentially within the polarized epithelium of the elimination organs.

The coordinated functioning of the phase 0, phase I, phase II, and phase III elimination mechanisms is a key determinant of xenobiotic systemic exposure. The four phases undergo a coordinated regulation such that regulation of phase I, phase II, and phase III mechanisms are generally positively correlated with each other (e.g., upregulated together) but negatively correlated with phase 0 cellular uptake mechanisms (e.g., downregulated when phase I, phase II, and phase III are upregulated) [18, 19]. Such coordination optimally limits xenobiotic exposures, particularly under significant xenobiotic exposure stress, as these processes work sequentially to restrict xenobiotic systemic exposure [30, 33]. For example, phase 0 uptake transporters enhance absorption and hepatocellular uptake but also enhance the availability of xenobiotics to the xenobiotic metabolizing enzymes inside the polarized epithelial cell, thereby increasing the rate and extent of their metabolism. Phase III transporters may limit oral bioavailability at the intestinal epithelium and ensure removal of polar phase II conjugates at the hepatocellular canalicular (apical) membrane to prevent their intracellular accumulation and ensure their elimination by the kidney. Furthermore, the concerted action of phase 0 and phase III transporters in the polarized epithelium ensures the vectorial transport (i.e., net movement in one direction) of xenobiotics across the epithelium thereby making the xenobiotic available either to the systemic circulation or enhancing its elimination by the kidney and liver [16]. Countless considerations can be made regarding the outcome of the interplay between the phase 0 – III mechanisms in the different elimination organs. An understanding of whether a xenobiotic is a substrate for the various transporters and enzymes of phase 0 – III elimination is necessary to fully appreciate the impact of the four phases of elimination on a xenobiotic.

Xenobiotic metabolising enzymes and transporters constitute a large family of proteins with highly versatile substrate specificities. Approximately 7% of the human genome encodes membrane transporters (~7% of the total genome) that transport a wide variety of water and lipid soluble endobiotics and xenobiotics, ions, metals, and other substances (http:/www.membranetransport.org) [34-36]. Xenobiotic transporters are divided into two large superfamilies, the Solute Carrier (SLC) Superfamily, which mediates phase 0 uptake [34, 35], and the ATP Binding Cassette (ABC) Superfamily, which mediates phase III efflux [36]. Uptake transporters facilitate entry into the epithelial barrier while efflux transporters limit xenobiotic entry into or enhance their removal from the polarized epithelium. The xenobiotic metabolising system is composed of two classes of enzymes, phase I and phase II, principally found in either the smooth endoplasmic reticulum or cytosol of the cell. Phase I elimination is largely mediated by a superfamily of enzymes, the cytochrome P450s, although other enzymes such as alcohol and aldehyde dehydrogenases, epoxide hydrolases, and flavin containing monooxygenases have importance for specific xenobiotics [37]. Phase II elimination is mediated by the conjugative enzymes [38-41], which combine an endogenous molecule to the xenobiotic or phase I metabolite of the xenobiotic to yield a metabolite that often requires phase III efflux from the polarized epithelium [42]. Glucuronidation, sulfation, glutathione conjugation, and acetylation are the principal phase II enzyme pathways, although methylation and amino acid conjugation has relevance to a limited number of xenobiotics. Table 1 summarizes the major families of xenobiotic metabolising enzymes and transporters.

Phase I and II Xenobiotic Metabolizing Enzymes

Xenobiotic metabolising enzyme system is responsible for enhancing the water solubility of hydrophobic xenobiotics to deactivate these molecules and promote their excretion from the body. Phase I enzymes function to add a polar functional group or expose a functional group. Phase II enzymes are conjugative enzymes, which typically conjugate an endogenous substrate to a parent xenobiotic or a xenobiotic metabolite to further increase water solubility and facilitate its excretion from the body by biliary or renal excretion. Often phase I reactions are sequentially followed by phase II reactions as the exposed functional group provides an acceptor group for addition of a highly polar molecule by phase II metabolism. The sequential metabolism of phase I to phase II significantly enhances water solubility of xenobiotic metabolites to facilitate their excretion from the body [43]. In the liver, higher molecular weight conjugates (usually >450 D) typically undergo phase III efflux excretion at the hepatocellular apical (canalicular) membrane into the bile with subsequent excretion into the feces. Smaller molecular weight conjugates are transported across the basolateral membrane by phase III efflux transporters into the blood supply for subsequent excretion by the kidney [44]. Phase I and phase II enzymes are subject to both saturation (i.e., when xenobiotic concentrations exceed the available enzyme sites) and inhibition in the presence of other xenobiotic or endobiotics.

Table 1. The major[a] families of human xenobiotic metabolising enzymes and transporters

Symbol*	Approved Name	Major Families
SLC	Solute Carrier Transporters	SLC1 – SLC52; SLCO1 – SLCO6[b]
ABC	ATP Binding Cassette Transporters	ABCA – ABCG
CYP	Cytochrome P450s	CYP1 – CYP3
UGT	UDP Glucuronosyltransferases	UGT1, UGT2
SULT	Cytosolic Sulfotransferases	SULT1, SULT2
GST	Glutathione-S-transferases	GSTA, GSTM, GSTO, GSTP, GSTT, GSTZ
NAT	N-Acetyltransferases	NAT1, NAT2
MT	Methyltransferases	TPMT, COMT

*Nomenclature taken from the Human Genome Organization Gene Nomenclature Committee website (http://www.genenames.org/).
[a]Minor contributing enzyme and transporter families not included in this list.
[b]SLCO = Solute Carrier Organic Anion Transporters.

Although their primary function is deactivation and enhancement of hydrophilicity, phase I and phase II enzyme reactions can result in the formation of an active metabolite or reactive intermediate (i.e., bioactivation), thereby increasing risk for xenobiotic toxicity [45]. A number of xenobiotics have been identified to undergo bioactivation by phase I or phase II enzyme mechanisms. This is usually considered an unfavourable outcome of the xenobiotic elimination processes due to ability of reactive intermediates to bind to cellular macromolecules (e.g., DNA, protein, lipid) and interfere with their normal function or cause the development of an immune response [46, 47]. Whether bioactivation results in xenobiotic toxicity depends upon the extent of reactive intermediate formation relative to the activity of other phase I and phase II pathways and cellular antioxidant defenses that function to detoxify the reactive intermediate and prevent oxidative stress.

Phase I Metabolism

The cytochrome P450 superfamily of enzymes constitute the largest family of phase I enzymes involved in xenobiotic metabolism [48-50]. Other phase I enzymes include the FAD-containing monooxygenases (FMO), monoamine oxidase (MAO), epoxide hydrolase (EH), and esterases. These latter enzymes typically play a minor role in xenobiotic metabolism relative to the cytochrome P450 enzymes. The cytochrome P450 (CYP) superfamily is composed of 18 families of which CYP1, CYP2, and CYP3 play important roles in xenobiotic elimination [51, 52]. Expression of CYP enzymes and other phase I xenobiotic metabolizing enzymes is highest in the hepatic polarized epithelium such that this organ is principally responsible for phase I elimination of xenobiotics. However, the intestinal epithelium and to a minor extent kidney and other tissue also express phase I enzymes, albeit at lower levels [53, 54].

The CYP enzymes are heme-containing proteins commonly referred to as mixed-function oxidases due to an ability to mediate mono-oxygenase, oxidase, or reductase activity [48, 50]. CYP enzymes are housed in the smooth endoplasmic reticulum although some members are found in the mitochondria [50]. Mono-oxygenase activity involves activation of molecular oxygen by electron transfer from NADPH to the heme prosthetic group in CYP by NADPH-CYP450 reductase. Subsequently, one oxygen molecule is incorporated into the xenobiotic while the other oxygen molecule is released as water resulting in various hydroxylation, epoxidation, dealkylation, deamination, N- or S-oxidation, and dehalogenation reactions [48, 55]. The oxidase activity produces superoxide anion radicals with subsequent production of hydrogen peroxide following an electron transfer from the reduced form of the CYP enzyme to molecular oxygen [56, 57]. Finally, the reductase activity follows from the direct transfer of electrons from the reduced CYP enzyme to the xenobiotic [57]. Such activity may result in formation of a reactive metabolite, which can subsequently interact with cellular macromolecules and result in toxicity. The type of activity depends upon the xenobiotic and CYP mediating the phase I reaction. In most cases, though, CYP metabolism renders the xenobiotic inactive.

The CYP enzymes metabolize a diverse array of xenobiotics. An individual CYP enzyme may have broad substrate specificity and therefore cause the biotransformation of a large variety of xenobiotics. As well, an individual xenobiotic may undergo metabolism by multiple CYP enzymes but with different affinity and capacity and at different locations on the xenobiotic's chemical structure. These features relate to a basic requirement of CYP enzymes for lipophilicity. Three CYP families and their respective subfamilies are largely responsible for the biotransformation of xenobiotics and discussion is limited to these families.

The CYP1 family is composed of two subfamilies, CYP1A and CYP1B. The CYP1A subfamily has two important members, CYP1A1 and CYP1A2, while CYP1B has one member, CYP1B1, involved in xenobiotic metabolism. CYP1A2 is constitutively expressed in high levels in the liver encompassing up to 16% of total CYP enzyme content, but has limited expression in other tissues [58-60]. Hepatic CYP1A1 levels are very low (except with induction) but CYP1A1 has constitutive expression in extrahepatic tissues [61, 62]. CYP1A1 metabolizes a range of xenobiotics that overlap with CYP1A2. However, aromatic amines and heterocyclic molecules are typical substrates of CYP1A2 while CYP1A1 favours planar aromatic hydrocarbons [50]. Notably, the CYP1A family of enzymes is known for their ability to bioactivate polycyclic aromatic hydrocarbons, aromatic amines, and heterocyclic amines. In the elimination organs, expression of CYP1B1 is low with few known xenobiotic substrates, but is important in the bioactivation of procarcinogens such as the polyaromatic hydrocarbons [61-63]. Given the role of CYP1 family in the metabolism of procarcinogens, mutagens, and signalling molecules, this family has received a great deal of interest in toxicological risk assessment and as susceptibility markers for cancer and other diseases.

The CYP2 family has eight subfamilies whose members are known to metabolize xenobiotics. CYP2A, CYP2B, CYP2C, CYP2D, and CYP2E subfamilies, though, are the key members of this family [51, 52]. In the CYP2A subfamily only one member, CYP2A6, has a role in the elimination of xenobiotics [64]. CYP2A6 is primarily expressed in the liver and constitutes up to 4% total hepatic CYP [58-60]. This enzyme metabolizes a limited range of xenobiotics with nicotine and coumarin being the classic examples [50]. However, CYP2A6 has an important role in the bioactivation of nitrosoamines and other procarcinogens [65].

The CYP2B6 enzyme of the CYP2B family is principally expressed in the liver comprising about 2% of total hepatic CYP enzyme content and metabolises an important range of xenobiotics including procarcinogens like aflatoxin B1 and pesticides [50, 60, 66]. Expression levels of CYP2B6 may vary with gender and in general shows up to 250-fold differences in expression amongst the population [67-69]. This extensive inter-individual variation in expression is due to genetic differences and the ability of this enzyme to undergo significant induction (increases in enzyme expression) following exposure to a variety of xenobiotics [66].

The CYP2C subfamily has four members, CYP2C8, CYP2C9, CYP2C18, and CYP2C19, and makes up approximately 25% of total hepatic CYP content, approximately 18% of total intestinal CYP content, and with minor expression in the kidney [49, 62, 70]. CYP2C18 and CYP2C19 are minor members and CYP2C8 and CYP2C9 constitute the majority of CYP2C expression in the liver [59]. Members of the CYP2C family tend to exhibit a more discrete substrate specificity with some overlap. CYP2C members also express functional genetic polymorphisms (i.e., differences in the nucleotide sequences that result in phenotypic changes in the activity of the enzyme) where a certain percentage of the population are poor metabolizers for certain CYP2C substrates [59].

The CYP2D subfamily has one enzyme, CYP2D6, which constitutes about 3% of total hepatic CYP content and has minor expression in the intestine and kidney [49]. Despite its minor hepatic content, CYP2D6 metabolizes up to 28% of marketed drugs [50]. Typical substrates of CYP2D6 contain an aromatic ring with a nitrogen atom and these lipophilic bases are typically ionized at physiological pH [71]. Interestingly, a number of xenobiotics may inhibit CYP2D6 yet are not substrates for this enzyme. Furthermore, its regulation is not typically affected by environmental xenobiotics unlike many of the other CYP enzymes [72].

This enzyme exhibits significant genetic polymorphisms resulting in a functional deficiency of the enzyme that divides the population into poor, intermediate, and extensive metabolizer phenotypes [71, 72].

CYP2E1 is the only member of the CYP2E subfamily and constitutes about 7% total CYP hepatic content and is widely expressed in other tissues [59, 70]. CYP2E1 has a limited substrate range. It metabolizes low molecular weight hydrophobic molecules (e.g., acetone, ethanol, chlorzoxazone) and is involved in the bioactivation of solvent carcinogens like benzene, carbon tetrachloride, and ethylene glycol [73]. CYP2E1 exhibits a strong tendency towards futile cycling (the uncoupling of oxygen consumption with electron transfer from NADPH), which results in the formation of reactive oxygen intermediates (superoxide radical, hydrogen peroxide) and possibly in cellular damage [74, 75].

The CYP3 family consists of one subfamily, CYP3A, which constitutes about 28% of total hepatic CYP content and 80% of total intestinal CYP content [58-60, 62, 70]. This subfamily metabolizes a substantial and diverse array of endobiotics and xenobiotics including approximately 50% of marketed drugs. CYP3A4, CYP3A5, CYP3A7, and CYP3A43 principally mediate the metabolism of xenobiotics. In the liver, CYP3A4 is the most significant member of this group as the other members are expressed at relatively low levels [59, 76]. The large and flexible active site of CYP3A4 likely accounts for the broadest array of lipophilic substrates metabolized by any of the enzymes in the CYP superfamily [77]. CYP3A4 and CYP3A5 have significant overlap in substrate specificities. However, only 20% of the human population expresses hepatic CYP3A5, although this enzyme is expressed in the intestine and kidney at similar levels to CYP3A4 in these tissues [50, 76]. Significant inter-individual differences (up to 100-fold) exist in the expression of CYP3A4 in the liver, which result in substantive variation in the rate and extent of xenobiotic presystemic and systemic elimination by this pathway [50]. The adult liver content of CYP3A7 is quite low as this enzyme is principally expressed during fetal and early neonatal life stages [78]. A developmental switch occurs within the first year of life such that CYP3A4 levels increase while CYP3A7 levels decrease during the postnatal period [79]. Some overlap exists in the substrate specificities of these two members but important differences in substrates do exist. CYP3A43 is expressed in low amounts in the liver and metabolizes a limited number of xenobiotics [76].

Other phase I enzymes that contribute to a minor extent to overall xenobiotic metabolism include the flavin mono-oxygenases (FMOs), epoxide hydrolases, and the esterases/amidases. The FMOs consist of five members (FMO1-5) that oxidize xenobiotics containing heteroatoms like nitrogen, sulphur, and phosphorous and requires the sequential transfer of two electrons [80]. The FMOs contain a flavin adenine dinucleotide (FAD) prosthetic group responsible for the oxidation of xenobiotic substrates. FMOs are highly expressed in the endoplasmic reticulum in the liver with minor expression in the kidney and intestine [80]. FMO3 is predominantly expressed in the liver and has broad substrate specificity. The remaining members also have tissue specific expression but metabolize a narrower range of xenobiotics. The epoxide hydrolases are involved in the hydrolysis of epoxides formed from CYP enzyme mediated metabolism to less reactive diols, but may also contribute to the bioactivation of certain xenobiotics [81]. The esterases and amidases are widely distributed and are responsible for hydrolysis of ester bonds and amide bonds, respectively.

Phase II Metabolism

The uridine diphosphate glucuronosyltransferases (UGTs) are an important family of phase II enzymes responsible for the metabolism of a wide range of xenobiotics. The UGT enzymes mediate the conjugation of glucuronic acid from the cofactor, UDP glucuronic acid, to nucleophilic heteroatoms such as O, N, and S on xenobiotics containing aliphatic alcohols or phenols [32]. These enzymes are housed in the smooth endoplasmic reticulum membrane (microsomes) such that their active sites face the lumen of this organelle [82]. The UGTs are considered high capacity but low affinity enzymes, thus showing ability to efficiently metabolize higher concentrations of xenobiotics and endobiotics [82]. Their high capacity for metabolism, their expression in the liver, kidney, and intestine, and their ability to metabolize a broad range of xenobiotics and endobiotics (that contain functional groups such as phenols, alcohols, aliphatic and aromatic amines, thiols, carboxylic acids) make these enzymes a major contributor to xenobiotic elimination in general [83]. In addition to xenobiotics, the UGT enzymes play a critical role in elimination of potentially toxic endobiotics including bilirubin, steroid hormones, bile acids, and fatty acids [83].

The UGTs consist of four families but only two, UGT1 and UGT2, are important in xenobiotic metabolism [84]. The UGT1 family has one subfamily, UGT1A, and nine functional members arise from multiple promoters at a single gene locus [85]. The UGT2 family is divided into two subfamilies, UGT2A and UGT2B. Members of the UGT2 family are encoded by different genes and contain multiple members [82, 85]. UGT1A8 and UGT1A10 are only expressed in the gastrointestinal tract but all other UGT members are expressed in the elimination organs. Although UGTs function to deactivate and enhance excretion of xenobiotics, these enzymes also are implicated in the formation of reactive acyl glucuronides that cause potential toxicity [85].

The cytosolic sulfotransferases (SULT) conjugate a sulfonyl group donated from the cosubstrate, 3'-phosphoadenosine 5'-phosphosulfate (PAPS), to a wide range of xenobiotics containing nucleophilic heteroatoms such as oxygen, sulphur and nitrogen on aliphatic alcohols, phenols, N-hydroxy arylamines, and heterocyclic amines with high affinity but low capacity [86-88]. The SULTs are widely distributed in the body and consist of 3 subfamilies, SULT1, SULT2, and SULT4, containing a large number of members with diverse and overlapping substrate specificities [89]. SULTs are instrumental in maintaining homeostasis of steroids, thyroid hormones, and catecholamines. SULT1 and SULT2 are most important for xenobiotic elimination [86, 90]. SULT1 has four subfamilies, but SULT1A, particularly SULT1A1, is principally involved in the metabolism of xenobiotics in liver and kidney, and SULT1B in the intestine [89, 90]. SULT1A1's broad substrate specificity makes it the most important SULT in xenobiotic elimination [90]. SULT2 has two subfamilies, SULT2A and SULT2B, which play a smaller role in xenobiotic metabolism and tend to carry out sulfonation of non-aromatic hydroxyl groups [90]. Like the UGT enzymes, SULTs may contribute to the production of toxic metabolites [91].

The UGTs and SULTs have overlapping substrate specificities, which allow these two metabolic pathways to function in a complementary fashion. As high affinity enzymes, SULTs contribution to xenobiotic metabolism predominates at low intracellular xenobiotic concentrations, while the lower affinity but high capacity UGT enzymes become more important as intracellular concentrations become greater. At sufficiently high intracellular concentrations, the low capacity SULTs become saturated (or their cosubstrate, PAPS, may become depleted) allowing the higher capacity UGTs to supplant the SULTs as the principal metabolizing enzymes at higher xenobiotic exposures [43, 92]. Furthermore, both pathways may be subject to reversible metabolism and recycling. Sulfatases in the liver may result in the deconjugation of sulfated xenobiotics making the xenobiotic available once again for metabolism by SULTs such that xenobiotics can cycle between parent and sulfate metabolite [92]. Glucuronide conjugates excreted into the bile by phase III transporters may encounter the beta-glucuronidases of the gastrointestinal microflora or mucosa. Deconjugation of the glucuronidated xenobiotic makes it available for reabsorption to undergo another possible cycle of glucuronidation and deconjugation in a process of enterohepatic circulation [93]. This process enhances and prolongs the duration of exposure of the gastrointestinal tract and liver to the xenobiotic, which can have important pharmacological or toxicological sequelae [44].

The glutathione S-transferases (GST) are ubiquitous, but in the liver these enzymes make up almost 4% of total soluble protein [94, 95]. In the gastrointestinal tract GST expression is high in the proximal small intestine and levels decrease more distally along the intestine [96]. The family is divided into membrane bound (endoplasmic reticulum), mitochondrial, and cytosolic enzymes. The 13 different enzymes are further divided into seven classes relevant to xenobiotic metabolism namely alpha (GSTA), mu (GSTM), omega (GSTO), pi (GSTP), sigma (GSTS), theta (GSTT), and zeta (GSTZ). In most cases cytosolic GST mediates xenobiotic metabolism. These enzymes catalyze the reaction of intracellular glutathione to electrophilic carbon, nitrogen, oxygen, and sulphur atoms often formed during CYP enzyme mediated metabolism of xenobiotics to detoxify these reactive electrophiles and enhance their excretion [97, 98]. Consequently, GSTs play a significant role in cellular protection and reduction in oxidative stress. The GST conjugated xenobiotic must exit the cell via phase III transporters and then typically undergoes further metabolism through sequential hydrolysis and N-acetylation reactions to form a mercapturate metabolite that is excreted into the urine [98, 99]. GST enzymes also contribute to xenobiotic intracellular transport and sequestration as they can bind to hydrophobic xenobiotics without catalyzing glutathione transfer to these molecules [97].

The N-acetyltransferases (NAT) consist of two enzymes, NAT1 and NAT2, which catalyze the conjugation of the N-acetyl group from N-acetyl-CoA to xenobiotics containing arylamines and arylhydrazine groups and heterocyclic amines [41]. As with other phase II enzymes, the NATs may cause bioactivation, specifically N-hydroxyarylamines, to reactive intermediates that can bind to cellular macromolecules and affect their function. NAT2 exhibits a significant genetic polymorphism such that the population is divided into rapid and slow acetylators and is implicated in xenobiotic toxicity [41]. The methyltransferases (MT) transfer a methyl group from S-adenosyl-L-methionine (SAM) to heteroatoms, oxygen, sulphur and nitrogen, of various xenobiotics. MTs play an important role in the regulation of the activity of proteins, genetic expression, and various endogenous molecules [100]. Unlike other phase I and phase II metabolic pathways, acetylation and methylation of xenobiotics usually decrease their aqueous solubility.

Phase 0 and Phase III Xenobiotic Transporters

Transporters are carrier proteins that span the plasma membrane and membranes of the various cellular organelles and mediate the translocation of xenobiotics into or out of the cell or organelle. These proteins contribute to the permeation of xenobiotics across these lipid barriers. Both passive diffusion and carrier-mediated transport processes often work together to assure vectorial transport (i.e., net movement in one direction) across the biological membrane but can work in opposition when a xenobiotic is a substrate of an efflux transporter. In the polarized epithelium, xenobiotics may require both uptake and efflux transporters on opposite sides of the epithelium to ensure vectorial movement across the epithelium [101, 102].

The rate of transporter-mediated movement of xenobiotics often exceeds passive diffusion rate and can therefore ensure an efficient uptake or efflux across the biological membrane. However, the relative rates of the transporter-mediated process and passive diffusion will define the contribution of the transporter to the overall membrane permeability of a xenobiotic [15, 103]. Being a substrate for a transporter does not guarantee that carrier-mediated transport is the predominant process in xenobiotic permeation across the membrane. Furthermore, being lipophilic does not guarantee that passive diffusion is the most significant component of membrane permeation as lipophilic xenobiotics are also substrates of various phase 0 and phase III transporters. When the contribution of a transporter is significant, intracellular concentrations and the concomitant concentration of xenobiotic at the metabolizing enzyme site may be quite different than concentrations expected from passive diffusion processes alone.

Transport by carrier proteins is characterized by the ability to be saturated (i.e., xenobiotic concentration exceeds the number of transporters available) and hence exhibit a maximal transport rate, as well as undergo competitive or noncompetitive inhibition by other xenobiotics and endobiotics. Many xenobiotics are known to inhibit phase 0 and phase III transporters thereby influencing the transport of key endobiotics and their homeostasis in general [30]. As with the phase I and phase II enzymes, carrier mediated transport is under the influence of both genetic and environmental factors that can result in substantive interindividual differences in xenobiotic transport and therefore an important mechanism underlying the variation in elimination capacity among the human population. The impact of transporters on xenobiotic elimination will depend upon whether they mediate xenobiotic uptake or efflux, their localization on the apical or basolateral membrane of the polarized epithelium, their expression within the various organs of elimination, and the impact of genetic and environmental factors on their overall function. When its role is critical in organ uptake or elimination, transporter distribution may account for organ specific sensitivity to xenobiotics, a situation akin to the distribution of phase I and phase II enzymes in the body. Figure 4 identifies expression of the major xenobiotic transporters in the polarized epithelia of each elimination organ [20].

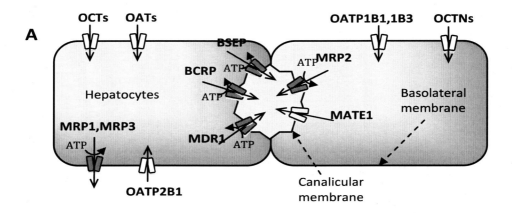
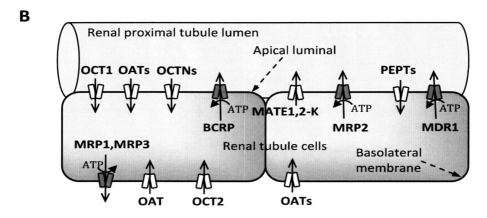
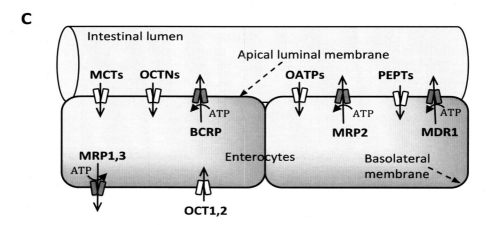

Figure 4. Localization of representative members of the Solute Carrier (SLC) and ATP Binding Cassette (ABC) transporter superfamilies within the polarized epithelia of liver (A), kidney (B), and intestine (C).

Solute Carrier Transporter Family

The Solute Carrier Transporter (SLC) superfamily is composed of 52 families with hundreds of individual transporters that mediate the uptake of xenobiotics across the biological membrane into the cell (or organelle). All uptake transporters fall within the SLC superfamily. Uptake is mediated through facilitated diffusion processes or secondary active transport that requires an energy coupling process [35, 104]. Facilitated diffusion involves movement of the xenobiotic down an electrochemical gradient. Secondary active transport requires the movement of an electrolyte or organic substrate in the same direction (symport) or opposite direction (antiport) as the xenobiotic. The xenobiotic is transported against a concentration gradient while the electrolyte or organic substrate moves down its electrochemical gradient, but at the expense of a separate energy consuming process that functions to maintain the ion gradient (e.g., Na^+/K^- ATPase pump present on all cell plasma membranes) [15]. In the polarized epithelium, SLC transporters are typically expressed on the basolateral, blood-facing side. The SLC transporters have broad and overlapping substrate specificities such that a xenobiotic can be transported by more than one type of transporter.

The SLC superfamily retains a large number of individual members. The following section highlights the key families involved in xenobiotic transport and provides a broad overview of their function. Those SLC transporters responsible for phase 0 uptake of xenobiotics largely fall within the SLCO (SLC21), SLC15, SLC16, SLC22, SLC28, SLC29, and SLC47 transporter families [25, 35, 105]. The International Transporter Consortium identifies these as the major families involved in xenobiotic transport [24].

SLCO Family

This family, formerly the SLC21 family renamed to SLCO (Solute Carrier Organic Anion Transporter), encompasses the organic anion transporting polypeptides (OATPs) [106]. SLCO consists of 6 subfamilies and 13 individual transporters [105]. OATPs generally mediate the uptake of large hydrophobic organic anions, zwitterionic compounds, and linear and cyclic peptides either by bidirectional facilitated diffusion or by the symport or antiport of bicarbonate, reduced glutathione, and glutathione conjugates [24, 107, 108]. Important endobiotics transported by the OATPs include bile acids and hormone conjugates [109]. Most members of this family are expressed in virtually every epithelium of the body at the apical or basolateral membrane depending upon the specific member. However, several members exhibit organ specific expression such as OATP1B1 and OATP1B3, which are expressed only in the basolateral membrane of hepatocytes [25, 110]. OATP1B1, OAT1B3, OATP1A2, and OATP2B1 are the key members involved in xenobiotic transport [26, 107]. OATP1A2 is expressed in the intestinal and renal epithelium, while OATP2B1 is widely distributed [107, 110]. These transporters have broad and overlapping substrate specificities and are often a site for xenobiotic interactions [111]. This is exemplified by the grapefruit component, naringen, known to inhibit the uptake and, hence, oral bioavailability of several important therapeutic agents such as fexofenadine transported by OATPs [112].

SLC15 Family

This family encompasses the oligopeptide transporters, PEPT1 and PEPT2. PEPTs are secondary active transporters that mediate the uptake of di- and tri-peptides and peptidomimetic substrates at the intestine and kidney and require the symport of a proton

[113]. PEPT1 is considered a high capacity, low affinity transporter of oligopeptides, while PEPT2 is a low capacity, high affinity transporter of these substrates [113]. PEPT1 has high expression in the apical membrane of the intestinal polarized epithelium where it is responsible for di- and tripeptide absorption. PEPT1 is also expressed in the early proximal part of the renal tubule luminal (apical) epithelium. PEPT2 is highly expressed in the kidney but in more distal portions of the proximal tubule epithelium [113]. These transporters are responsible for the reabsorption of filtered oligopeptides. PEPT2 also exhibits some expression in the hepatocellular canalicular (apical) membrane [114].

SLC16 Family

The SLC16 family is referred to as the monocarboxylate transporters. The family comprises the proton-coupled monocarboxylate transporters (MCTs) and the sodium-dependent monocarboxylate transporters (SMCTs) [115]. MCT1, MCT2, MCT3, and MCT4 require the cooperation of glycoproteins, basigin or embigin, which act as chaperones and ensure appropriate insertion of these MCTs into the plasma membrane for their proper activity [115, 116]. The SLC16 members have ubiquitous expression due to their significant involvement in a number of metabolic pathways such as energy homeostasis [115]. The MCTs transport a broad range of short chain monocarboxylates, particularly L-lactate, pyruvate, and ketone bodies, but are key to the uptake of a few important xenobiotics like nicotinic acid and gamma-hydroxybutyrate.

SLC22 Family

The SLC22 family is composed of the organic anion transporters and organic cation transporters. Members of the SLC22 family are expressed on almost every epithelium of the body. The organic anion transporters are responsible for the influx of a diverse range of low molecular weight organic anions by organic anion exchange (e.g., exchange with alpha-ketoglutarate) (secondary active transport) and comprise the organic anion transporters (OAT) and urate transporters (URAT1) [102, 110, 117-119]. The SLC22 family has over 10 OAT members. OAT1, OAT2, and OAT3 are highly expressed on the basolateral membrane of the renal tubular epithelium and therefore have an important role in the renal excretion of many xenobiotic anions [120]. OAT4 and OAT10 are expressed in the luminal apical membrane of the renal tubule epithelium, while OAT2 and OAT7 have high expression in the hepatocellular basolateral membrane and are important in hepatocellular uptake of xenobiotic anions [107, 110, 117]. URAT1 is found in the luminal apical membrane of the renal proximal tubular epithelium and is responsible for the uptake of urate from the renal filtrate [121].

Organic cation uptake is mediated by the organic cation transporters (OCT) and the carnitine/organic cation transporters (OCTN) [25, 110, 122]. The key SLC22 family members for xenobiotic transport are 4 OCT members, OCT1, OCT2, OCT3, and OCT6, and two OCTN members, OCTN1 and OCTN2. OCTs are bidirectional facilitated diffusion transporters that transport a diverse range of low molecular weight, hydrophilic organic cations [123]. OCT1 tends to have higher expression in the basolateral membrane of the hepatic polarized epithelium, OCT2 in the basolateral membrane of the renal proximal tubule cells, and OCT3 with more ubiquitous expression [107, 120, 123]. OCT1 is also expressed in the apical luminal membrane of the proximal and distal renal tubule epithelium and participates in the uptake of cations from the urinary filtrate [124]. OCT1's high expression in the hepatocellular basolateral membrane positions this transporter to play a key role in the hepatic presystemic elimination of many cationic xenobiotics. OCT2 expression in the basolateral surface of the renal epithelium suggests an important role for this transporter in the renal excretion of various positively charged xenobiotics.

The *novel* transporters, OCTNs, have rather narrow substrate selectivities and their mechanism of transport depends on the xenobiotic substrate. Transport may involve cation/proton exchange, cation/cation exchange, or sodium-dependent or sodium-independent transport [120, 125, 126]. The OCTN transporters are characterized by overlapping substrate specificity, but some xenobiotics undergo specific transport such as the transport of the dietary plant antioxidant, ergothioeine, by OCTN1 but not OCTN2 [127]. The principal role of these transporters is maintenance of L-carnitine homeostasis, a key amino acid in the oxidation of fatty acids for cellular energy production, through their regulation of intestinal absorption and renal reabsorption, as these transporters are expressed in the apical membranes of the respective organ polarized epithelia [126].

The SLC22 family plays a particularly important role in the elimination of xenobiotics due to their ability to transport very structurally diverse organic anions and cations (both endobiotics and xenobiotics) and to their high expression in the polarized epithelium of the liver and kidney [119, 123]. Their broad substrate specificities also provide an opportunity for significant xenobiotic interactions where two xenobiotics compete with the same transporter or a nonsubstrate xenobiotic may inhibit SLC22 transport by noncompetitive mechanisms [110, 117, 120].

SLC28 and SLC29 Families

The concentrative nucleoside transporters (CNTs) and equilibrative nucleoside transporters (ENTs) comprise the SLC28 and SLC29 families, respectively [128]. The human concentrative nucleoside transporters consist of three members, CNT1, CNT2, and CNT3. These transporters mediate the uptake of xenobiotics with structural similarity to nucleosides that involves a secondary active transport mechanism through coupling with cation gradients. The CNTs are widely expressed in polarized epithelia and primarily at the apical luminal membrane of the intestine and kidney, but at both the apical luminal and basolateral membranes of the hepatic polarized epithelium [129]. The four members of the equilibrative nucleoside transporters, ENT1, ENT2, ENT3, and ENT4, are also widely expressed with apical luminal and basolateral expression in the polarized epithelia of liver, kidney, and intestine. The ENTs mediate bidirectional facilitated diffusion of xenobiotics with structural similarity to nucleosides and nucleobases [129]. The CNTs and ENTs are responsible for the cellular uptake of several important xenobiotics, but have very important endobiotic substrates that play significant physiological roles in the body [128].

SLC47 Family

The multidrug and toxin extrusion proteins (MATEs) make up the SLC47 family [130, 131]. Two members, MATE1 and MATE2-K, mediate the efflux of cations, as well as some zwitterions and anions. MATE1 is expressed at the luminal membrane of the liver (canalicular) and kidney proximal tubule epithelial cells and use a proton gradient operating in the opposite direction as the driving force [132]. MATE2-K uses a similar driving force for transport and is expressed only in the kidney [131]. As proton/cation exchangers, MATEs maintain the gradient for excretion of cations and are often coupled with OCTs expressed at the basolateral membrane to allow vectorial transcellular transport and elimination of organic cations by the kidney and liver via the urinary filtrate and bile, respectively [123].

The ATP Binding Cassette Transporter Family

The ABC transporter family represents a large family of transport proteins responsible for the active efflux of lipophilic and amphipathic xenobiotics and their metabolites from the polarized epithelia of the elimination organs [133]. These transporters utilize direct ATP hydrolysis to provide the energy to transport xenobiotics against a concentration gradient (i.e., primary active transport) [133]. This characteristic is significant as many of the ABC transporter substrates have high passive diffusion characteristics, which competes with the active efflux mechanisms and impacts overall net vectorial movement of a xenobiotic across the polarized epithelial barrier. The ABC transporters also exhibit tissue specific expression and specific localization in the polarized epithelium and have rather wide and overlapping substrate specificities making generalizable characterizations of their role in phase III elimination very difficult [13].

In the elimination organs, ABC transporters are usually expressed on the apical membrane of the polarized epithelium, although several important ABC transporter members are expressed on the basolateral membrane of the intestinal and hepatic epithelia. The expression of ABC transporters on the apical luminal membrane results in the active excretion of xenobiotics into the gastrointestinal lumen, hepatic biliary system, and renal urinary filtrate. Hence, this family of efflux transporters are responsible for the ultimate removal (phase III) of xenobiotics and xenobiotic metabolites from the body. In the intestine and liver, ABC transporter expression on the basolateral membrane facilitates xenobiotic or xenobiotic metabolite entrance into the systemic blood supply. The ABC superfamily is divided into 7 known families, ABCA to ABCG (http://nutrigene.4t.com/humanabc.htm) [134]. Discussion of ABC transporter families will be limited to those key transporters involved in xenobiotic transport as identified by the International Transporter Consortium [24].

ABCB Family

This family consists of 11 members and includes the first discovered and most well-studied ABC transporter, p-glycoprotein or multidrug resistance protein 1 (MDR1; ABCB1). MDR1 represents an important mechanism limiting organ and cellular exposure to xenobiotics [13, 135]. It effluxes a very broad range of structurally diverse xenobiotics that are hydrophobic, amphipathic in nature [107]. MDR1 has at least three xenobiotic binding sites and these sites work in a positive cooperative fashion [136]. Its localization to the apical luminal membrane of the entire length of the intestinal epithelium [137] and apical canalicular epithelial membrane of the liver indicates MDR1 has an excretory function to limit xenobiotic systemic exposure by limiting oral bioavailability or enhancing hepatic presystemic or systemic elimination [13, 133, 138]. MDR1 expression in the luminal membrane of the renal tubular epithelium indicates an additional role in systemic elimination by the kidney and reductions in overall systemic exposure to xenobiotics and xenobiotic metabolites [138].

The bile salt excretory protein (BSEP; ABCB11) is expressed in the hepatocellular canalicular epithelial membrane (as well as in the intestinal mucosa) and is responsible for the excretion of conjugated and unconjugated bile salts into the bile, which aids in the maintenance of bile-salt dependent bile flow [139-141]. Few xenobiotics undergo BSEP-mediated transport but it is significant as it serves as an important site of xenobiotic inhibition [142, 143]. BSEP inhibition is a common cause of cholestasis and liver failure, which led to the market withdrawal of a number of therapeutic xenobiotics [144].

ABCC Family

The multidrug resistance-associated proteins, or MRPs, are the largest family in the ABC superfamily of transporters. These transporters efflux a broad range of hydrophobic xenobiotics and organic anions including glucuronide, sulfate, and glutathione conjugates of various endobiotics and xenobiotics [133]. Depending upon the member, MRPs either localize to the basolateral or apical membranes of polarized epithelia [13, 107, 145]. Key members include MRP1, MRP2, and MRP3. MRP2 is expressed at the apical luminal membrane of the liver, kidney, and intestinal polarized epithelia [146]. MRP1 (ABCC1) is widely expressed and has an important role in limiting systemic exposure of a wide variety of xenobiotics particularly hydrophilic conjugated metabolites of xenobiotics [147]. Notably, the co-transport of glutathione is required for the MRP1-mediated efflux of a number of xenobiotics and xenobiotic conjugates and MRP1 may efflux both oxidized and reduced glutathione in the absence of xenobiotics [147]. MRP2 (ABCC2) is responsible for the efflux of many xenobiotics as well as phase II xenobiotic conjugate metabolites, in particular glucuronide, glutathione, and sulfate conjugates [13, 148]. In this role, MRP2 also plays a key function in limiting systemic exposure to a xenobiotic by enhancing systemic elimination or limiting oral bioavailability, and provides a mechanism for the intracellular removal of polar xenobiotic conjugates for ultimate elimination in the feces or urine. Notable endogenous substrates include glucuronidated bilirubin and estradiol [107]. MRP3 (ABCC3) expressed at the basolateral epithelial membrane of liver and intestine also is responsible for xenobiotic conjugate efflux into the blood circulatory system [133, 134, 149]. The key endogenous role of MRP3 is the maintenance of bile salt enterohepatic circulation [150].

ABCG Family

This family includes the breast cancer resistance protein (BCRP, ABCG2) involved in the active efflux of many structurally divergent xenobiotics from cells, in particular neutral and negatively charged ions and sulphate and glucuronide conjugates of organic anion xenobiotics [109, 151, 152]. Important endogenous substrates include estrone-3-sulfate, dehydroepiandrosterone sulfate, and uric acid [107, 133]. BCRP exists as a half-transporter and activity requires formation of oligomers [25]. This transporter localizes to the apical membrane in polarized epithelia of the elimination organs and shows significant overlap with MDR1 with respect to its tissue expression and substrate specificity [107, 133]. As with other ABC transporters, BCRP has a similar function to limit systemic exposure via reductions in oral bioavailability and enhancements in systemic elimination through biliary and renal excretion. Additional members, ABCG5 and ABCG8, are involved in plant sterol excretion into bile and the intestinal lumen to prevent their absorption, but do not play a significant role in xenobiotic elimination [153].

KEY FACTORS CONTRIBUTING TO INTER-INDIVIDUAL VARIABILITY IN XENOBIOTIC ELIMINATION

Considerable inter-individual differences exist in the expression of phase 0, phase I, phase II, and phase III proteins in the elimination organs. Such differences result in highly variable rates and patterns of xenobiotic elimination that can lead to quite dissimilar xenobiotic systemic exposures and a spectrum of possible responses (i.e., toxicity to no effect) to a particular xenobiotic exposure. Various physiological and environmental factors contribute to the inter-individual variation in xenobiotic elimination. These factors include age, gender, ethnicity, disease, diet, xenobiotic interactions (where the elimination of the xenobiotic is influenced by the presence of an endobiotic or another xenobiotic), epigenetic regulation, transcriptional regulation, and genetic polymorphisms in the enzymes, transporters, and transcription factors regulating enzyme and transporter expression. Knowledge of these factors and their influence on xenobiotic presystemic and systemic elimination is necessary to explain population differences in xenobiotic exposure outcomes.

Epigenetic Factors and Nongenetic Host Factors

The impact of epigenetic factors, changes in gene function due to mechanisms not associated with alterations in DNA sequence, has received limited attention until recently. A growing number of studies suggest a role for DNA methylation and histone deacetylation in the transcriptional upregulation or downregulation of expression of a number of xenobiotic metabolizing enzymes and transporters [154-158]. MicroRNAs, noncoding RNAs that bind to target mRNAs to inhibit translation or enhance degradation of the target mRNA, also impact enzyme and transporter expression and are increasingly identified as underlying causes of xenobiotic metabolizing enzyme and transporter variability in disease [159-161]. Gender related differences in expression of enzymes and transporters have been acknowledged and some clinically used xenobiotics show evidence that females may metabolize xenobiotics faster than males [162-164]. Ontogeny of enzymes and transporters typically result in reduced capacity for neonates to eliminate xenobiotics, while normal aging changes in the physiological determinants of xenobiotic elimination may account for reduced capacities for xenobiotic elimination in the elderly [79, 162]. Disease can have variable influences depending upon the pathology [165]. For example, inflammation is known to downregulate the expression of most xenobiotic metabolizing enzymes and transporters [166]. Dietary influences also have variable effects that may be mediated through alterations in transcriptional regulation mechanisms or direct inhibition of xenobiotic metabolizing enzymes and transporters [167].

Xenobiotic Interactions with Other Xenobiotics and Endobiotics

Phase 0 through to phase III mechanisms have a significant role in maintaining body homeostasis. Phase I and phase II enzymes are critical mechanisms of xenobiotic elimination, but also regulate cellular and systemic levels of important endobiotics, such as hormones, vitamins, antioxidants, signalling molecules, and nutrients as examples [102]. Phase 0 and phase 3 transporters are responsible for the transport of many endobiotics that either support cellular function or require transport out of the cell and the body to avoid their accumulation and subsequent toxicity. Xenobiotics exploit the same transporters originally evolved to support endobiotic transport across cellular membranes. Consequently, phase 0 through to phase III mechanisms become a target for important xenobiotic interactions, either through xenobiotic-endobiotic or xenobiotic-xenobiotic interactions at the same enzyme or transporter or via the transcriptional regulatory mechanisms [40, 102, 107].

Several factors determine whether a xenobiotic interaction will result in significant alterations in xenobiotic elimination. Any significant interaction will alter systemic exposures, which have important consequences on xenobiotic effect or alterations in body homeostasis due to interference with the endogenous function of these enzymes and transporters. Such factors include the relative concentrations of the xenobiotics/endobiotics at the site of interaction, the site of the elimination mechanism, and the extent to which other elimination mechanisms contribute to presystemic and systemic elimination. A significant interaction is most plausible when a single enzyme or transporter principally determines the elimination of a xenobiotic. Hundreds of clinically significant xenobiotic interactions have been reported when elimination is principally mediated by a single CYP enzyme or by a phase 0 or phase III transporter. Only a few important interactions have been reported for high capacity systems such as the UGTs. A clear example follows from the grapefruit juice interaction with a number of drugs that exhibit low oral bioavailability and are principally metabolized by CYP3A4 or undergo OATP mediated uptake. The juice component bergamotten potently inhibits intestinal CYP3A4 while naringin (actually the aglycone, naringenin) inhibits intestinal OATP1A2 to cause reductions in presystemic elimination, enhanced oral bioavailability, enhanced systemic exposure, and hence an increased risk of toxicity for these drugs [112, 168, 169].

Genetic Factors

Genetic factors are a significant underlying cause of inter-individual variation. A single nucleotide change that occurs in the promoter, coding region, or noncoding regulatory portion of a gene may result in an amino acid sequence modification with subsequent functional alterations in enzyme and transporter activity or alteration in their respective expression levels. These single nucleotide polymorphism (SNPs) may result in loss of function or a gain of function due to an increase in gene copies, promoter variants, or variants within the encoded portion of the gene that increase catalytic rate [50, 170, 171]. Numerous SNPs have been identified in the phase 0 – III mechanisms and the transcription factors regulating these processes [68, 72, 170-173]. Many of these SNPs have either no phenotypic effect or cause decreases in enzyme or transporter activity. In general, SNPs involving phase I and phase II enzymes can result in substantive inter-individual variation. For example, the SNPs of CYP2D6 and CYP2C19 generally divide the population into two distinct phenotypes, poor metabolizers and extensive metabolisers, with further variability within these distinct phenotypic populations due to the presence of multiple SNPs in these genes [71, 72, 174]. The role of SNPs in transporters is less well characterized. However, SNPs of phase 0 and phase III transporters usually account for a smaller proportion of the observed inter-individual variation in xenobiotic elimination [27, 175].

Transcriptional Regulation (Induction)

Environmental or pathophysiological factors are known to affect the levels of enzymes and transporters through pathways that regulate gene expression. Many xenobiotic metabolizing enzymes and transporters are under transcriptional regulation by the once orphaned type II nuclear receptors, the aryl hydrocarbon receptor (AhR), the nuclear factor-erythroid 2 p45-related factor (Nrf2), and other transcription factors such as hepatocyte nuclear factor 1α and 4 (HNF1α, HNF4) [105, 110, 120, 176-180]. These transcription factors are expressed in the intestine, liver, and kidney and upon activation bind to xenobiotic response elements in the promoter region of target genes to increase transcription rate and the protein level of xenobiotic metabolising enzymes and transporters, a process called induction. Induction is an adaptive response and may be considered a protective mechanism when it leads to enhanced systemic elimination or reduced bioavailability and systemic exposure [180]. However, induction can result in enhanced bioactivation of xenobiotics to reactive intermediates. Alternatively, the induced protein may become a more significant site for xenobiotic interactions. In both cases, an increased risk for adverse effects and organ toxicity is an undesired outcome of induction [181].

The principal nuclear receptors involved in regulation of xenobiotic metabolism and transport include the constitutive androstane receptor (CAR), pregnane X receptor (PXR), farnesoid X receptor (FXR), peroxisome proliferator-activated receptor alpha (PPARα), and retinoic acid receptor (RAR) [173]. These are often referred to as the 'xenosensing' receptors as they function to 'sense' potential toxic xenobiotics and their metabolites to cause induction of those elimination pathways responsible to enhance their removal [182]. Many xenobiotics (natural products and drugs) are known ligands of the nuclear receptors [183]. The nuclear receptors are composed of a ligand binding domain and a DNA binding domain and exist in the cytoplasm until their activation [178]. The binding of a ligand (endobiotic or xenobiotic) to the ligand binding domain results in nuclear receptor transactivation and translocation to the nucleus. Here, the nuclear receptors heterodimerize with 9-cis-retinoic acid receptor (RXR) and subsequently bind to the consensus sequence in the promoter regions of the genes encoding transporters and enzymes to increase transcription rate [177, 178].

PXR is highly expressed in the liver and intestine, while CAR has highest expression in liver and significant expression in the intestine and kidney [178]. Unlike other nuclear receptors, CAR does not require ligand binding for activation as it exists in a constitutively active state. Androstenol and androstanol are endogenous antagonists of CAR that inhibit its transactivation. In their absence, CAR adopts an active conformation [184, 185]. Ligand binding to CAR may actually reduce CAR activity and behave as inverse agonists of CAR [178, 183]. PPARα is highly expressed in the liver and kidney. Although it regulates expression of phase 0 – III enzymes and transporters, PPARα is best known for its role in regulating expression of enzymes in fatty acid metabolism [186, 187]. FXR regulates bile acid homeostasis and is expressed in liver, intestine, and kidney [188]. Since many of the enzymes and transporters involved in bile acid homeostasis are also xenobiotic metabolizing enzymes and transporters, FXR plays a role in xenobiotic elimination [178]. Hepatic nuclear factors (HNF) principally regulate expression of genes involved in the maintenance of hepatic homeostasis [189]. Nonetheless, HNFs are expressed in liver, intestinal, and renal polarized epithelia and play a role in the regulation of xenobiotic elimination pathways [190].

The AhR is a ligand activated soluble Per-Sim-ARNT (Pas) domain receptor with rather broad ligand specificities and regulates a number of the phase I and phase II enzymes and phase 0 and phase III transporters [63, 173, 179, 191]. The AhR is present in the cytoplasm complexed with a heat shock protein (Hsp90) dimer that keeps it inactive but ready to bind various ligands. Ligand binding causes a conformation change in the AhR resulting in the release of the Hsp90, nuclear translocation of the AhR, and its heterodimerization with aryl hydrocarbon receptor nuclear translocator (ARNT) [191]. The heterodimer then binds to DNA consensus sequences in the promoter regions of genes influenced by this transcription factor.

The transcription factor, Nrf2, is often considered a key factor in cellular protection against oxidative stress [19, 192]. Nrf2 is a member of the basic region-leucine zipper family and becomes activated by electrophiles and reactive oxygen species [46]. In the cytoplasm Nrf2 is bound to Kelch like ECH-associated protein 1 (Keap1), a cytoskeletal anchoring protein that keeps Nrf2 within the cytoplasm [193]. The presence of electrophiles or reactive oxygen species causes the modification of sulfhydryl groups in the cysteine residues of Keap1. This results in the subsequent release of Nrf2, which then translocates to the nucleus and heterodimerizes with activator protein (AP-1) family members like Maf, or other regulatory proteins. The heterodimer binds to the antioxidant response elements (ARE) in the promoter region of genes regulated by this transcription factor [19, 194]. The interaction between Keap1 and Nrf2 also can be disrupted via activation of kinase signalling cascades including the MAPK pathway by reactive electrophiles [19]. Many of these gene targets include phase I and II enzymes, phase III transporters, reactive oxygen species scavenging proteins, glutathione homeostasis, and other enzymes involved in cellular protection. Consequently, those xenobiotics responsible for the activation of Nrf2 are considered as cytoprotective agents [19, 94, 194].

The nuclear receptors, AhR, and Nrf2 generally have broad and overlapping gene targets such that a single phase 0, phase I, phase II, or phase III member can undergo transcriptional regulation by several different transcription factors. As well, a single transcription factor may regulate a number of xenobiotic enzymes and transporters simultaneously. The transcription factors also have overlapping ligand binding specificities. This overlap between transcriptional targets and ligand specificities results in an extensive cross-talk between the transcriptional regulatory pathways such that alterations in xenobiotic elimination mechanisms may result from a variety of xenobiotic exposures through a variety of mechanisms [178]. The overlap and cross talk between the different transcriptional activation pathways results in a highly coordinated pattern of regulation of the xenobiotic elimination system in general [46, 178, 195, 196].

CONCLUSION

The xenobiotic elimination system is a highly versatile and adaptable system designed to capably manage xenobiotic exposures and prevent untoward effects. Elimination is achieved through a plethora of xenobiotic metabolizing enzymes and transporters in the polarized epithelia of the key organs of elimination, liver, kidney, and intestine. Although identification of the individual enzymes and/or transporters involved in the presystemic and systemic elimination of a xenobiotic is important, xenobiotic elimination is the end product of a number of competing, collaborating, and interacting processes that ultimately determines the nature and pattern of elimination and the outcome of an exposure. The widely held historical understanding that most xenobiotics simply undergo passive diffusion has undergone repeated interrogation as our understanding of phase 0 and phase III transporter processes grow. The phase I and phase II xenobiotic metabolizing enzymes often work in concert with the phase 0 and phase III transporters to effectively eliminate xenobiotics and limit their systemic exposures. The extensive cross talk between the different transcriptional activation pathways ensures a highly coordinated pattern of regulation and ability of the xenobiotic elimination system to quickly adapt to changing xenobiotic exposures. Our foremost challenge remains the ability to predict the quantitative impact of the various xenobiotic elimination processes on xenobiotic systemic exposures and of the genetic and environmental factors that influence the xenobiotic elimination system.

REFERENCES

[1] Nebert, D. W., (1991). Proposed role of drug-metabolizing enzymes: regulation of steady state levels of the ligands that effect growth, homeostasis, differentiation, and neuroendocrine functions. *Mol Endocrinol*. 5, 1203-1214.

[2] Kaminsky, L. S., Zhang, Q. Y., (2003). The small intestine as a xenobiotic-metabolizing organ. *Drug Metab Dispos*. 31, 1520-1525.

[3] Schrattenholz, A., Soskic, V., (2008). What does systems biology mean for drug development? *Curr Med Chem*. 15, 1520-1528.

[4] Paine, M. F., Oberlies, N. H., (2007). Clinical relevance of the small intestine as an organ of drug elimination: drug-fruit juice interactions. *Expert Opin Drug Metab Toxicol*. 3, 67-80.

[5] Oinonen, T., Lindros, K. O., (1998). Zonation of hepatic cytochrome P-450 expression and regulation. *Biochem J*. 329 (Pt 1), 17-35.

[6] Kwon, Y., Morris, M. E., (1997). Membrane transport in hepatic clearance of drugs. II: Zonal distribution patterns of concentration-dependent transport and elimination processes. *Pharm Res*. 14, 780-785.

[7] Soars, M. G., Burchell, B., Riley, R. J., (2002). In vitro analysis of human drug glucuronidation and prediction of in vivo metabolic clearance. *J Pharmacol Exp Ther*. 301, 382-390.

[8] Lohr, J. W., Willsky, G. R., Acara, M. A., (1998). Renal drug metabolism. *Pharmacol Rev*. 50, 107-141.

[9] Masereeuw, R., Russel, F. G., (2001). Mechanisms and clinical implications of renal drug excretion. *Drug Metab Rev*. 33, 299-351.

[10] Pacha, J., (2000). Development of intestinal transport function in mammals. *Physiol Rev*. 80, 1633-1667.

[11] van de Kerkhof, E. G., de Graaf, I. A., Groothuis, G.M., (2007). In vitro methods to study intestinal drug metabolism. *Curr Drug Metab*. 8, 658-675.

[12] Doherty, M. M., Charman, W. N., (2002). The mucosa of the small intestine: how clinically relevant as an organ of drug metabolism? *Clin Pharmacokinet*. 41, 235-253.

[13] Chan, L. M., Lowes, S., Hirst, B. H., (2004). The ABCs of drug transport in intestine and liver: efflux proteins limiting drug absorption and bioavailability. *Eur J Pharm Sci.* 21, 25-51.

[14] Mouly, S., Paine, M. F., (2003). P-glycoprotein increases from proximal to distal regions of human small intestine. *Pharm Res.* 20, 1595-1599.

[15] Sugano, K., Kansy, M., Artursson, P., Avdeef, A., Bendels, S., Di, L., Ecker, G. F., Faller, B., Fischer, H., Gerebtzoff, G., Lennernaes, H., Senner, F., (2010). Coexistence of passive and carrier-mediated processes in drug transport. *Nat Rev Drug Discov.* 9, 597-614.

[16] Ito, K., Suzuki, H., Horie, T., Sugiyama, Y., (2005). Apical/basolateral surface expression of drug transporters and its role in vectorial drug transport. *Pharm Res.* 22, 1559-1577.

[17] Benet, L. Z., Cummins, C. L., Wu, C. Y., (2004). Unmasking the dynamic interplay between efflux transporters and metabolic enzymes. *Int J Pharm.* 277, 3-9.

[18] Olinga, P., Elferink, M. G., Draaisma, A. L., Merema, M. T., Castell, J. V., Perez, G., Groothuis, G. M., (2008). Coordinated induction of drug transporters and phase I and II metabolism in human liver slices. *Eur J Pharm Sci.* 33, 380-389.

[19] Shen, G., Kong, A. N., (2009). Nrf2 plays an important role in coordinated regulation of Phase II drug metabolism enzymes and Phase III drug transporters. *Biopharm Drug Dispos.* 30, 345-355.

[20] Doring, B., Petzinger, E., (2014). Phase 0 and phase III transport in various organs: combined concept of phases in xenobiotic transport and metabolism. *Drug Metab Rev.* 46, 261-282.

[21] Williams, R. T. Detoxification Mechanisms: The Metabolism and Detoxification of Drugs, Toxic Substances and Other Organic Compounds. 2nd Edition ed. London: Chapman and Hall Ltd.; 1959.

[22] Dobson, P. D., Kell, D. B., (2008). Carrier-mediated cellular uptake of pharmaceutical drugs: an exception or the rule? *Nat Rev Drug Discov.* 7, 205-220.

[23] Oostendorp, R. L., Beijnen, J. H., Schellens, J. H., (2009). The biological and clinical role of drug transporters at the intestinal barrier. *Cancer Treat Rev.* 35, 137-147.

[24] Giacomini, K. M., Huang, S. M., Tweedie, D. J., Benet, L. Z., Brouwer, K. L., Chu, X., Dahlin, A., Evers, R., Fischer, V., Hillgren, K. M., Hoffmaster, K. A., Ishikawa, T., Keppler, D., Kim, R. B., Lee, C. A., Niemi, M., Polli, J. W., Sugiyama, Y., Swaan, P. W., Ware, J. A., Wright, S. H., Yee, S. W., Zamek-Gliszczynski, M. J., Zhang, L., (2010). Membrane transporters in drug development. *Nat Rev Drug Discov.* 9, 215-236.

[25] Klaassen, C. D., Aleksunes, L. M., (2010). Xenobiotic, bile acid, and cholesterol transporters: function and regulation. *Pharmacol Rev.* 62, 1-96.

[26] Shitara, Y., Maeda, K., Ikejiri, K., Yoshida, K., Horie, T., Sugiyama, Y., (2013). Clinical significance of organic anion transporting polypeptides (OATPs) in drug disposition: their roles in hepatic clearance and intestinal absorption. *Biopharm Drug Dispos.* 34, 45-78.

[27] Zolk, O., Fromm, M. F., (2011). Transporter-mediated drug uptake and efflux: important determinants of adverse drug reactions. *Clin Pharmacol Ther.* 89, 798-805.

[28] Benet, L. Z., (2009). The drug transporter-metabolism alliance: uncovering and defining the interplay. *Mol Pharm.* 6, 1631-1643.

[29] Pang, K. S., Maeng, H. J., Fan, J., (2009). Interplay of transporters and enzymes in drug and metabolite processing. *Mol Pharm*. 6, 1734-1755.

[30] Li, Y., Lu, J., Paxton, J. W., (2012). The role of ABC and SLC transporters in the pharmacokinetics of dietary and herbal phytochemicals and their interactions with xenobiotics. *Curr Drug Metab*. 13, 624-639.

[31] Shitara, Y., Horie, T., Sugiyama, Y., (2006). Transporters as a determinant of drug clearance and tissue distribution. *Eur J Pharm Sci*. 27, 425-446.

[32] Iyanagi, T., (2007). Molecular mechanism of phase I and phase II drug-metabolizing enzymes: implications for detoxification. *Int Rev Cytol*. 260, 35-112.

[33] Kruijtzer, C. M., Beijnen, J. H., Schellens, J. H., (2002). Improvement of oral drug treatment by temporary inhibition of drug transporters and/or cytochrome P450 in the gastrointestinal tract and liver: an overview. *Oncologist*. 7, 516-530.

[34] He, L., Vasiliou, K., Nebert, D. W., (2009). Analysis and update of the human solute carrier (SLC) gene superfamily. *Hum Genomics*. 3, 195-206.

[35] Hediger, M. A., Clemencon, B., Burrier, R. E., Bruford, E. A., (2013). The ABCs of membrane transporters in health and disease (SLC series): introduction. *Mol Aspects Med*. 34, 95-107.

[36] Vasiliou, V., Vasiliou, K., Nebert, D. W., (2009). Human ATP-binding cassette (ABC) transporter family. *Hum Genomics*. 3, 281-290.

[37] Guengerich, F. P., (2008). Cytochrome p450 and chemical toxicology. *Chem Res Toxicol*. 21, 70-83.

[38] Gamage, N., Barnett, A., Hempel, N., Duggleby, R. G., Windmill, K. F., Martin, J. L., McManus, M. E., (2006). Human sulfotransferases and their role in chemical metabolism. *Toxicol Sci*. 90, 5-22.

[39] Hayes, J. D., Flanagan, J. U., Jowsey, I. R., (2005). Glutathione transferases. *Annu Rev Pharmacol Toxicol*. 45, 51-88.

[40] Rowland, A., Miners, J. O., Mackenzie, P. I., (2013). The UDP-glucuronosyltransferases: their role in drug metabolism and detoxification. *Int J Biochem Cell Biol*. 45, 1121-1132.

[41] Sim, E., Westwood, I., Fullam, E., (2007). Arylamine N-acetyltransferases. *Expert Opin Drug Metab Toxicol*. 3, 169-184.

[42] Nies, A. T., Schwab, M., Keppler, D., (2008). Interplay of conjugating enzymes with OATP uptake transporters and ABCC/MRP efflux pumps in the elimination of drugs. *Expert Opin Drug Metab Toxicol*. 4, 545-568.

[43] Zamek-Gliszczynski, M. J., Hoffmaster, K. A., Nezasa, K., Tallman, M. N., Brouwer, K. L., (2006). Integration of hepatic drug transporters and phase II metabolizing enzymes: mechanisms of hepatic excretion of sulfate, glucuronide, and glutathione metabolites. *Eur J Pharm Sci*. 27, 447-486.

[44] Sallustio, B. C., Sabordo, L., Evans, A. M., Nation, R. L., (2000). Hepatic disposition of electrophilic acyl glucuronide conjugates. *Curr Drug Metab*. 1, 163-180.

[45] Hinson, J. A., Pumford, N. R., Nelson, S. D., (1994). The role of metabolic activation in drug toxicity. *Drug Metab Rev*. 26, 395-412.

[46] Aleksunes, L. M., Manautou, J. E., (2007). Emerging role of Nrf2 in protecting against hepatic and gastrointestinal disease. *Toxicol Pathol*. 35, 459-473.

[47] Zhou, S., Chan, E., Duan, W., Huang, M., Chen, Y. Z., (2005). Drug bioactivation, covalent binding to target proteins and toxicity relevance. *Drug Metab Rev*. 37, 41-213.

[48] Danielson, P. B., (2002). The cytochrome P450 superfamily: biochemistry, evolution and drug metabolism in humans. *Curr Drug Metab.* 3, 561-597.

[49] Rendic, S., (2002). Summary of information on human CYP enzymes: human P450 metabolism data. *Drug Metab Rev.* 34, 83-448.

[50] Zanger, U. M., Schwab, M., (2013). Cytochrome P450 enzymes in drug metabolism: regulation of gene expression, enzyme activities, and impact of genetic variation. *Pharmacol Ther.* 138, 103-141.

[51] Nelson, D. R., (2006). Cytochrome P450 nomenclature, 2004. *Methods Mol Biol.* 320, 1-10.

[52] Nelson, D. R., (2009). The cytochrome p450 homepage. *Hum Genomics.* 4, 59-65.

[53] Galetin, A., Houston, J. B., (2006). Intestinal and hepatic metabolic activity of five cytochrome P450 enzymes: impact on prediction of first-pass metabolism. *J Pharmacol Exp Ther.* 318, 1220-1229.

[54] Knights, K. M., Rowland, A., Miners, J.O., (2013). Renal drug metabolism in humans: the potential for drug-endobiotic interactions involving cytochrome P450 (CYP) and UDP-glucuronosyltransferase (UGT). *Br J Clin Pharmacol.* 76, 587-602.

[55] Urlacher, V. B., Girhard, M., (2012). Cytochrome P450 monooxygenases: an update on perspectives for synthetic application. *Trends Biotechnol.* 30, 26-36.

[56] Bast, A., Brenninkmeijer, J. W., Savenije-Chapel, E. M., Noordhoek, J., (1983). Cytochrome P450 oxidase activity and its role in NADPH dependent lipid peroxidation. *FEBS Lett.* 151, 185-188.

[57] Goeptar, A. R., Scheerens, H., Vermeulen, N. P., (1995). Oxygen and xenobiotic reductase activities of cytochrome P450. *Crit Rev Toxicol.* 25, 25-65.

[58] Kawakami, H., Ohtsuki, S., Kamiie, J., Suzuki, T., Abe, T., Terasaki, T., (2011). Simultaneous absolute quantification of 11 cytochrome P450 isoforms in human liver microsomes by liquid chromatography tandem mass spectrometry with in silico target peptide selection. *J Pharm Sci.* 100, 341-352.

[59] Ohtsuki, S., Schaefer, O., Kawakami, H., Inoue, T., Liehner, S., Saito, A., Ishiguro, N., Kishimoto, W., Ludwig-Schwellinger, E., Ebner, T., Terasaki, T., (2012). Simultaneous absolute protein quantification of transporters, cytochromes P450, and UDP-glucuronosyltransferases as a novel approach for the characterization of individual human liver: comparison with mRNA levels and activities. *Drug Metab Dispos.* 40, 83-92.

[60] Shimada, T., Yamazaki, H., Mimura, M., Inui, Y., Guengerich, F. P., (1994). Interindividual variations in human liver cytochrome P-450 enzymes involved in the oxidation of drugs, carcinogens and toxic chemicals: studies with liver microsomes of 30 Japanese and 30 Caucasians. *J Pharmacol Exp Ther.* 270, 414-423.

[61] Ding, X., Kaminsky, L. S., (2003). Human extrahepatic cytochromes P450: function in xenobiotic metabolism and tissue-selective chemical toxicity in the respiratory and gastrointestinal tracts. *Annu Rev Pharmacol Toxicol.* 43, 149-173.

[62] Paine, M. F., Hart, H. L., Ludington, S. S., Haining, R. L., Rettie, A. E., Zeldin, D. C., (2006). The human intestinal cytochrome P450 "pie." *Drug Metab Dispos.* 34, 880-886.

[63] Nebert, D. W., Dalton, T. P., Okey, A. B., Gonzalez, F. J., (2004). Role of aryl hydrocarbon receptor-mediated induction of the CYP1 enzymes in environmental toxicity and cancer. *J Biol Chem.* 279, 23847-23850.

[64] Honkakoski, P., Negishi, M., (1997). The structure, function, and regulation of cytochrome P450 2A enzymes. *Drug Metab Rev*. 29, 977-996.

[65] Rao, Y., Hoffmann, E., Zia, M., Bodin, L., Zeman, M., Sellers, E. M., Tyndale, R. F., (2000). Duplications and defects in the CYP2A6 gene: identification, genotyping, and in vivo effects on smoking. *Mol Pharmacol*. 58, 747-755.

[66] Wang, H., Tompkins, L. M., (2008). CYP2B6: new insights into a historically overlooked cytochrome P450 isozyme. *Curr Drug Metab*. 9, 598-610.

[67] Code, E. L., Crespi, C. L., Penman, B. W., Gonzalez, F. J., Chang, T. K., Waxman, D. J., (1997). Human cytochrome P4502B6: interindividual hepatic expression, substrate specificity, and role in procarcinogen activation. *Drug Metab Dispos*. 25, 985-993.

[68] Lamba, V., Lamba, J., Yasuda, K., Strom, S., Davila, J., Hancock, M. L., Fackenthal, J. D., Rogan, P. K., Ring, B., Wrighton, S. A., Schuetz, E. G., (2003). Hepatic CYP2B6 expression: gender and ethnic differences and relationship to CYP2B6 genotype and CAR (constitutive androstane receptor) expression. *J Pharmacol Exp Ther*. 307, 906-922.

[69] Lang, T., Klein, K., Fischer, J., Nussler, A. K., Neuhaus, P., Hofmann, U., Eichelbaum, M., Schwab, M., Zanger, U. M., (2001). Extensive genetic polymorphism in the human CYP2B6 gene with impact on expression and function in human liver. *Pharmacogenetics*. 11, 399-415.

[70] Thelen, K., Dressman, J. B., (2009). Cytochrome P450-mediated metabolism in the human gut wall. *J Pharm Pharmacol*. 61, 541-558.

[71] Wang, B., Yang, L. P., Zhang, X. Z., Huang, S. Q., Bartlam, M., Zhou, S. F., (2009). New insights into the structural characteristics and functional relevance of the human cytochrome P450 2D6 enzyme. *Drug Metab Rev*. 41, 573-643.

[72] Ingelman-Sundberg, M., (2005). Genetic polymorphisms of cytochrome P450 2D6 (CYP2D6): clinical consequences, evolutionary aspects and functional diversity. *Pharmacogenomics J*. 5, 6-13.

[73] Kessova, I., Cederbaum, A. I., (2003). CYP2E1: biochemistry, toxicology, regulation and function in ethanol-induced liver injury. *Curr Mol Med*. 3, 509-518.

[74] Caro, A. A., Cederbaum, A. I., (2004). Oxidative stress, toxicology, and pharmacology of CYP2E1. *Annu Rev Pharmacol Toxicol*. 44, 27-42.

[75] Hochstein, P., (1983). Futile redox cycling: implications for oxygen radical toxicity. *Fundam Appl Toxicol*. 3, 215-217.

[76] Daly, A. K., (2006). Significance of the minor cytochrome P450 3A isoforms. *Clin Pharmacokinet*. 45, 13-31.

[77] Scott, E. E., Halpert, J. R., (2005). Structures of cytochrome P450 3A4. *Trends Biochem Sci*. 30, 5-7.

[78] Leeder, J. S., Gaedigk, R., Marcucci, K. A., Gaedigk, A., Vyhlidal, C. A., Schindel, B. P., Pearce, R. E., (2005). Variability of CYP3A7 expression in human fetal liver. *J Pharmacol Exp Ther*. 314, 626-635.

[79] Alcorn, J., McNamara, P. J., (2002). Ontogeny of hepatic and renal systemic clearance pathways in infants: part I. *Clin Pharmacokinet*. 41, 959-998.

[80] Cashman, J. R., Zhang, J., (2006). Human flavin-containing monooxygenases. *Annu Rev Pharmacol Toxicol*. 46, 65-100.

[81] Shimada, T., (2006). Xenobiotic-metabolizing enzymes involved in activation and detoxification of carcinogenic polycyclic aromatic hydrocarbons. *Drug Metab Pharmacokinet.* 21, 257-276.

[82] Tripathi, S. P., Bhadauriya, A., Patil, A., Sangamwar, A. T., (2013). Substrate selectivity of human intestinal UDP-glucuronosyltransferases (UGTs): in silico and in vitro insights. *Drug Metab Rev.* 45, 231-252.

[83] Wells, P. G., Mackenzie, P. I., Chowdhury, J. R., Guillemette, C., Gregory, P. A., Ishii, Y., Hansen, A. J., Kessler, F. K., Kim, P. M., Chowdhury, N. R., Ritter, J. K., (2004). Glucuronidation and the UDP-glucuronosyltransferases in health and disease. *Drug Metab Dispos.* 32, 281-290.

[84] Mackenzie, P. I., Bock, K. W., Burchell, B., Guillemette, C., Ikushiro, S., Iyanagi, T., Miners, J. O., Owens, I. S., Nebert, D. W., (2005). Nomenclature update for the mammalian UDP glycosyltransferase (UGT) gene superfamily. *Pharmacogenet Genomics.* 15, 677-685.

[85] Tukey, R. H., Strassburg, C. P., (2000). Human UDP-glucuronosyltransferases: metabolism, expression, and disease. *Annu Rev Pharmacol Toxicol.* 40, 581-616.

[86] Coughtrie, M. W., (2002). Sulfation through the looking glass--recent advances in sulfotransferase research for the curious. *Pharmacogenomics J.* 2, 297-308.

[87] Kauffman, F. C., (2004). Sulfonation in pharmacology and toxicology. *Drug Metab Rev.* 36, 823-843.

[88] Negishi, M., Pedersen, L. G., Petrotchenko, E., Shevtsov, S., Gorokhov, A., Kakuta, Y., Pedersen, L. C., (2001). Structure and function of sulfotransferases. *Arch Biochem Biophys.* 390, 149-157.

[89] Riches, Z., Stanley, E. L., Bloomer, J. C., Coughtrie, M. W., (2009). Quantitative evaluation of the expression and activity of five major sulfotransferases (SULTs) in human tissues: the SULT "pie." *Drug Metab Dispos.* 37, 2255-2261.

[90] James, M. O., Ambadapadi, S., (2013). Interactions of cytosolic sulfotransferases with xenobiotics. *Drug Metab Rev.* 45, 401-414.

[91] Glatt, H., (2000). Sulfotransferases in the bioactivation of xenobiotics. *Chem Biol Interact.* 129, 141-170.

[92] Pang, K. S., Schwab, A. J., Goresky, C. A., Chiba, M., (1994). Transport, binding, and metabolism of sulfate conjugates in the liver. *Chem Biol Interact.* 92, 179-207.

[93] Roberts, M. S., Magnusson, B. M., Burczynski, F. J., Weiss, M., (2002). Enterohepatic circulation: physiological, pharmacokinetic and clinical implications. *Clin Pharmacokinet.* 41, 751-790.

[94] Bousova, I., Skalova, L., (2012). Inhibition and induction of glutathione S-transferases by flavonoids: possible pharmacological and toxicological consequences. *Drug Metab Rev.* 44, 267-286.

[95] van Bladeren, P. J., (2000). Glutathione conjugation as a bioactivation reaction. *Chem Biol Interact.* 129, 61-76.

[96] Coles, B. F., Chen, G., Kadlubar, F. F., Radominska-Pandya, A., (2002). Interindividual variation and organ-specific patterns of glutathione S-transferase alpha, mu, and pi expression in gastrointestinal tract mucosa of normal individuals. *Arch Biochem Biophys.* 403, 270-276.

[97] Hayes, J. D., Pulford, D. J., (1995). The glutathione S-transferase supergene family: regulation of GST and the contribution of the isoenzymes to cancer chemoprotection and drug resistance. *Crit Rev Biochem Mol Biol.* 30, 445-600.
[98] Oakley, A., (2011). Glutathione transferases: a structural perspective. *Drug Metab Rev.* 43, 138-151.
[99] Salinas, A. E., Wong, M. G., (1999). Glutathione S-transferases--a review. *Curr Med Chem.* 6, 279-309.
[100] Lan, J., Hua, S., He, X., Zhang, Y., (2010). DNA methyltransferases and methyl-binding proteins of mammals. *Acta Biochim Biophys Sin (Shanghai).* 42, 243-252.
[101] Cui, Y., Konig, J., Keppler, D., (2001). Vectorial transport by double-transfected cells expressing the human uptake transporter SLC21A8 and the apical export pump ABCC2. *Mol Pharmacol.* 60, 934-943.
[102] Nigam, S. K., (2015). What do drug transporters really do? *Nat Rev Drug Discov.* 14, 29-44.
[103] Oswald, S., Grube, M., Siegmund, W., Kroemer, H. K., (2007). Transporter-mediated uptake into cellular compartments. *Xenobiotica.* 37, 1171-1195.
[104] Schlessinger, A., Yee, S. W., Sali, A., Giacomini, K. M., (2013). SLC classification: an update. *Clin Pharmacol Ther.* 94, 19-23.
[105] Hagenbuch, B., Stieger, B., (2013). The SLCO (former SLC21) superfamily of transporters. *Mol Aspects Med.* 34, 396-412.
[106] Hagenbuch, B., Meier, P. J., (2004). Organic anion transporting polypeptides of the OATP/ SLC21 family: phylogenetic classification as OATP/ SLCO superfamily, new nomenclature and molecular/functional properties. *Pflugers Arch.* 447, 653-665.
[107] Konig, J., Muller, F., Fromm, M. F., (2013). Transporters and drug-drug interactions: important determinants of drug disposition and effects. *Pharmacol Rev.* 65, 944-966.
[108] Li, L., Meier, P. J., Ballatori, N., (2000). Oatp2 mediates bidirectional organic solute transport: a role for intracellular glutathione. *Mol Pharmacol.* 58, 335-340.
[109] Meyer zu Schwabedissen, H.E., Kroemer, H.K., (2011). In vitro and in vivo evidence for the importance of breast cancer resistance protein transporters (BCRP/MXR/ABCP/ABCG2). *Handb Exp Pharmacol.* 325-371.
[110] Roth, M., Obaidat, A., Hagenbuch, B., (2012). OATPs, OATs and OCTs: the organic anion and cation transporters of the SLCO and SLC22A gene superfamilies. *Br J Pharmacol.* 165, 1260-1287.
[111] Stieger, B., Hagenbuch, B., (2014). Organic anion-transporting polypeptides. *Curr Top Membr.* 73, 205-232.
[112] Bailey, D. G., Dresser, G. K., Leake, B. F., Kim, R. B., (2007). Naringin is a major and selective clinical inhibitor of organic anion-transporting polypeptide 1A2 (OATP1A2) in grapefruit juice. *Clin Pharmacol Ther.* 81, 495-502.
[113] Smith, D. E., Clemencon, B., Hediger, M. A., (2013). Proton-coupled oligopeptide transporter family SLC15: physiological, pharmacological and pathological implications. *Mol Aspects Med.* 34, 323-336.
[114] Rubio-Aliaga, I., Daniel, H., (2008). Peptide transporters and their roles in physiological processes and drug disposition. *Xenobiotica.* 38, 1022-1042.
[115] Halestrap, A. P., (2013). The SLC16 gene family - structure, role and regulation in health and disease. *Mol Aspects Med.* 34, 337-349.

[116] Philp, N. J., Ochrietor, J. D., Rudoy, C., Muramatsu, T., Linser, P. J., (2003). Loss of MCT1, MCT3, and MCT4 expression in the retinal pigment epithelium and neural retina of the 5A11/basigin-null mouse. *Invest Ophthalmol Vis Sci.* 44, 1305-1311.

[117] Burckhardt, G., (2012). Drug transport by Organic Anion Transporters (OATs). *Pharmacol Ther.* 136, 106-130.

[118] Nigam, S. K., Bush, K. T., Martovetsky, G., Ahn, S. Y., Liu, H. C., Richard, E., Bhatnagar, V., Wu, W., (2015). The organic anion transporter (OAT) family: a systems biology perspective. *Physiol Rev.* 95, 83-123.

[119] Pelis, R. M., Wright, S. H., (2014). SLC22, SLC44, and SLC47 transporters--organic anion and cation transporters: molecular and cellular properties. *Curr Top Membr.* 73, 233-261.

[120] Koepsell, H., (2013). The SLC22 family with transporters of organic cations, anions and zwitterions. *Mol Aspects Med.* 34, 413-435.

[121] Enomoto, A., Kimura, H., Chairoungdua, A., Shigeta, Y., Jutabha, P., Cha, S. H., Hosoyamada, M., Takeda, M., Sekine, T., Igarashi, T., Matsuo, H., Kikuchi, Y., Oda, T., Ichida, K., Hosoya, T., Shimokata, K., Niwa, T., Kanai, Y., Endou, H., (2002). Molecular identification of a renal urate anion exchanger that regulates blood urate levels. *Nature.* 417, 447-452.

[122] Ciarimboli, G., (2008). Organic cation transporters. *Xenobiotica.* 38, 936-971.

[123] Nies, A. T., Koepsell, H. K., Damme, K., Schwab, M. Organic cation transporters (OCTs, MATEs), in vitro and in vivo evidence for the importance in drug therapy. Fromm, M.F., Kim, R.B., editors. Berlin Heidelberg: Springer-Verlag; 2011.

[124] Tzvetkov, M. V., Vormfelde, S. V., Balen, D., Meineke, I., Schmidt, T., Sehrt, D., Sabolic, I., Koepsell, H., Brockmoller, J., (2009). The effects of genetic polymorphisms in the organic cation transporters OCT1, OCT2, and OCT3 on the renal clearance of metformin. *Clin Pharmacol Ther.* 86, 299-306.

[125] Meier-Abt, F., Faulstich, H., Hagenbuch, B., (2004). Identification of phalloidin uptake systems of rat and human liver. *Biochim Biophys Acta.* 1664, 64-69.

[126] Tamai, I., (2013). Pharmacological and pathophysiological roles of carnitine/organic cation transporters (OCTNs: SLC22A4, SLC22A5 and Slc22a21). *Biopharm Drug Dispos.* 34, 29-44.

[127] Grundemann, D., Harlfinger, S., Golz, S., Geerts, A., Lazar, A., Berkels, R., Jung, N., Rubbert, A., Schomig, E., (2005). Discovery of the ergothioneine transporter. *Proc Natl Acad Sci U S A.* 102, 5256-5261.

[128] Young, J. D., Yao, S. Y., Baldwin, J. M., Cass, C. E., Baldwin, S. A., (2013). The human concentrative and equilibrative nucleoside transporter families, SLC28 and SLC29. *Mol Aspects Med.* 34, 529-547.

[129] Govindarajan, R., Bakken, A. H., Hudkins, K. L., Lai, Y., Casado, F. J., Pastor-Anglada, M., Tse, C. M., Hayashi, J., Unadkat, J. D., (2007). In situ hybridization and immunolocalization of concentrative and equilibrative nucleoside transporters in the human intestine, liver, kidneys, and placenta. *Am J Physiol Regul Integr Comp Physiol.* 293, R1809-1822.

[130] Damme, K., Nies, A. T., Schaeffeler, E., Schwab, M., (2011). Mammalian MATE (SLC47A) transport proteins: impact on efflux of endogenous substrates and xenobiotics. *Drug Metab Rev.* 43, 499-523.

[131] Motohashi, H., Inui, K., (2013). Multidrug and toxin extrusion family SLC47: physiological, pharmacokinetic and toxicokinetic importance of MATE1 and MATE2-K. *Mol Aspects Med.* 34, 661-668.
[132] Tanihara, Y., Masuda, S., Sato, T., Katsura, T., Ogawa, O., Inui, K., (2007). Substrate specificity of MATE1 and MATE2-K, human multidrug and toxin extrusions/H(+)-organic cation antiporters. *Biochem Pharmacol.* 74, 359-371.
[133] Schinkel, A. H., Jonker, J. W., (2003). Mammalian drug efflux transporters of the ATP binding cassette (ABC) family: an overview. *Adv Drug Deliv Rev.* 55, 3-29.
[134] Borst, P., Elferink, R. O., (2002). Mammalian ABC transporters in health and disease. *Annu Rev Biochem.* 71, 537-592.
[135] Juliano, R. L., Ling, V., (1976). A surface glycoprotein modulating drug permeability in Chinese hamster ovary cell mutants. *Biochim Biophys Acta.* 455, 152-162.
[136] Martin, C., Berridge, G., Higgins, C. F., Mistry, P., Charlton, P., Callaghan, R., (2000). Communication between multiple drug binding sites on P-glycoprotein. *Mol Pharmacol.* 58, 624-632.
[137] Canaparo, R., Finnstrom, N., Serpe, L., Nordmark, A., Muntoni, E., Eandi, M., Rane, A., Zara, G. P., (2007). Expression of CYP3A isoforms and P-glycoprotein in human stomach, jejunum and ileum. *Clin Exp Pharmacol Physiol.* 34, 1138-1144.
[138] Thiebaut, F., Tsuruo, T., Hamada, H., Gottesman, M. M., Pastan, I., Willingham, M. C., (1987). Cellular localization of the multidrug-resistance gene product P-glycoprotein in normal human tissues. *Proc Natl Acad Sci U S A.* 84, 7735-7738.
[139] Noe, J., Kullak-Ublick, G. A., Jochum, W., Stieger, B., Kerb, R., Haberl, M., Mullhaupt, B., Meier, P. J., Pauli-Magnus, C., (2005). Impaired expression and function of the bile salt export pump due to three novel ABCB11 mutations in intrahepatic cholestasis. *J Hepatol.* 43, 536-543.
[140] Strautnieks, S. S., Bull, L. N., Knisely, A. S., Kocoshis, S. A., Dahl, N., Arnell, H., Sokal, E., Dahan, K., Childs, S., Ling, V., Tanner, M. S., Kagalwalla, A. F., Nemeth, A., Pawlowska, J., Baker, A., Mieli-Vergani, G., Freimer, N. B., Gardiner, R. M., Thompson, R. J., (1998). A gene encoding a liver-specific ABC transporter is mutated in progressive familial intrahepatic cholestasis. *Nat Genet.* 20, 233-238.
[141] Torok, M., Gutmann, H., Fricker, G., Drewe, J., (1999). Sister of P-glycoprotein expression in different tissues. *Biochem Pharmacol.* 57, 833-835.
[142] Hirano, M., Maeda, K., Hayashi, H., Kusuhara, H., Sugiyama, Y., (2005). Bile salt export pump (BSEP/ABCB11) can transport a nonbile acid substrate, pravastatin. *J Pharmacol Exp Ther.* 314, 876-882.
[143] Morgan, R. E., Trauner, M., van Staden, C. J., Lee, P. H., Ramachandran, B., Eschenberg, M., Afshari, C. A., Qualls, C. W., Jr., Lightfoot-Dunn, R., Hamadeh, H. K., (2010). Interference with bile salt export pump function is a susceptibility factor for human liver injury in drug development. *Toxicol Sci.* 118, 485-500.
[144] Pedersen, J. M., Matsson, P., Bergstrom, C. A., Hoogstraate, J., Noren, A., LeCluyse, E. L., Artursson, P., (2013). Early identification of clinically relevant drug interactions with the human bile salt export pump (BSEP/ABCB11). *Toxicol Sci.* 136, 328-343.
[145] Jonker, J. W., Smit, J. W., Brinkhuis, R. F., Maliepaard, M., Beijnen, J. H., Schellens, J. H., Schinkel, A. H., (2000). Role of breast cancer resistance protein in the bioavailability and fetal penetration of topotecan. *J Natl Cancer Inst.* 92, 1651-1656.

[146] Keppler, D., (2011). Multidrug resistance proteins (MRPs, ABCCs): importance for pathophysiology and drug therapy. *Handb Exp Pharmacol*. 299-323.

[147] Cole, S. P., (2014). Multidrug resistance protein 1 (MRP1, ABCC1), a "multitasking" ATP-binding cassette (ABC) transporter. *J Biol Chem*. 289, 30880-30888.

[148] Nies, A. T., Keppler, D., (2007). The apical conjugate efflux pump ABCC2 (MRP2). *Pflugers Arch*. 453, 643-659.

[149] Ortiz, D. F., Li, S., Iyer, R., Zhang, X., Novikoff, P., Arias, I. M., (1999). MRP3, a new ATP-binding cassette protein localized to the canalicular domain of the hepatocyte. *Am J Physiol*. 276, G1493-1500.

[150] Kullak-Ublick, G. A., Stieger, B., Meier, P. J., (2004). Enterohepatic bile salt transporters in normal physiology and liver disease. *Gastroenterology*. 126, 322-342.

[151] Mao, Q., Unadkat, J. D., (2005). Role of the breast cancer resistance protein (ABCG2) in drug transport. *AAPS J*. 7, E118-133.

[152] Suzuki, M., Suzuki, H., Sugimoto, Y., Sugiyama, Y., (2003). ABCG2 transports sulfated conjugates of steroids and xenobiotics. *J Biol Chem*. 278, 22644-22649.

[153] Graf, G. A., Yu, L., Li, W. P., Gerard, R., Tuma, P. L., Cohen, J. C., Hobbs, H. H., (2003). ABCG5 and ABCG8 are obligate heterodimers for protein trafficking and biliary cholesterol excretion. *J Biol Chem*. 278, 48275-48282.

[154] Anttila, S., Hakkola, J., Tuominen, P., Elovaara, E., Husgafvel-Pursiainen, K., Karjalainen, A., Hirvonen, A., Nurminen, T., (2003). Methylation of cytochrome P4501A1 promoter in the lung is associated with tobacco smoking. *Cancer Res*. 63, 8623-8628.

[155] Beedanagari, S. R., Taylor, R. T., Bui, P., Wang, F., Nickerson, D. W., Hankinson, O., (2010). Role of epigenetic mechanisms in differential regulation of the dioxin-inducible human CYP1A1 and CYP1B1 genes. *Mol Pharmacol*. 78, 608-616.

[156] Schaeffeler, E., Hellerbrand, C., Nies, A. T., Winter, S., Kruck, S., Hofmann, U., van der Kuip, H., Zanger, U. M., Koepsell, H., Schwab, M., (2011). DNA methylation is associated with downregulation of the organic cation transporter OCT1 (SLC22A1) in human hepatocellular carcinoma. *Genome Med*. 3, 82.

[157] Ichihara, S., Kikuchi, R., Kusuhara, H., Imai, S., Maeda, K., Sugiyama, Y., (2010). DNA methylation profiles of organic anion transporting polypeptide 1B3 in cancer cell lines. *Pharm Res*. 27, 510-516.

[158] Rodriguez-Antona, C., Gomez, A., Karlgren, M., Sim, S. C., Ingelman-Sundberg, M., (2010). Molecular genetics and epigenetics of the cytochrome P450 gene family and its relevance for cancer risk and treatment. *Hum Genet*. 127, 1-17.

[159] Pan, Y. Z., Gao, W., Yu, A. M., (2009). MicroRNAs regulate CYP3A4 expression via direct and indirect targeting. *Drug Metab Dispos*. 37, 2112-2117.

[160] Rieger, J. K., Reutter, S., Hofmann, U., Schwab, M., Zanger, U. M., (2015). Inflammation-Associated MicroRNA-130b Down-Regulates Cytochrome P450 Activities and Directly Targets CYP2C9. *Drug Metab Dispos*. 43, 884-888.

[161] Takagi, S., Nakajima, M., Kida, K., Yamaura, Y., Fukami, T., Yokoi, T., (2010). MicroRNAs regulate human hepatocyte nuclear factor 4alpha, modulating the expression of metabolic enzymes and cell cycle. *J Biol Chem*. 285, 4415-4422.

[162] Cotreau, M. M., von Moltke, L. L., Greenblatt, D. J., (2005). The influence of age and sex on the clearance of cytochrome P450 3A substrates. *Clin Pharmacokinet*. 44, 33-60.

[163] Zhang, Y., Klein, K., Sugathan, A., Nassery, N., Dombkowski, A., Zanger, U. M., Waxman, D. J., (2011). Transcriptional profiling of human liver identifies sex-biased genes associated with polygenic dyslipidemia and coronary artery disease. *PLoS One*. 6, e23506.

[164] Liu, W., Kulkarni, K., Hu, M., (2013). Gender-dependent differences in uridine 5'-diphospho-glucuronosyltransferase have implications in metabolism and clearance of xenobiotics. *Expert Opin Drug Metab Toxicol*. 9, 1555-1569.

[165] Gandhi, A., Moorthy, B., Ghose, R., (2012). Drug disposition in pathophysiological conditions. *Curr Drug Metab*. 13, 1327-1344.

[166] Aitken, A. E., Richardson, T. A., Morgan, E. T., (2006). Regulation of drug-metabolizing enzymes and transporters in inflammation. *Annu Rev Pharmacol Toxicol*. 46, 123-149.

[167] Murray, M., (2006). Altered CYP expression and function in response to dietary factors: potential roles in disease pathogenesis. *Curr Drug Metab*. 7, 67-81.

[168] Bailey, D. G., Malcolm, J., Arnold, O., Spence, J. D., (1998). Grapefruit juice-drug interactions. *Br J Clin Pharmacol*. 46, 101-110.

[169] Guengerich, F. P., Kim, D. H., (1990). In vitro inhibition of dihydropyridine oxidation and aflatoxin B1 activation in human liver microsomes by naringenin and other flavonoids. *Carcinogenesis*. 11, 2275-2279.

[170] Sadee, W., Wang, D., Papp, A. C., Pinsonneault, J. K., Smith, R. M., Moyer, R. A., Johnson, A. D., (2011). Pharmacogenomics of the RNA world: structural RNA polymorphisms in drug therapy. *Clin Pharmacol Ther*. 89, 355-365.

[171] Meyer, U. A., Zanger, U. M., Schwab, M., (2013). Omics and drug response. *Annu Rev Pharmacol Toxicol*. 53, 475-502.

[172] Bruhn, O., Cascorbi, I., (2014). Polymorphisms of the drug transporters ABCB1, ABCG2, ABCC2 and ABCC3 and their impact on drug bioavailability and clinical relevance. *Expert Opin Drug Metab Toxicol*. 10, 1337-1354.

[173] De Mattia, E., Dreussi, E., Cecchin, E., Toffoli, G., (2013). Pharmacogenetics of the nuclear hormone receptors: the missing link between environment and drug effects? *Pharmacogenomics* 14, 2035-2054.

[174] Helsby, N. A., Burns, K. E., (2012). Molecular mechanisms of genetic variation and transcriptional regulation of CYP2C19. *Front Genet*. 3, 206.

[175] Lai, Y., Varma, M., Feng, B., Stephens, J. C., Kimoto, E., El-Kattan, A., Ichikawa, K., Kikkawa, H., Ono, C., Suzuki, A., Suzuki, M., Yamamoto, Y., Tremaine, L., (2012). Impact of drug transporter pharmacogenomics on pharmacokinetic and pharmacodynamic variability - considerations for drug development. *Expert Opin Drug Metab Toxicol*. 8, 723-743.

[176] Handschin, C., Meyer, U. A., (2003). Induction of drug metabolism: the role of nuclear receptors. *Pharmacol Rev*. 55, 649-673.

[177] Mangelsdorf, D. J., Evans, R. M., (1995). The RXR heterodimers and orphan receptors. *Cell*. 83, 841-850.

[178] Xu, C., Li, C. Y., Kong, A. N., (2005). Induction of phase I, II and III drug metabolism/transport by xenobiotics. *Arch Pharm Res*. 28, 249-268.

[179] Denison, M. S., Nagy, S. R., (2003). Activation of the aryl hydrocarbon receptor by structurally diverse exogenous and endogenous chemicals. *Annu Rev Pharmacol Toxicol*. 43, 309-334.

[180] Urquhart, B. L., Tirona, R. G., Kim, R. B., (2007). Nuclear receptors and the regulation of drug-metabolizing enzymes and drug transporters: implications for interindividual variability in response to drugs. *J Clin Pharmacol*. 47, 566-578.

[181] Fuhr, U., (2000). Induction of drug metabolising enzymes: pharmacokinetic and toxicological consequences in humans. *Clin Pharmacokinet*. 38, 493-504.

[182] Timsit, Y. E., Negishi, M., (2007). CAR and PXR: the xenobiotic-sensing receptors. *Steroids*. 72, 231-246.

[183] Chang, T. K., Waxman, D. J., (2006). Synthetic drugs and natural products as modulators of constitutive androstane receptor (CAR) and pregnane X receptor (PXR). *Drug Metab Rev*. 38, 51-73.

[184] Forman, B. M., Tzameli, I., Choi, H. S., Chen, J., Simha, D., Seol, W., Evans, R. M., Moore, D. D., (1998). Androstane metabolites bind to and deactivate the nuclear receptor CAR-beta. *Nature*. 395, 612-615.

[185] Honkakoski, P., Sueyoshi, T., Negishi, M., (2003). Drug-activated nuclear receptors CAR and PXR. *Ann Med*. 35, 172-182.

[186] Barbier, O., Fontaine, C., Fruchart, J. C., Staels, B., (2004). Genomic and non-genomic interactions of PPARalpha with xenobiotic-metabolizing enzymes. *Trends Endocrinol Metab*. 15, 324-330.

[187] Desvergne, B., Wahli, W., (1999). Peroxisome proliferator-activated receptors: nuclear control of metabolism. *Endocr Rev*. 20, 649-688.

[188] Lu, T. T., Repa, J. J., Mangelsdorf, D. J., (2001). Orphan nuclear receptors as eLiXiRs and FiXeRs of sterol metabolism. *J Biol Chem*. 276, 37735-37738.

[189] Li, J., Ning, G., Duncan, S. A., (2000). Mammalian hepatocyte differentiation requires the transcription factor HNF-4alpha. *Genes Dev*. 14, 464-474.

[190] Kamiyama, Y., Matsubara, T., Yoshinari, K., Nagata, K., Kamimura, H., Yamazoe, Y., (2007). Role of human hepatocyte nuclear factor 4alpha in the expression of drug-metabolizing enzymes and transporters in human hepatocytes assessed by use of small interfering RNA. *Drug Metab Pharmacokinet*. 22, 287-298.

[191] Hahn, M. E., (2002). Aryl hydrocarbon receptors: diversity and evolution. *Chem Biol Interact*. 141, 131-160.

[192] Ramos-Gomez, M., Kwak, M. K., Dolan, P. M., Itoh, K., Yamamoto, M., Talalay, P., Kensler, T. W., (2001). Sensitivity to carcinogenesis is increased and chemoprotective efficacy of enzyme inducers is lost in nrf2 transcription factor-deficient mice. *Proc Natl Acad Sci U S A*. 98, 3410-3415.

[193] Kang, M. I., Kobayashi, A., Wakabayashi, N., Kim, S. G., Yamamoto, M., (2004). Scaffolding of Keap1 to the actin cytoskeleton controls the function of Nrf2 as key regulator of cytoprotective phase 2 genes. *Proc Natl Acad Sci U S A*. 101, 2046-2051.

[194] Nguyen, T., Sherratt, P. J., Pickett, C. B., (2003). Regulatory mechanisms controlling gene expression mediated by the antioxidant response element. *Annu Rev Pharmacol Toxicol*. 43, 233-260.

[195] Kohle, C., Bock, K. W., (2007). Coordinate regulation of Phase I and II xenobiotic metabolisms by the Ah receptor and Nrf2. *Biochem Pharmacol*. 73, 1853-1862.

[196] Kohle, C., Bock, K. W., (2009). Coordinate regulation of human drug-metabolizing enzymes, and conjugate transporters by the Ah receptor, pregnane X receptor and constitutive androstane receptor. *Biochem Pharmacol*. 77, 689-699.

In: Broccoli
Editor: Bernhard H. J. Juurlink

ISBN: 978-1-63484-313-3
© 2016 Nova Science Publishers, Inc.

Chapter 5

CELLULAR REDOX, AGING AND DIET

*Lida Sadeghinejad[1], Hossein Noyan[2]
and Bernhard H. J. Juurlink[3],**

[1]Department of Biomaterials, Faculty of Dentistry,
University of Toronto, Toronto, ON, Canada
[2]Keenan Research Centre, Li Ka Shing Knowledge Institute,
St Michael's Hospital, Toronto, ON, Canada
[3]Department of Anatomy & Cell Biology, College of Medicine,
University of Saskatchewan, Saskatoon, SK, Canada

ABSTRACT

A brief overview of cellular oxidant production and scavenging is presented along with the evidence for oxidative stress playing a role in aging. Oxidative stress is associated with dysregulated kinase signalling and increased generalized inflammation. The dysregulated kinase signalling that is also associated with increased NFkappaB activation is likely due to oxidation of cysteine residues in protein and lipid phosphatases. Although transient phosphatase inactivation is a normal part of many signal transduction pathways an increase in overall oxidative stress will result in inappropriate spatial and temporal activation of kinase signalling pathways, likely accounting for many of the problems associated with aging such as an increase in generalized inflammation. Dietary interventions that include increased cysteine intake and intake of Nrf2 activators that promote the expression of dozens of anti-oxidant genes will decrease oxidative stress resulting in more normalized cellular signalling.

Keywords: aging, cysteine, diet, glutathione, inflammation; oxidative stress, redox, kinases, Nrf2, phosphatases

---

* Corresponding author, Email: bernhard.juurlink@usask.ca.

INTRODUCTION

Oxidants and Aging

Historical perspective: In 1956 Denman Harman proposed that aging was due to free radical-mediated damage of cellular macromolecules [1]. This hypothesis has generated great debate with many taking the attitude that free radical and other oxidant-mediated damage is a by-product of aging rather than being a causal factor [2]. In support of this idea of free radicals being a consequence of aging is that there is little evidence that increasing intake of anti-oxidants (e.g., beta-carotene, ascorbic acid, alpha-tocopherol) [3] or increasing expression of oxidant scavenging enzymes (specifically Cu-Zn superoxide dismutase, Mn-superoxide dismutase or catalase) [4] influences aging. However, what the authors of these studies do not appreciate is the limited, albeit important, roles such anti-oxidants and anti-oxidant enzymes play in oxidant scavenging (see Juurlink [5]). Thus, for example, alpha-tocopheral plays an important role in inactivating lipid peroxyl radicals but it leaves behind lipid hydroperoxides that can be readily converted to strong oxidants - lipid hydroperoxides are converted to innocuous lipid alcohols and water by the actions of glutathione peroxidase using glutathione (GSH) as the electron donor. Ascorbic acid also has a limited role in oxidant scavenging - it reduces oxidized alpha-tocopherol allowing alpha-tocopherol to again be in a position to inactivate lipid peroxyl radicals. Both Cu-Zn- and Mn-superoxide dismutases convert superoxide free radicals to hydrogen peroxide. The hydrogen peroxide formed can be converted by transition metal ions to the very powerful oxidant, the hydroxyl radical. Unless the hydrogen peroxide is scavenged, the effect of the superoxide dismutases in free radical scavenging is to produce an oxidant with the potential to do far more damage than the parent superoxide radicals. Overexpression of catalase, an enzyme that converts hydrogen peroxide to water and molecular oxygen does not influence the aging of mice [4]; however, one should not make too much of this since catalase is mainly restricted to peroxisomes and, most importantly, catalase has a low affinity for hydrogen peroxide with a K_m of 80 mM [6], i.e., catalase efficiently scavenges hydrogen peroxide only at millimolar concentrations but not at submillimolar concentrations where the cell is reliant upon the selenoprotein family of glutathione peroxidases that uses GSH as an electron donor in peroxide reduction. Glutathione peroxidases have a much higher affinity (K_m of ~25 µM) for hydrogen peroxide [7] and, hence, can effectively reduce sub-millimolar concentrations of hydrogen peroxide whereas catalase cannot. Glutathione peroxidases will also reduce a wide variety of organic peroxides, including lipid hydroperoxides. There are a number of different isoforms of glutathione peroxidase [8] widely distributed throughout the cell, including a membrane-associated peroxidase, and in extracellular fluids. The V_{max} of the glutathione peroxidases, on the other hand, is much lower (more than 6 orders of magnitude) than that of catalase, i.e., the rate of reaction is very much slower. For the many roles of GSH (Figure 1) in scavenging oxidants please see Juurlink [5].

Oxidative Stress & Aging: Both in rodents and in humans oxidative stress increases in tissues with age [10]. Oxidative stress is defined as a deficiency in oxidant scavenging by tissues and/or an increase in oxidant production by tissues. The end result is an imbalance between production and scavenging of oxidants. In the rat there is an aging-associated decline in most of the anti-oxidant enzymes [11] and in tissue GSH [12, 13].

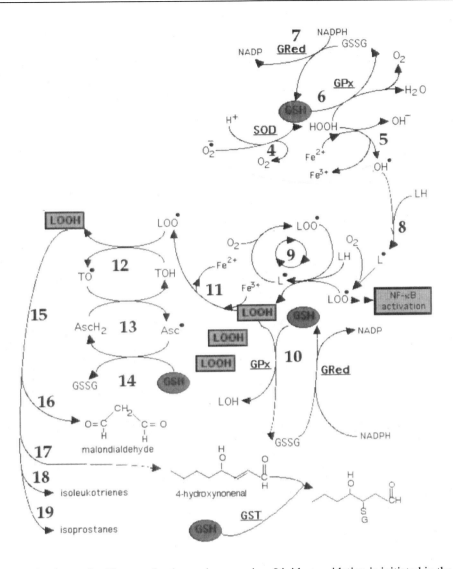

Figure 1. Mechanisms of oxidant production and scavenging. Lipid peroxidation is initiated in the presence of a strong oxidant like the hydroxyl radical (step 8) and once initiated continues as long is there is molecular oxygen and unsaturated fatty acids (LH) forming lipid hydroperoxides (LOOH). The lipid hydroperoxides formed can break down to other oxidants as well as pro-inflammatory lipid molecules. Vitamin E (TOH) plays an important role in inactivating the lipid peroxyl radicals (LOO·) formed (step 12) and ascorbic acid (AscH$_2$) reduces the oxidized vitamin E (step 13) while GSH reduces the oxidized ascorbate (step 14). It is clear from these sets of reactions that vitamins E and C play important but limited roles in inhibiting lipid peroxidation. As important is the scavenging of the lipid hydroperoxides by glutathione peroxidase and peroxiredoxins (step 10). Also included in this diagram are the roles of superoxide dismutases (step 4), glutathione reductase (steps 7 and 10) in these oxidant scavenging processes. Note the many roles of GSH in oxidant scavenging. Taken from Figure 18 in Juurlink [9].

As noted above, GSH plays a central role in the anti-oxidant defense system [5]. There is an increase in oxidant levels in brain tissue of a variety of mammalian and avian species with age and lifespan is inversely correlated with tissue oxidant levels [14]. Furthermore, aging in the aorta of Fisher 344-Brown Norway rat crosses is associated with increased superoxide anion production and decreased ability to synthesize GSH that appears to be related to suboptimal functioning of the nuclear factor (erythroid-derived 2) like-2 (Nrf2) signalling pathway [15]. The Nrf2 signalling system dominates many chapters in this book since one of the therapeutic compounds obtained from broccoli is sulforaphane, a potent activator of the Nrf2 signalling pathway. An overview of this pathway is given in Chapter 6. Impairment of the Nrf2 signalling pathway is seen not only in the aging rodent but also seen in the primate *Macaca mulatta* [15] and, thus, most likely in the aging human.

The decline in GSH seen with aging correlates well with a decline in the expression of the rate-limiting enzyme for GSH synthesis, γ-glutamyl-cysteine synthase [16, 17]: this enzyme, comprised of 2 subunits can be upregulated by activation of the Nrf2 signalling pathway (see Chapter 6). Of note is that here is an aging-associated decline in Nrf2 transcriptional activity with age [18, 19]. Furthermore, lifespan in 10 species of rodents examined is positively correlated with Nrf2 signalling levels [20].

One measure of oxidative stress is to examine the relationship between cysteine and its oxidized form, cystine (cysteine disulfide), as well as GSH and its oxidized disulfide form (GSSG) in extracellular fluids. There is a progressive increase in the ratio of cystine to cysteine in aging healthy humans with an increase of GSSG to GSH from the mid forties onwards [21]. An aging-associated increase in GSSG has also been reported by Samiec and colleagues [22] as well as an aging-associated increase in cystine by Droge and colleagues [23].

Furthermore, increased plasma malondialdehyde and protein carbonyls associated with decreased plasma redox capacity are seen in aged humans (61-85 years) compared to young (21-40 years) [24]. Similar findings in humans have been reported by other groups, e.g., [25, 26]. In line with changes in plasma oxidative stress measures during aging, GSH levels in human fibroblasts obtained from older individuals are lower than those obtained from younger individuals [27]. Thus, in humans as in rodents there is an increase in oxidative stress with age (Figure 2).

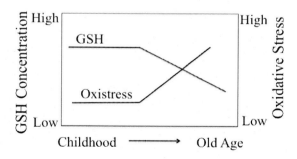

Figure 2. Graph representing schematically the typical decline in the average person of tissue GSH levels from the forties onwards and the associated increase in oxidative stress. Taken from Figure 18 in Juurlink [9].

Finally, not only is there a gradual increase in oxidative stress during aging but frail elderly are under greater oxidative stress than non-frail elderly [28, 29].

KINASE SIGNALLING PATHWAYS AND AGING-RELATED PROBLEMS

Kinases are a very large family of evolutionarily-related proteins [30] that add phosphate groups to substrates. These substrates may be quaternary ammonia salts such as choline, sugars such as inositol, nucleosides such as adenosine, amino acid residues such as serine, threonine or tyrosine. Kinase cascades dominate intracellular signalling pathways.

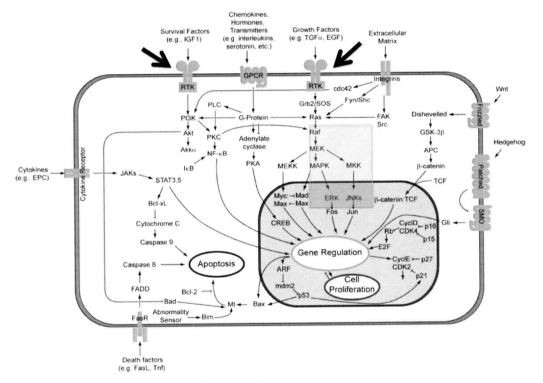

Figure 3. Diagram illustrating a number of signalling pathways. Many of the signalling pathways converge (indicated by light coloured rectangle) onto mitogen-activated protein (MAP) kinase pathways (represented in this diagram by ERK and JNKs). The MAP kinases ERK and Jun as well as p38 MAP kinase (not represented in this diagram) are regulated by upstream kinases. Image is in the public domain and taken from the Wikimedia Commons (http://en.wikipedia.org/wiki/ Cell_signalling). Author is Roadnottaken.

Many kinases involved in cellular signalling add a phosphate to either serine/threonine or to tyrosine residues in target proteins. A signalling group of kinases that dominate intracellular signalling is known as mitogen-activated protein (MAP) kinases [31].

There are three major families of MAP kinases: amino-terminal jun kinase (JNK, also known as stress-associated protein kinases [SAPK]); extracellular receptor kinase (ERK, also known as p42/p44 MAP kinases); and p38 MAP kinase (Figure 3). These MAP kinases are activated by specific upstream dual specificity kinases that phosphorylate on serine/threonine as well as tyrosine residues known as MAP/ERK kinases (MEK or MKK). These MEK/MKK kinases in turn are activated by a set of very diverse kinases known as MEK kinases (MEKK). These MAP kinase cascades allow for amplification as well as integration of a large number of signalling pathways. Major downstream targets of MAP kinases are transcription factors, e.g., Waas et al. [32], thus allowing MAP kinase cascades to influence gene expression.

Phosphorylation of proteins on tyrosine and/or serine/threonine residues alters protein charge and therefore conformation and function. Phosphorylation generally activates, but sometimes inactivates kinase activities. Protein kinase actions are counteracted by phosphatase activities. Phosphatase activities influence the amplitude and duration of kinase activities. Many problems of aging are associated with increased activation states of kinases, likely due, at least in part, to decreased phosphatase activities. A few examples of such dysregulated kinase activities are outlined below.

Nuclear Factor Kappa B

Overactivation of the transcription factor complex nuclear factor kappa B (NFκB) is associated with aging-related problems. NFκB is normally sequestered in the cytoplasm as a heterotrimer generally comprised of p65, p50 and inhibitory protein Bα (IκBα) [33]. Activation of an upstream kinase, IκB kinase (IKK) causes phosphorylation of IκBα that leads to ubiquitination and subsequent proteasomal degradation of IκBα. Loss of IκBα leads to the exposure of the nuclear localization signal on p65 resulting in the translocation of the p65/p50 heterodimer to the nucleus where it can bind to κB elements in the promoter region of a number of genes (Figure 4).

Genes with κB elements in their promoter region tend to be pro-inflammatory genes [33-35]. Activation of NFκB is redox sensitive with an oxidizing environment tending to promote activation [33, 36]. This redox sensitivity likely is related to activation of IKK as will be discussed below.

Increased activation of NFκB is seen in a number of animal models of aging [37, 38], as well there is age-related increased activation of NFκB in human tissues including human vascular endothelium [38-40] and muscle [41]. This fits in well with a general increase in the expression of pro-inflammatory genes in tissues examined, including human kidney [42-45] and aging-related inflammatory problems such as atherosclerosis [46]. Over-activation of IKK has been shown to lead to over-activation of NFκB that results in muscle wasting in a mouse model [47].

Both generalized inflammation [48] and muscle wasting [49] are problems seen in many aging humans. This association of generalized inflammation with aging is often referred to as inflamm-aging [50].

NFkB Is Central In Inflammation

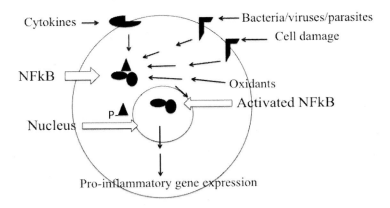

Figure 4. The heterotrimeric nuclear factor kappa B (NFκB) plays a central role in inflammation. Activation of NFκB is initiated by phosphorylation of the I kappa B (IκB) member (solid triangle) of the heterotrimer resulting in polyubiquitination and degradation of IκB allowing the p50/p65 heterodimer to translocate to the nucleus promoting the expression of genes with kappa B elements in their promoter regions - these are mostly pro-inflammatory genes. Normally, NFκB is activated in response to Toll-like receptor activation by microorganism macromolecules and/or cell damage products or by cytokine receptor activation. However, oxidative stress, likely by inactivating protein phosphatases, can also activate NFκB. Figure taken from Figure 14 in Juurlink [9].

Other Kinases and Aging-Related Disorders

Hypertension in spontaneously hypertensive stroke-prone rat (SHRsp) is associated with over-activation of endothelial p38 MAP kinase while p38 MAP kinase inhibitors prevent the development of hypertension in SHRsp [51]. Over-activation of ERK1,2 and JNK has been demonstrated in aorta in the Dahl salt-sensitive hypertensive rats with JNK increasing before ERK [52]. Increased activation of Rho kinase plays a causal role in pulmonary hypertension and insulin resistance [53, 54]; furthermore, inhibition of Rho kinase ameliorates pulmonary hypertension [55].

Adipocytes from Type 2 diabetic patients have high basal levels of activated ERK1,2, JNK and p38 MAP kinase [56]; furthermore, there is little further activation of these kinases upon exposure to insulin. This may be due to decreased protein phosphatase activities (see below) since knock-down of Leukocyte Antigen-Related (LAR) tyrosine phosphatase induces post-receptor insulin resistance while insulin induced activation of PKB/AKT and MAP kinases is markedly inhibited [57]. Inhibitors of Rho kinase allow regain of insulin sensitivity in Zucker obese rats [53].

In the brain increased JNK and ERK activity has been associated with increased phosphorylation of tau protein and increased amyloid deposition [58, 59]. This increased kinase activity may be due to impairment of protein phosphatase 2A [60, 61]. Increased activities of protein kinase B (AKT) [62] and cyclin-dependent kinase 5 [63] are also seen in brain tissue from Alzheimer's patients.

It is likely that dysregulation of protein kinases plays a causal role in many aging-related diseases processes. Although non-steroidal anti-inflammatory drugs (NSAIDs) have been shown to decrease the probability of having Alzheimer's disease, treatment of patients with Alzheimer's disease with NSAIDs have shown no therapeutic effect [64], suggesting possibly that inflammation plays a role in the onset, but not in the progression, of Alzheimer's disease. On the other hand, it has been shown that those NSAIDs as well as the statins are associated with decreased probability of developing Alzheimer's disease by inhibiting Rho kinase activity [65, 66] and there is interest in how statin-associated inhibition of Rho kinase may prevent complications of diabetes [67].

What may cause such dysregulation of protein kinase activity?

REDOX-SENSITIVE SIGNALLING PATHWAYS

The dysregulation of protein kinase activity outlined above is likely due to increased tissue oxidative stress. Oxidative stress is known to upregulate kinase activity in a number of contexts [68-70].

What is the relationship between oxidative stress and dysregulation of kinase activity? Major targets of redox regulation are cysteine residues.

Protein Cysteine Residues Are Readily Oxidized

Cysteine residues, particularly when ionized (thiolates), in proteins are readily oxidized and, thereby, act as redox sensors [71-73]. Chapter 6 describes how the thiols of the protein Keap1 act as a generalized cellular redox sensor and how this protein is involved in the cellular anti-oxidant response.

Proteins that have cysteine residues in sites critical for function include such diverse proteins as the calcium-binding protein calbindin D28k [74], cysteine-dependent protein phosphatases [75-77], ubiquitin-conjugating enzymes [65], various proteases [78], the oxidized protein repair system methionine sulfoxide reductase A [79]. Not surprisingly, because of the ease with which thiols are oxidized and reduced, a number of proteins important in oxidant scavenging also have cysteines in their catalytic site: these include the thioredoxin family [80] and glutathione reductase [81]. Also important in oxidant scavenging are proteins with the easily oxidized selenocysteines in their catalytic sites: these include the glutathione peroxidase family [81, 82] and the thioredoxin reductase family [83]. Because of the susceptibility of these anti-oxidant enzymes to oxidative inactivation if oxidant scavenging does not match oxidant production the cell can rapidly enter an oxidative stress spiral from which it is difficult to exit (Figure 5).

Cellular redox states can both directly and indirectly influence gene expression. Many transcription factors contain cysteine residues and binding to DNA is redox-dependent, for example NFκB and the AP1 complex [84]. Furthermore, many transcription factors contain zinc finger motifs [85] and the cysteine residues in such zinc fingers are susceptible to oxidation [86]. In addition, epigenetic control of gene expression is redox susceptible. Both class I histone deacetylases [87] and DNA methylases [88, 89] can be oxidatively inactivated thus increasing transcription of genes that normally would not be expressed or expressed at lower rates. Oxidative stress is associated with hypomethylation and normalizing redox states can normalize DNA methylation states [90].

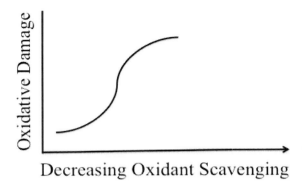

Figure 5. Graph illustrating that oxidative damage can quickly spiral out of control when there is decreased oxidant scavenging abilities.

The functions of many transcription factors are modulated by reversible phosphorylation and a major means whereby oxidative stress influences gene expression is by altering normal kinase cascades. Many protein phosphatases that play an important role in shaping kinase cascades are susceptible to oxidative inactivation.

Protein Phosphatases

Most protein phosphatases can be divided into two broad groupings: i) Fe^{2+}-based phosphatases and ii) Cysteine-based phosphatases. The former is represented by the serine/threonine phosphatases that have a dimetal ion cluster with one of the metal ions being Fe^{2+} and the other metal often being Zn^{2+} or Mn^{2+} [91, 92]. Fe^{2+} is readily oxidized [93] and oxidation of Fe^{2+} to Fe^{3+} would obviate the catalytic function of this family of enzymes. Fe^{2+}-based phosphatases can be inactivated by increased cellular oxidant production [94] and in the case of calcineurin it appears to be due to oxidation of Fe^{2+} to Fe^{3+} [95] although with other enzymes, such as protein phosphatase 1, 2A or 2B, it may also involve oxidation of cysteine residues outside of catalytic sites [94].

The cysteine-based phosphatases can be divided into the following families [96, 97]: i) the conventional (high molecular weight) protein tyrosine phosphatases comprised of the tyrosine-specific phosphatases, the dual specificity phosphatases that dephosphorylate at both tyrosine and serine/threonine residues, and the lipid phosphatases such as the phosphatase and tensin homologue (PTEN), ii) the cdc25 phosphatases that are dual specificity phosphatase in activity, and iii) the low molecular weight protein tyrosine phosphatases. These three cysteine-based phosphatases have little in common other than the CysXXXXXArg protein phosphatase motif in their catalytic region. This cysteine residue is deprotonated to form a thiolate ion that is very susceptible to being oxidized [98, 99]. Reversible oxidation of such thiolate ions is part of normal intracellular signalling [98-101]. Such thiolates are generally irreversibly oxidized by strong oxidants such as peroxynitrate [102].

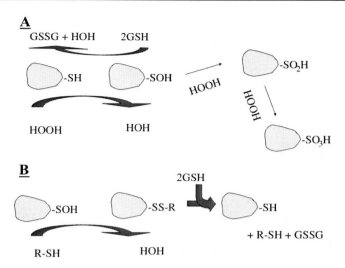

Figure 6. A: Diagram illustrating the oxidation of thiol groups by hydrogen peroxide giving rise to sulfenic (-SOH) that in turn can be oxidized to sulfinic acid (-SO$_2$H) that in turn can be oxidized to sulfonic acid (-SO$_3$H). Sulfenic acid can be reduced directly (A) or indirectly (B) by GSH. Figure taken from Figure 9 in Juurlink [9].

Oxidation of a cysteine residue results in a sulfenic acid residue (Figure 6A) inactivating the catalytic function of the protein. This reaction can be reversed using GSH as the electron donor (Figure 6A); hence, the higher the GSH concentration, the more rapidly is the sulfenic acid residue reduced back to the thiol. Selenic acid residues can also interact with other thiols giving rise to mixed disulfides that in turn can be reduced by GSH (Figure 6B). The mixed disulfide may involve another protein thiol or may involve GSH itself. Parenthetically, glutathiolation of the cysteine residue in the ATP-binding domain appears to be a mechanism used to transiently inactivate certain MAP kinases (e.g., MEKK1) [103].

If oxidative stress is severe, the selenic acid residues can be further oxidized to sulfinic and then to sulfonic acid residues. With most proteins, oxidation to sulfinic acid is irreversible; however, with certain peroxiredoxins (PrxI, II, III and IV), sulfinic acid residues can be reduced to thiols by sulfiredoxin [104, 105].

Protein Phosphatases and Kinase Signalling

Phosphorylation of protein kinases modulate their activity, generally activating but sometimes inactivating. Phosphatases limit the duration and amplitude of altered kinase activity [106]. One can promote kinase signalling either by increasing the phosphorylation state of the kinases or decreasing the activity of protein phosphatases. As noted above, protein phosphatases are readily inactivated by oxidants. Indeed, the transient inactivation of protein phosphatases through generation of reactive oxygen species by NAD(P)H oxidase are components of many signalling pathways [96]. The superoxide anion generated by NAD(P)H oxidase may oxidize cysteine residues or the superoxide generated may be dismutated to hydrogen peroxide that in turn oxidizes critical cysteine residues. Three examples will be given.

One example is signalling via platelet-derived growth factor (PDGF) signalling where one of the results of PDGF receptor activation is activation of NAD(P)H oxidase that transiently inactivates the protein tyrosine phosphatase SHP-2 thereby allowing the phosphorylation state (active state) of PDGF receptor to be maintained [98]. Activated PDGF receptor activates phosphatidylinosital-3 kinase (PI3K). PI3K then phosphorylates phosphatidylinositol-4,5-phosphate on the 3 position forming PtdIns3,4,5(P3). This allows components of the NAD(P)H complex to dock to PtdIns3,4,5(P3) allowing activation and production of superoxide anions [107].

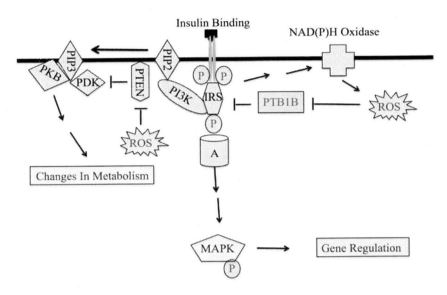

Figure 7. Schematic diagram outlining several aspects of insulin signalling. In the middle are some of the molecular players that include the dimeric insulin receptor, insulin, phosphatidylinositol-4,5-phosphate (PIP2), insulin receptor substrate protein (IRS), phosphoinositide-3-phosphate kinase (PI3K), phosphoinositide-dependent protein kinase (PDK), protein kinase B (PKB), any of a number of adapter proteins (A) and mitogen-activated protein kinase (MAPK). When insulin binds to its receptor it results in receptor autophosphorylation and subsequent phosphorylation and binding of IRS. The phosphorylated IRS binds and activates PI3K resulting in formation of PIP3 that leads to activation of PDK and PKB. Activation of PKB results in signalling cascades that results in changes in metabolism. Phosphorylated IRS also interacts with a variety of adaptor proteins (A) some of which will initiate a signalling cascade that activates MAP kinases that in turn alters the phosphorylation of transcription factors that will influence gene expression. Protein phosphatases involved in the insulin signalling pathways include the lipid phosphatase PTEN that converts PIP3 back to PIP2, PTP1B that dephosphorylates the insulin receptor and IRS proteins as well as phosphatases that act downstream of PKB and the MAP kinase cascades (not shown). PTB1B dephosphorylates the phosphorylated IRS. These phosphatases can be inactivated by oxidants. Also shown in this diagram is NAD(P)H oxidase that is activated in some yet unknown manner by insulin signalling. Activation of NAD(P)H oxidase results in oxidant production that prolongs the insulin signalling. Taken from Figure 12 in Juurlink [9].

A second example is transient inactivation of the lipid phosphatase PTEN by oxidants produced during insulin signalling [108] allowing a longer period of signalling. Here insulin binding to the insulin receptor (a receptor tyrosine kinase) causes receptor autophosphorylation allowing the binding of the insulin receptor substrate that in turn binds and activates PI3K. PI3K then phosphorylates PtdIns4,5(P2) forming PtdIns3,4,5(P3). This allows protein kinase B (or AKT) to bind to PtdIns3,4,5(P3) and become activated. Oxidants inhibiting PTEN allows a longer period of activation of downstream signalling (Figure 7). Oxidants also inhibit the action of PTB1B that normally dephosphorylates insulin substrate protein.

The third example is signalling by transforming growth factor-β (TGFβ) promoting plasminogen activator-1 protein expression. TGFβ signalling promotes nuclearly-localized NAD(P)H oxidase activity resulting in the inhibition of MAP kinase phosphatase-1 (MPK1) [109]. Inhibition of MPK1 results in more prolonged activation of JNK and p38 MAP kinase thereby promoting expression of plasminogen activator-1 protein.

Such physiological examples of transient oxidant-mediated inactivation of phosphatases is dependent upon precise spatial localization of the phosphatase to the receptor and the localization of the NAD(P)H oxidase in the membrane adjacent to the receptor. Only with such close neighbouring localizations can sufficiently high but transient levels of oxidants be present to oxidize thiols.

Oxidative Stress and Kinase Signalling

Normally cellular signalling is present in only localized regions of the cell governed by location of the specific receptor and the presence of specific scaffolding proteins allowing docking of components of the signalling pathway [110]. Oxidants temporarily inactivating phosphatase activity would govern the shape and duration of the activated state of the signalling pathway. Under conditions of oxidative stress this is no longer the case. Here, there is an increase in oxidant concentration over much of the cell where oxidants can inactivate phosphatases involved in many different signalling pathways over long periods of time. Now one would expect that that inhibition of MAP kinase phosphatases would result in the conversion of acute MAP kinase signals to a prolonged signal (Figure 8).

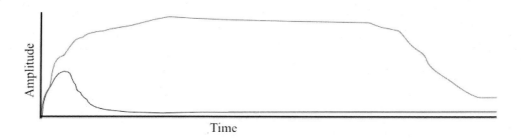

Figure 8. Influence of oxidative stress on kinase-dependent signalling. Increased oxidative stress converts normal signalling (bottom line) into an abnormal prolonged signalling with increased amplitude and with increased basal signalling activity (upper line). Taken from Figure 13 in Juurlink [9].

This certainly is the case in experimental systems where oxidative stress is increased. For example, tumour necrosis factor-α (TNFα) signalling can cause apoptotic cell death. Kamata and colleagues have shown that TNFα receptor activation in NFκB deficient fibroblasts causes a large increase in oxidant production that results in oxidation of the JNK phosphatases MKP1, MKP3 and MKP7 to sulfenic, sulfinic and even sulfonic residues [111]. The consequence of this is that JNK signalling in response to TNFα receptor activation was changed from the normal peaking at 15 minutes and terminating completely by one hour to a sustained signalling for more than 8 hours.

DIET AND OXIDATIVE STRESS

Historical Perspective of B. H. J. Juurlink

In the early 1990s, unbeknownst to me, Facilities management at the University of Saskatchewan decided not to air condition research laboratories on weekends during the summer. One of the consequences to me was that the oligodendrocyte precursor cells in culture died during that first weekend as incubator temperatures went into the low forty degrees Celsius. Curiosity as to why these cells were susceptible to elevated temperature and not the astrocytes that were in the same incubator led to a very fruitful area of research where members of the Juurlink lab dissected the differences in oxidant production and scavenging between these two lineages of cells [112-118].

By the latter part of the 1990s we noticed that GSH synthesis in astrocytes increased following exposure to the redox cycler menadione, whereas, this did not occur with the oligodendrocyte lineage of cells. These findings suggested that GSH synthesis was somehow under the control of an anti-oxidant response element, at least in astrocytes. A quick perusal of the literature showed that the two subunits of the rate-limiting enzyme in GSH synthesis, γ-glutamylcysteine ligase, did indeed contain anti-oxidant response elements (electrophile responsive element) as demonstrated by Mulcahy and colleagues (see Chapter 6). This literature search also resulted in our coming across the work of Dr Paul Talalay and colleagues on dietary phase 2 protein inducers, now commonly referred to as Nrf2 activators (see Chapter 1). At the time Dr Talalay and colleagues had a major interest in phase 2 enzyme inducers as a means to protect against carcinogenic agents, whereas the Juurlink lab was becoming very interested in the role of oxidative stress in promoting generalized inflammation [116, 119, 120]. This literature search led to the publication of an article on potential health benefits of phase 2 protein inducers [121]. Subsequent to this, together with colleagues, we have published a series of papers demonstrating that dietary intake of phase 2 protein inducers can ameliorate a variety of problems that have an underlying oxidative stress and inflammation to them both in *in vitro* systems and in animal systems [90, 122-127].

Nrf2 Activators and Health

Many laboratories have now examined the ability of sulforaphane to ameliorate oxidative stress and associated inflammation in a number of cell culture and animal models of disease. For example, Dr Talalay and colleagues have demonstrated the ability of sulforaphane to protect against spinal cord injury in a rat model [128]. Other laboratories have demonstrated the ability of sulforaphane to protect against: ischemia-reperfusion injury of the retina [129], systemic inflammation and renal injury following cardiovascular bypass surgery [130] and the development of experimental autoimmune encephalomyelitis [131]. There are many other studies in the literature and it would be too exhaustive to mention them all. There are also a number of human studies examining the effects of broccoli sprouts high in sulforaphane glucosinolate: see Chapters 12 and 13.

Does dietary upregulation of the Nrf2 signalling pathway lead to healthier aging? One approach that leads to healthier aging is caloric restriction [132]. It is known that the Nrf2-dependent protection against oxidative stress declines with age and that this can be corrected by caloric restriction [133]. The decreased oxidative stress associated with caloric restriction is associated with decreased NFκB activation and associated decreased generalized inflammation [133]. Our laboratory has shown that mice consuming tertiary-butylated hydroxyanisole (tBHA), whose metabolites are Nrf2 activators, had both increased Nrf2 protein as well as activated Nrf2 (i.e., nuclearly-localized Nrf2) in the liver and spinal cords of aged mice compared to mice on control diet [127]. This was associated with less oxidative stress and less generalized inflammation in the organs tested as well as greater physical agility at 18 months of age and much less weight gain despite the fact that mouse chow consumption was identical in the two groups. A small group of mice on control and experimental diet were allowed to live out their natural lifespan: the mice on the tBHA-containing diet lived 30% longer than the mice on control diet (Figure 9), this is similar to the effect seen with caloric restriction.

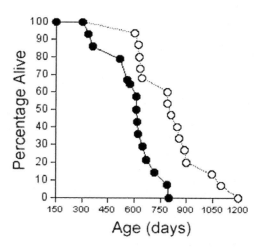

Figure 9. C57BL/6Ncri which, from weaning, were either on a control mouse chow (solid circles, n = 16) or rat chow containing tertiary butylated hydroxyanisole (open circles, n = 15) and allowed to live out their natural lifespan. These are previously unpublished data from the experiments described in [127].

The above findings suggest that increased intake of dietary Nrf2 activators may well positively influence aging. It may also be that basal levels of Nrf2 expression varies amongst human populations with populations that have a long agricultural history consuming few fruits and vegetables being selected for higher basal Nrf2 expression. It has been speculated that the reason for Type 2 diabetes and other chronic diseases becoming very common amongst indigenous populations when they consume a Western-style diet is that these populations are very dependent upon dietary Nrf2 activators for adequate Nrf2 signalling

[134]. Indeed, a recent study has shown correlations between Nrf2 polymorphisms and blood pressure in a Japanese population [135], suggesting that basal levels of Nrf2 expression may vary amongst individuals, and possibly populations.

Other Dietary Factors That Influence Oxidative Stress and Inflammation

Broccoli also contains a number of flavonoids, in particular quercetin and kaempferol. These flavonoids also influence kinase signalling pathways as well as the Nrf2 signalling pathway as outlined in Chapters 6 and 7. The promotion of the synthesis of GSH is a major means of decreasing oxidative stress. As noted above the rate-limiting enzyme for GSH synthesis, γ-glutamylcysteine ligase, is Nrf2-inducible. Furthermore, glutathione reductase that reduces GSSG using NADPH as the electron donor and glucose-6-phosphate dehydrogenase that generates much of the cellular NADPH are induced by Nrf2 activators [136, 137]. Thus, as noted above, one means of increasing cellular GSH content is to consume dietary Nrf2 activators such as sulforaphane and we have demonstrated this in both mouse [127] and rat [90, 124-126] models of disease and aging.

Dietary protein is the major source of cysteine. Cysteine is the rate-limiting amino acid for GSH synthesis [138]. The majority of 'cysteine' in the plasma and other extracellular fluids is present in the oxidized form of cystine. Cystine is taken up by the glutamate-cystine antiporter: the glutamate-cystine antiporter is also inducible by Nrf2 activators [139]. Unfortunately, one of the undesired consequences of cooking is a reduction in cysteine content of the proteins due to oxidation of cysteine residues as well as reactions of cysteine residues with reducing sugars [140]. One way to overcome this is to consume cysteine-rich proteins exposed to minimal temperature increases. A particularly rich source of cysteine is whey protein. Clinical studies have shown that undenatured whey proteins, that are rich in cysteine residues, can markedly increase GSH in lymphocytes [141], and presumably other cells.

Glutathione peroxidases and the thioredoxin reductases are critical in maintaining normal redox states in the cell. These enzymes use a selenocysteine residue in their catalytic sites [142]; hence, it is important to have adequate selenium in one's diet. Finally, as noted in Figure 1, ascorbic acid and tocopherols play important roles in the oxidant scavenging processes; hence, it is important to have adequate levels of these vitamins in one's diet.

CONCLUSION

There is much interest in how diet can positively affect chronic diseases associated with aging. In 1990, Dr Dale Ornish and colleagues described a very rigorous dietary and exercise regime that reversed coronary artery lesions [143]. Very few people are able to carry out the Ornish lifestyle regime year after year. Coronary artery disease is simply an example of one of the chronic diseases associated with aging that is driven by oxidative stress and inflammation. Our laboratory has demonstrated that effects similar to caloric restriction or the Ornish diet can be obtained by incorporating Nrf2 activators in the diet. Many other laboratories have shown that Nrf2 activators improve outcomes in animal models of disease and, as well, there are several clinical trials published showing Nrf2 activators such as sulforaphane have shown promise in ameliorating a number of human conditions where homeostasis is disrupted (see Chapters 12 and 13).

We trust that this review has better enabled the reader to understand some of the mechanisms of oxidative stress and inflammation associated with chronic disease and how a dietary intervention can ameliorate the conditions that lead to chronic disease.

REFERENCES

[1] Harman D. Aging: a theory based on free radical and radiation chemistry. *J. Gerontol.* 1956; 11: 298-300.

[2] Hekimi S, Lapointe J, Wen Y. Taking a "good" look at free radicals in the aging process. *Trends Cell Biol.* 2011; 21: 569-76.

[3] Howes RM. The free radical fantasy: a panoply of paradoxes. *Ann. N. Y. Acad. Sci.* 2006; 1067: 22-6.

[4] Perez VI, Van Remmen H, Bokov A, Epstein CJ, Vijg J, Richardson A. The overexpression of major antioxidant enzymes does not extend the lifespan of mice. *Aging Cell* 2009; 8: 73-5.

[5] Juurlink BH. Management of oxidative stress in the CNS: the many roles of glutathione. *Neurotox Res.* 1999; 1: 119-40.

[6] Switala J, Loewen PC. Diversity of properties among catalases. *Arch. Biochem. Biophys.* 2002; 401: 145-54.

[7] Carsol MA, Pouliquen-Sonaglia I, Lesgards G, Marchis-Mouren G, Puigserver A, Santimone M. A new kinetic model for the mode of action of soluble and membrane-immobilized glutathione peroxidase from bovine erythrocytes-effects of selenium. *Eur. J. Biochem.* 1997; 247: 248-55.

[8] Margis R, Dunand C, Teixeira FK, Margis-Pinheiro M. Glutathione peroxidase family - an evolutionary overview. *FEBS J.* 2008; 275: 3959-70.

[9] Juurlink BHJ. Molecular medicine is where chronic diseases, nutrition and physical activity interset: A suggestion on how to deal with chronic diseases in the medical curriculum. In: Ganguly P, editor. Health and Disease: Curriculum for the 21st Century. Hauppauge, N.Y.: Nova Science; 2014. p. 105-37.

[10] Junqueira VB, Barros SB, Chan SS, et al. Aging and oxidative stress. *Mol. Aspects Med.* 2004; 25: 5-16.

[11] Tian L, Cai Q, Wei H. Alterations of antioxidant enzymes and oxidative damage to macromolecules in different organs of rats during aging. *Free Radic. Biol. Med.* 1998; 24: 1477-84.

[12] Hazelton GA, Lang CA. Glutathione contents of tissues in the aging mouse. *Biochem. J.* 1980; 188: 25-30.

[13] Armeni T, Pieri C, Marra M, Saccucci F, Principato G. Studies on the life prolonging effect of food restriction: glutathione levels and glyoxalase enzymes in rat liver. *Mech. Ageing Dev.* 1998; 101: 101-10.

[14] Sasaki T, Unno K, Tahara S, Kaneko T. Age-related increase of reactive oxygen generation in the brains of mammals and birds: is reactive oxygen a signaling molecule

to determine the aging process and life span? *Geriatr Gerontol. Int.* 2010; 10 Suppl 1: S10-24.

[15] Ungvari Z, Bailey-Downs L, Gautam T, et al. Age-associated vascular oxidative stress, Nrf2 dysfunction, and NF-{kappa}B activation in the nonhuman primate Macaca mulatta. *J. Gerontol. A. Biol. Sci. Med. Sci.* 2011; 66: 866-75.

[16] Liu R, Choi J. Age-associated decline in gamma-glutamylcysteine synthetase gene expression in rats. *Free Radic. Biol. Med.* 2000; 28: 566-74.

[17] Liu RM. Down-regulation of gamma-glutamylcysteine synthetase regulatory subunit gene expression in rat brain tissue during aging. *J. Neurosci. Res.* 2002; 68: 344-51.

[18] Suh JH, Shenvi SV, Dixon BM, et al. Decline in transcriptional activity of Nrf2 causes age-related loss of glutathione synthesis, which is reversible with lipoic acid. *Proc. Natl. Acad. Sci. USA* 2004; 101: 3381-6.

[19] Sykiotis GP, Habeos IG, Samuelson AV, Bohmann D. The role of the antioxidant and longevity-promoting Nrf2 pathway in metabolic regulation. *Curr. Opin. Clin. Nutr. Metab. Care* 2011; 14: 41-8.

[20] Lewis KN, Wason E, Edrey YH, Kristan DM, Nevo E, Buffenstein R. Regulation of Nrf2 signaling and longevity in naturally long-lived rodents. *Proc. Natl. Acad. Sci. USA* 2015; 112: 3722-7.

[21] Jones DP, Mody VC, Jr., Carlson JL, Lynn MJ, Sternberg P, Jr. Redox analysis of human plasma allows separation of pro-oxidant events of aging from decline in antioxidant defenses. *Free Radic. Biol. Med.* 2002; 33: 1290-300.

[22] Samiec PS, Drews-Botsch C, Flagg EW, et al. Glutathione in human plasma: decline in association with aging, age- related macular degeneration, and diabetes. *Free Radic. Biol. Med.* 1998; 24: 699-704.

[23] Droge W. Aging-related changes in the thiol/disulfide redox state: implications for the use of thiol antioxidants. *Exp. Gerontol.* 2002; 37: 1333-45.

[24] Mutlu-Turkoglu U, Ilhan E, Oztezcan S, Kuru A, Aykac-Toker G, Uysal M. Age-related increases in plasma malondialdehyde and protein carbonyl levels and lymphocyte DNA damage in elderly subjects. *Clin. Biochem.* 2003; 36: 397-400.

[25] Mendoza-Nunez VM, Ruiz-Ramos M, Sanchez-Rodriguez MA, Retana-Ugalde R, Munoz-Sanchez JL. Aging-related oxidative stress in healthy humans. *Tohoku J. Exp. Med.* 2007; 213: 261-8.

[26] Chehab O, Ouertani M, Souiden Y, Chaieb K, Mahdouani K. Plasma antioxidants and human aging: a study on healthy elderly Tunisian population. *Mol. Biotechnol.* 2008; 40: 27-37.

[27] Keogh BP, Allen RG, Pignolo R, Horton J, Tresini M, Cristofalo VJ. Expression of hydrogen peroxide and glutathione metabolizing enzymes in human skin fibroblasts derived from donors of different ages. *J. Cell Physiol.* 1996; 167: 512-22.

[28] Serviddio G, Romano AD, Greco A, et al. Frailty syndrome is associated with altered circulating redox balance and increased markers of oxidative stress. *Int. J. Immunopathol. Pharmacol.* 2009; 22: 819-27.

[29] Saum KU, Dieffenbach AK, Jansen EH, et al. Association between Oxidative Stress and Frailty in an Elderly German Population: Results from the ESTHER Cohort Study. Gerontology 2015.

[30] Scheeff ED, Bourne PE. Structural evolution of the protein kinase-like superfamily. *PLoS Comput. Biol.* 2005; 1: e49.

[31] Hommes DW, Peppelenbosch MP, van Deventer SJ. Mitogen activated protein (MAP) kinase signal transduction pathways and novel anti-inflammatory targets. *Gut* 2003; 52: 144-51.

[32] Waas WF, Lo HH, Dalby KN. The kinetic mechanism of the dual phosphorylation of the ATF2 transcription factor by p38 mitogen-activated protein (MAP) kinase alpha. Implications for signal/response profiles of MAP kinase pathways. *J. Biol. Chem. 2001*; 276: 5676-84.

[33] Christman JW, Sadikot RT, Blackwell TS. The role of nuclear factor-kappa B in pulmonary diseases. *Chest* 2000; 117: 1482-7.

[34] Baeuerle PA. Pro-inflammatory signaling: last pieces in the NF-kappaB puzzle? *Curr. Biol.* 1998; 8: R19-22.

[35] Tian B, Brasier AR. Identification of a nuclear factor kappa B-dependent gene network. *Recent Prog. Horm Res.* 2003; 58: 95-130.

[36] Flohé L, Brigelius-Flohe R, Saliou C, Traber MG, Packer L. Redox regulation of NF-kappa B activation. *Free Radic. Biol. Med.* 1997; 22: 1115-26.

[37] Kim HJ, Jung KJ, Yu BP, Cho CG, Choi JS, Chung HY. Modulation of redox-sensitive transcription factors by calorie restriction during aging. *Mech. Ageing Dev.* 2002; 123: 1589-95.

[38] Radak Z, Chung HY, Naito H, et al. Age-associated increase in oxidative stress and nuclear factor kappaB activation are attenuated in rat liver by regular exercise. *FASEB J.* 2004; 18: 749-50.

[39] Donato AJ, Black AD, Jablonski KL, Gano LB, Seals DR. Aging is associated with greater nuclear NF kappa B, reduced I kappa B alpha, and increased expression of proinflammatory cytokines in vascular endothelial cells of healthy humans. *Aging Cell* 2008; 7: 805-12.

[40] Pierce GL, Lesniewski LA, Lawson BR, Beske SD, Seals DR. Nuclear factor-{kappa}B activation contributes to vascular endothelial dysfunction via oxidative stress in overweight/obese middle-aged and older humans. *Circulation* 2009; 119: 1284-92.

[41] Buford TW, Cooke MB, Manini TM, Leeuwenburgh C, Willoughby DS. Effects of age and sedentary lifestyle on skeletal muscle NF-kappaB signaling in men. *J. Gerontol. A. Biol. Sci. Med. Sci.* 2010; 65: 532-7.

[42] Cao SX, Dhahbi JM, Mote PL, Spindler SR. Genomic profiling of short- and long-term caloric restriction effects in the liver of aging mice. *Proc. Natl. Acad. Sci. USA* 2001; 98: 10630-5.

[43] Prolla TA. DNA microarray analysis of the aging brain. *Chem Senses* 2002; 27: 299-306.

[44] Csiszar A, Ungvari Z, Koller A, Edwards JG, Kaley G. Aging-induced proinflammatory shift in cytokine expression profile in coronary arteries. *FASEB J.* 2003; 17: 1183-5.

[45] Melk A, Mansfield ES, Hsieh SC, et al. Transcriptional analysis of the molecular basis of human kidney aging using cDNA microarray profiling. *Kidney Int.* 2005; 68: 2667-79.

[46] Ungvari Z, Csiszar A, Kaley G. Vascular inflammation in aging. *Herz 2004*; 29: 733-40.

[47] Cai D, Frantz JD, Tawa NE, Jr., et al. IKKbeta/NF-kappaB activation causes severe muscle wasting in mice. *Cell* 2004; 119: 285-98.

[48] Tracy RP. Emerging relationships of inflammation, cardiovascular disease and chronic diseases of aging. *Int. J. Obes. Relat. Metab. Disord.* 2003; 27 Suppl 3: S29-34.
[49] Lang PO, Michel JP, Zekry D. Frailty syndrome: a transitional state in a dynamic process. *Gerontology* 2009; 55: 539-49.
[50] Michaud M, Balardy L, Moulis G, et al. Proinflammatory cytokines, aging, and age-related diseases. *J. Am. Med. Dir. Assoc.* 2013; 14: 877-82.
[51] Ju H, Behm DJ, Nerurkar S, et al. p38 MAPK inhibitors ameliorate target organ damage in hypertension: Part 1. p38 MAPK-dependent endothelial dysfunction and hypertension. *J. Pharmacol. Exp. Ther.* 2003; 307: 932-8.
[52] Kim S, Murakami T, Izumi Y, et al. Extracellular signal-regulated kinase and c-Jun NH2-terminal kinase activities are continuously and differentially increased in aorta of hypertensive rats. *Biochem. Biophys. Res. Commun.* 1997; 236: 199-204.
[53] Kanda T, Wakino S, Homma K, et al. Rho-kinase as a molecular target for insulin resistance and hypertension. *FASEB J.* 2005.
[54] Do e Z, Fukumoto Y, Takaki A, et al. Evidence for Rho-kinase activation in patients with pulmonary arterial hypertension. *Circ. J.* 2009; 73: 1731-9.
[55] Guilluy C, Sauzeau V, Rolli-Derkinderen M, et al. Inhibition of RhoA/Rho kinase pathway is involved in the beneficial effect of sildenafil on pulmonary hypertension. *Br. J. Pharmacol.* 2005; 146: 1010-8.
[56] Carlson CJ, Koterski S, Sciotti RJ, Poccard GB, Rondinone CM. Enhanced basal activation of mitogen-activated protein kinases in adipocytes from Type 2 diabetes: potential role of p38 in the downregulation of GLUT4 expression. *Diabetes* 2003; 52: 634-41.
[57] Mander A, Hodgkinson CP, Sale GJ. Knock-down of LAR protein tyrosine phosphatase induces insulin resistance. *FEBS Lett.* 2005; 579: 3024-8.
[58] Ferrer I, Blanco R, Carmona M, et al. Phosphorylated map kinase (ERK1, ERK2) expression is associated with early tau deposition in neurones and glial cells, but not with increased nuclear DNA vulnerability and cell death, in Alzheimer disease, Pick's disease, progressive supranuclear palsy and corticobasal degeneration. *Brain Pathol.* 2001; 11: 144-58.
[59] Okazawa H, Estus S. The JNK/c-Jun cascade and Alzheimer's disease. *Am. J. Alzheimers Dis. Other Demen.* 2002; 17: 79-88.
[60] Zhao WQ, Feng C, Alkon DL. Impairment of phosphatase 2A contributes to the prolonged MAP kinase phosphorylation in Alzheimer's disease fibroblasts. *Neurobiol. Dis.* 2003; 14: 458-69.
[61] Torrent L, Ferrer I. PP2A and Alzheimer Disease. *Curr. Alzheimer Res.* 2012.
[62] Griffin RJ, Moloney A, Kelliher M, et al. Activation of Akt/PKB, increased phosphorylation of Akt substrates and loss and altered distribution of Akt and PTEN are features of Alzheimer's disease pathology. *J. Neurochem.* 2005; 93: 105-17.
[63] Monaco EA, 3rd. Recent evidence regarding a role for Cdk5 dysregulation in Alzheimer's disease. *Curr. Alzheimer Res.* 2004; 1: 33-8.
[64] Eikelenboom P, van Gool WA. Neuroinflammatory perspectives on the two faces of Alzheimer's disease. *J. Neural Transm.* 2004; 111: 281-94.
[65] Zhou Y, Su Y, Li B, et al. Nonsteroidal anti-inflammatory drugs can lower amyloidogenic Abeta42 by inhibiting Rho. *Science* 2003; 302: 1215-7.

[66] Tang BL. Alzheimer's disease: channeling APP to non-amyloidogenic processing. *Biochem. Biophys. Res. Commun.* 2005; 331: 375-8.

[67] Zhou H, Li Y. Long-term diabetic complications may be ameliorated by targeting Rho kinase. *Diabetes Metab. Res. Rev.* 2011; 27: 318-30.

[68] Chakraborti S, Chakraborti T. Oxidant-mediated activation of mitogen-activated protein kinases and nuclear transcription factors in the cardiovascular system: a brief overview. *Cell Signal* 1998; 10: 675-83.

[69] Griendling KK, Sorescu D, Lassegue B, Ushio-Fukai M. Modulation of protein kinase activity and gene expression by reactive oxygen species and their role in vascular physiology and pathophysiology. *Arterioscler Thromb Vasc. Biol.* 2000; 20: 2175-83.

[70] Barthel A, Klotz LO. Phosphoinositide 3-kinase signaling in the cellular response to oxidative stress. *Biol. Chem.* 2005; 386: 207-16.

[71] Claiborne A, Yeh JI, Mallett TC, et al. Protein-sulfenic acids: diverse roles for an unlikely player in enzyme catalysis and redox regulation. *Biochemistry* 1999; 38: 15407-16.

[72] Poole LB, Karplus PA, Claiborne A. Protein sulfenic acids in redox signaling. *Annu. Rev. Pharmacol. Toxicol.* 2004; 44: 325-47.

[73] Barford D. The role of cysteine residues as redox-sensitive regulatory switches. *Curr. Opin. Struct. Biol.* 2004; 14: 679-86.

[74] Cedervall T, Berggard T, Borek V, Thulin E, Linse S, Akerfeldt KS. Redox sensitive cysteine residues in calbindin D28k are structurally and functionally important. *Biochemistry* 2005; 44: 684-93.

[75] Xu D, Rovira, II, Finkel T. Oxidants painting the cysteine chapel: redox regulation of PTPs. *Dev Cell* 2002; 2: 251-2.

[76] van Montfort RL, Congreve M, Tisi D, Carr R, Jhoti H. Oxidation state of the active-site cysteine in protein tyrosine phosphatase 1B. *Nature* 2003; 423: 773-7.

[77] Levinthal DJ, Defranco DB. Reversible oxidation of ERK-directed protein phosphatases drives oxidative toxicity in neurons. *J. Biol. Chem.* 2005; 280: 5875-83.

[78] Barrett AJ, Rawlings ND. Evolutionary lines of cysteine peptidases. *Biol. Chem.* 2001; 382: 727-33.

[79] Lopez-Berenguer C, Martinez-Ballesta Mdel C, Moreno DA, Carvajal M, Garcia-Viguera C. Growing hardier crops for better health: Salinity tolerance and the nutritional value of broccoli. *J. Agric. Food Chem.* 2009; 57: 572-78.

[80] Tanaka T, Nakamura H, Nishiyama A, et al. Redox regulation by thioredoxin superfamily; protection against oxidative stress and aging. *Free Radic. Res.* 2000; 33: 851-5.

[81] Tabatabaie T, Floyd RA. Susceptibility of glutathione peroxidase and glutathione reductase to oxidative damage and the protective effect of spin trapping agents. *Arch. Biochem. Biophys.* 1994; 314: 112-9.

[82] Cho CS, Lee S, Lee GT, Woo HA, Choi EJ, Rhee SG. Irreversible inactivation of glutathione peroxidase 1 and reversible inactivation of peroxiredoxin II by H_2O_2 in red blood cells. *Antioxid Redox Signal* 2010; 12: 1235-46.

[83] Mustacich D, Powis G. Thioredoxin reductase. *Biochem. J.* 2000; 346 Pt 1: 1-8.

[84] Biswas S, Chida AS, Rahman I. Redox modifications of protein-thiols: emerging roles in cell signaling. *Biochem. Pharmacol.* 2006; 71: 551-64.

[85] Klug A. The discovery of zinc fingers and their applications in gene regulation and genome manipulation. *Annu. Rev. Biochem.* 2010; 79: 213-31.

[86] Kroncke KD, Klotz LO. Zinc fingers as biologic redox switches? *Antioxid. Redox Signal* 2009; 11: 1015-27.

[87] Doyle K, Fitzpatrick FA. Redox signaling, alkylation (carbonylation) of conserved cysteines inactivates class I histone deacetylases 1, 2, and 3 and antagonizes their transcriptional repressor function. *J. Biol. Chem.* 2010; 285: 17417-24.

[88] Chen L, MacMillan AM, Chang W, Ezaz-Nikpay K, Lane WS, Verdine GL. Direct identification of the active-site nucleophile in a DNA (cytosine-5)-methyltransferase. *Biochemistry* 1991; 30: 11018-25.

[89] Svedruzic ZM, Reich NO. The mechanism of target base attack in DNA cytosine carbon 5 methylation. *Biochemistry* 2004; 43: 11460-73.

[90] Senanayake GV, Banigesh A, Wu L, Lee P, Juurlink BH. The dietary phase 2 protein inducer sulforaphane can normalize the kidney epigenome and improve blood pressure in hypertensive rats. *Am. J. Hypertens* 2012; 25: 229-35.

[91] Jia Z. Protein phosphatases: structures and implications. *Biochem. Cell Biol.* 1997; 75: 17-26.

[92] Swingle MR, Honkanen RE, Ciszak EM. Structural basis for the catalytic activity of human serine/threonine protein phosphatase-5. *J. Biol. Chem.* 2004; 279: 33992-9.

[93] Halliwell B, Gutteridge JMC. Free Radicals in Biology and Medicine. Second ed. Oxford: Clarendon Press; 1989. 543 p.

[94] Sommer D, Coleman S, Swanson SA, Stemmer PM. Differential susceptibilities of serine/threonine phosphatases to oxidative and nitrosative stress. *Arch. Biochem. Biophys.* 2002; 404: 271-8.

[95] Ullrich V, Namgaladze D, Frein D. Superoxide as inhibitor of calcineurin and mediator of redox regulation. *Toxicol. Lett.* 2003; 139: 107-10.

[96] den Hertog J, Groen A, van der Wijk T. Redox regulation of protein-tyrosine phosphatases. *Arch. Biochem. Biophys.* 2005; 434: 11-5.

[97] Salmeen A, Barford D. Functions and mechanisms of redox regulation of cysteine-based phosphatases. *Antioxid Redox Signal* 2005; 7: 560-77.

[98] Meng TC, Fukada T, Tonks NK. Reversible oxidation and inactivation of protein tyrosine phosphatases in vivo. *Mol. Cell* 2002; 9: 387-99.

[99] Meng TC, Hsu SF, Tonks NK. Development of a modified in-gel assay to identify protein tyrosine phosphatases that are oxidized and inactivated in vivo. *Methods* 2005; 35: 28-36.

[100] Ostman A, Frijhoff J, Sandin A, Bohmer FD. Regulation of protein tyrosine phosphatases by reversible oxidation. *J. Biochem.* 2011; 150: 345-56.

[101] Tanner JJ, Parsons ZD, Cummings AH, Zhou H, Gates KS. Redox regulation of protein tyrosine phosphatases: structural and chemical aspects. *Antioxid. Redox Signal* 2011; 15: 77-97.

[102] Takakura K, Beckman JS, MacMillan-Crow LA, Crow JP. Rapid and irreversible inactivation of protein tyrosine phosphatases PTP1B, CD45, and LAR by peroxynitrite. *Arch. Biochem. Biophys.* 1999; 369: 197-207.

[103] Cross JV, Templeton DJ. Oxidative stress inhibits MEKK1 by site-specific glutathionylation in the ATP-binding domain. *Biochem. J.* 2004; 381: 675-83.

[104] Woo HA, Jeong W, Chang TS, et al. Reduction of cysteine sulfinic acid by sulfiredoxin is specific to 2-cys peroxiredoxins. *J. Biol. Chem.* 2005; 280: 3125-8.

[105] Jonsson TJ, Murray MS, Johnson LC, Lowther WT. Reduction of cysteine sulfinic acid in peroxiredoxin by sulfiredoxin proceeds directly through a sulfinic phosphoryl ester intermediate. *J. Biol. Chem.* 2008; 283: 23846-51.

[106] Theodosiou A, Ashworth A. MAP kinase phosphatases. *Genome Biol. 2002*; 3: REVIEWS3009.

[107] Baumer AT, Ten Freyhaus H, Sauer H, et al. Phosphatidylinositol 3-kinase-dependent membrane recruitment of Rac-1 and p47phox is critical for alpha-platelet-derived growth factor receptor-induced production of reactive oxygen species. *J. Biol. Chem.* 2008; 283: 7864-76.

[108] Seo JH, Ahn Y, Lee SR, Yeol Yeo C, Chung Hur K. The major target of the endogenously generated reactive oxygen species in response to insulin stimulation is phosphatase and tensin homolog and not phosphoinositide-3 kinase (PI-3 kinase) in the PI-3 kinase/Akt pathway. *Mol. Biol. Cell* 2005; 16: 348-57.

[109] Liu RM, Choi J, Wu JH, et al. Oxidative modification of nuclear mitogen-activated protein kinase phosphatase 1 is involved in transforming growth factor beta1-induced expression of plasminogen activator inhibitor 1 in fibroblasts. *J. Biol. Chem.* 2010; 285: 16239-47.

[110] Morrison DK, Davis RJ. Regulation of MAP kinase signaling modules by scaffold proteins in mammals. *Annu. Rev. Cell Dev. Biol.* 2003; 19: 91-118.

[111] Kamata H, Honda S, Maeda S, Chang L, Hirata H, Karin M. Reactive oxygen species promote TNFalpha-induced death and sustained JNK activation by inhibiting MAP kinase phosphatases. *Cell* 2005; 120: 649-61.

[112] Juurlink BH. Type-2 astrocytes have much greater susceptibility to heat stress than type-1 astrocytes. *J. Neurosci. Res.* 1994; 38: 196-201.

[113] Juurlink BH, Husain J. Hyperthermic injury of oligodendrocyte precursor cells: implications for dysmyelination disorders. *Brain Res.* 1994; 641: 353-6.

[114] Husain J, Juurlink BH. Oligodendroglial precursor cell susceptibility to hypoxia is related to poor ability to cope with reactive oxygen species. *Brain Res.* 1995; 698: 86-94.

[115] Thorburne SK, Juurlink BH. Low glutathione and high iron govern the susceptibility of oligodendroglial precursors to oxidative stress. *J. Neurochem.* 1996; 67: 1014-22.

[116] Juurlink BH, Sweeney MI. Mechanisms that result in damage during and following cerebral ischemia. *Neurosci. Biobehav. Rev.* 1997; 21: 121-8.

[117] Juurlink BH, Thorburne SK, Hertz L. Peroxide-scavenging deficit underlies oligodendrocyte susceptibility to oxidative stress. *Glia* 1998; 22: 371-8.

[118] Jelinski SE, Yager JY, Juurlink BH. Preferential injury of oligodendroblasts by a short hypoxic-ischemic insult. *Brain Res.* 1999; 815: 150-3.

[119] Juurlink BH, Paterson PG. Review of oxidative stress in brain and spinal cord injury: suggestions for pharmacological and nutritional management strategies. *J. Spinal Cord Med.* 1998; 21: 309-34.

[120] Christman JW, Blackwell TS, Juurlink BH. Redox regulation of nuclear factor kappa B: therapeutic potential for attenuating inflammatory responses. *Brain Pathol.* 2000; 10: 153-62.

[121] Juurlink BH. Therapeutic potential of dietary phase 2 enzyme inducers in ameliorating diseases that have an underlying inflammatory component. *Can. J. Physiol. Pharmacol.* 2001; 79: 266-82.

[122] Wu L, Juurlink BH. The impaired glutathione system and its up-regulation by sulforaphane in vascular smooth muscle cells from spontaneously hypertensive rats. *J. Hypertens* 2001; 19: 1819-25.

[123] Mohamed AA, Avila JG, Schultke E, et al. Amelioration of experimental allergic encephalitis (EAE) through phase 2 enzyme induction. *Biomed. Sci. Instrum.* 2002; 38: 9-13.

[124] Wu L, Noyan Ashraf MH, Facci M, et al. Dietary approach to attenuate oxidative stress, hypertension, and inflammation in the cardiovascular system. *Proc. Natl. Acad. Sci. USA* 2004; 101: 7094-9.

[125] Noyan-Ashraf MH, Sadeghinejad Z, Juurlink BH. Dietary approach to decrease aging-related CNS inflammation. *Nutr. Neurosci.* 2005; 8: 101-10.

[126] Noyan-Ashraf MH, Wu L, Wang R, Juurlink BH. Dietary approaches to positively influence fetal determinants of adult health. *FASEB J.* 2006; 20: 371-3.

[127] Noyan-Ashraf MH, Sadeghinejad Z, Davies GF, et al. Phase 2 protein inducers in the diet promote healthier aging. *J. Gerontol. A. Biol. Sci. Med. Sci.* 2008; 63: 1168-76.

[128] Benedict AL, Mountney A, Hurtado A, et al. Neuroprotective effects of sulforaphane after contusive spinal cord injury. *J. Neurotrauma* 2012; 29: 2576-86.

[129] Pan H, He M, Liu R, Brecha NC, Yu AC, Pu M. Sulforaphane protects rodent retinas against ischemia-reperfusion injury through the activation of the Nrf2/HO-1 antioxidant pathway. *PLoS One* 2014; 9: e114186.

[130] Nguyen B, Luong L, Naase H, et al. Sulforaphane pretreatment prevents systemic inflammation and renal injury in response to cardiopulmonary bypass. *J. Thorac. Cardiovasc. Surg.* 2014; 148: 690-7 e3.

[131] Li B, Cui W, Liu J, et al. Sulforaphane ameliorates the development of experimental autoimmune encephalomyelitis by antagonizing oxidative stress and Th17-related inflammation in mice. *Exp. Neurol.* 2013; 250: 239-49.

[132] Anderson RM, Weindruch R. Metabolic reprogramming, caloric restriction and aging. *Trends Endocrinol. Metab.* 2010; 21: 134-41.

[133] Csiszar A, Gautam T, Sosnowska D, et al. Caloric restriction confers persistent anti-oxidative, pro-angiogenic, and anti-inflammatory effects and promotes anti-aging miRNA expression profile in cerebromicrovascular endothelial cells of aged rats. *Am. J. Physiol. Heart Circ. Physiol.* 2014; 307: H292-306.

[134] Juurlink BH. Can dietary intake of phase 2 protein inducers affect the rising epidemic of diseases such as Type 2 diabetes? *MedGenMed* 2003; 5: 25.

[135] Badimon L, Vilahur G, Padro T. Nutraceuticals and atherosclerosis: human trials. *Cardiovasc. Ther.* 2010; 28: 202-15.

[136] Thimmulappa RK, Mai KH, Srisuma S, Kensler TW, Yamamoto M, Biswal S. Identification of Nrf2-regulated genes induced by the chemopreventive agent sulforaphane by oligonucleotide microarray. *Cancer Res.* 2002; 62: 5196-203.

[137] Li J, Pankratz M, Johnson JA. Differential gene expression patterns revealed by oligonucleotide versus long cDNA arrays. *Toxicol. Sci.* 2002; 69: 383-90.

[138] Meister A. Metabolism and function of glutathione. In: Dolphin D, Avramovic O, Poulson R, editors. Glutathione Chemical, Biochemical, and Medical Aspects. A. New York: John Wiley & Sons; 1989. p. 367-474.

[139] Ishii T, Itoh K, Takahashi S, et al. Transcription factor Nrf2 coordinately regulates a group of oxidative stress-inducible genes in macrophages. *J. Biol. Chem.* 2000; 275: 16023-9.

[140] Jayasena DD, Jung S, Kim HJ, Yong HI, Nam KC, Jo C. Taste-active compound levels in Korean native chicken meat: The effects of bird age and the cooking process. *Poult Sci.* 2015.

[141] Grey V, Mohammed SR, Smountas AA, Bahlool R, Lands LC. Improved glutathione status in young adult patients with cystic fibrosis supplemented with whey protein. *J. Cyst. Fibros* 2003; 2: 195-8.

[142] Shchedrina VA, Zhang Y, Labunskyy VM, Hatfield DL, Gladyshev VN. Structure-function relations, physiological roles, and evolution of mammalian ER-resident selenoproteins. *Antioxid. Redox Signal* 2010; 12: 839-49.

[143] Ornish D, Brown SE, Scherwitz LW, et al. Can lifestyle changes reverse coronary heart disease? The Lifestyle Heart Trial. *Lancet* 1990; 336: 129-33.

In: Broccoli
Editor: Bernhard H. J. Juurlink

ISBN: 978-1-63484-313-3
© 2016 Nova Science Publishers, Inc.

Chapter 6

THE NRF2 SIGNALLING SYSTEM

*Bernhard H. J. Juurlink**
Department of Anatomy and Cell Biology,
University of Saskatchewan, Saskatoon, SK, Canada

ABSTRACT

This chapter gives a brief review of the Nrf2 signalling system and how it promotes redox and metabolic homeostasis. Included is a description of many of the genes with anti-oxidant response elements; the role of Keap1 and associated ubiquitin ligase complex as well as the role of glycogen synthase 3β in regulating the half-life of Nrf2; the role of Keap1 oxidation as well as phosphorylation of Nrf2 in Nrf2 signalling; the newly discovered consequences of Nrf2 signalling such as promoting mitochondrial and intermediary metabolism homeostasis; and finally, a caveat that promoting redox homeostasis is not necessarily desired where cancer is involved.

Keywords: anti-oxidant response element, intermediary metabolism, Keap1, kinases, phase 2 enzymes, proteasome, redox, small maf

INTRODUCTION

The purpose of this chapter is to give a brief introduction to the role of the transcription factor Nuclear factor (erythroid-derived-2) like-2 (Nrf2) in homeostatic regulatory mechanisms. The first defined role of Nrf2 was in redox homeostasis, in particular in activation of the anti-oxidant response. Activation of the anti-oxidant response increases the ability of cells to inactivate oxidants or decrease the ability to produce strong oxidants. The anti-oxidant response typically is activated once cells can no longer efficiently deal with an increasing cellular oxidizing environment. The anti-oxidant response is initiated by the binding of a transcription factor complex to anti-oxidant response elements (AREs) present in

---

* Email: bernhard.juurlink@usask.ca.

many genes. An excellent review of the history of discoveries that elucidated the role of Nrf2 in redox homeostasis is given by Itoh and colleagues [1].

THE ANTI-OXIDANT RESPONSE

The ARE, also known as the electrophile response element (EpRE), was first identified as promoter elements in the NAD(P)H:quinone oxireductase (NQO1) gene as well as in glutathione S-transferase genes in the early 1990s [2], i.e., in phase 2 enzyme genes (for phase 2 enzymes see Chapter 4). The core sequence has been described as 5'-TGACnnnGCn [3]; however, upstream and downstream sequences as well as variants within the core sequence can affect binding of the transcription factor complexes and, thus, affect the efficacy of gene transcription (see Nerland for more details [3]). Binding of a heterodimer comprised of Nrf2 and small Musculo-aponeurotic fibrosarcoma (Maf) proteins to AREs was first described in 1997 [4].

Genes with AREs

Phase 2 enzymes are involved in xenobiotic metabolism (see Chapter 4) and these genes contain AREs. Xenobiotic metabolism typically involves the actions of phase 1 enzymes to produce a reactive product from the xenobiotic (drug or phytochemical). Phase 2 enzymes then often form a water-soluble conjugate with the reactive xenobiotic. The final stage in xenobiotic metabolism is the export of the water-soluble conjugate from the cell via phase 3 protein exporters.

The phase 2 proteins that form conjugates with the reactive products of phase 1 enzyme action include genes whose protein products are involved in the formation of glutathione conjugates via the glutathione S-transferases [5, 6]; of sulfate conjugates via sulfotransferases [7]; as well as glucoronic acid conjugates via UDP-glucoronosyltransferase [8]. In addition, other enzymes include NAD(P)H quinone oxireductase-1 [9] involved in the reduction of quinones to hydroquinones, thus bypassing the formation of highly reactive semi-quinones, and epoxide hydrolase [6, 10] that converts highly reactive epoxides to diols.

AREs are also present in many phase 3 proteins involved in transporting large molecules, such as conjugates derived from phase 2 enzyme action, across the plasmalemma. These include: the ATP-Binding Cassette C Multidrug Resistance Proteins (Mrps)-1, 2, 3, 4, 5 and 6 involved in the transport of organic anions [7, 11, 12], Organic Anion Transporting Polypeptide 2B1 (OATP2B1) [7], as well as the Transporter Associated with Antigen Processing-1B (TAP-1B) [13].

A number of anti-oxidant mechanisms utilize GSH, for example, glutathione S-transferases, glutathione peroxidases as well as the glyoxalase system that inactivates dicarbonyls [14]. The rate-limiting enzyme for GSH synthesis, γ-glutamyl-cysteine ligase (GCL), is a heterodimer, comprised of a regulatory and catalytic subunit [15]. Both the regulatory and catalytic subunit of GCL have AREs in their promoter regions and are Nrf2-inducible [16]. Other genes whose protein products are related to formation of GSH also contain AREs in their promoter regions. These include: the cystine-glutamate antiporter that is the main mechanism taking up cystine into cells [17]. Cystine is the oxidized form of cysteine and about 90% of cysteine residues in the extracellular fluid is in the form of cystine. The cystine, taken up by the antiporter, is then reduced to cysteine, the rate-limiting amino acid in GSH synthesis [15]. In addition, glutathione reductase gene contains an ARE [10]: glutathione reductase reduces oxidized-glutathione back to GSH. Other genes that contain AREs include glucose-6-phosphate dehydrogenase, 6-phosphogluconate dehydrogenase and malic enzyme [10] that provides the NADPH necessary for glutathione reductase action; the selenoprotein glutathione peroxidase-2 [10] that uses GSH as an electron donor to convert the reactive hydroperoxides to inactive alcohols or water and molecular oxygen in the case of hydrogen peroxide; and peroxiredoxin-1, 3 and 5 [17] that are GSH-dependent enzymes that convert alkylhydroperoxides to inactive alcohols.

Furthermore, many other proteins important in redox regulation are Nrf2-inducible. These include both thioredoxin and thioredoxin reductase, proteins that are important in redox regulation of protein thiols [11, 18]; aldo-keto reductase, which is important in, amongst other things, the reduction of the dialdehyde metabolite of Aflatoxin B$_1$ [11, 18]; and carbonyl reductase [18] that inactivates reactive carbonyls.

Many metal-binding proteins, that decrease the probability of strong oxidant formation, also contain AREs in their promoter regions. For example, ferritin H and L chains that sequester redox-active Fe^{2+} as Fe^{3+} [19] and metallothioneins [20] that sequester other redox active metal ions such as copper. Furthermore, the iron in the heme of damaged heme proteins can mediate the formation of strong oxidants [21]. Hence, it is not surprising that heme oxygenase-1, which converts heme to biliverdin and Fe^{2+} has an ARE in its promoter region [17]; the Fe^{2+} can be safely sequestered as Fe^{3+} in ferritin while biliverdin has anti-oxidant properties. Oxidative stress also denatures proteins and it is, hence, not surprising that many stress proteins and proteosomal proteins have AREs in their promoter regions as well as a number of chaperones/stress proteins [18].

Finally, as noted in Chapter 5, with aging there is increased oxidative stress that is associated with a decreased expression of Nrf2. Of particular significance to the field of nutrigenomics is the fact that Nrf2 gene [22] as well as the small Maf protein Maf-G [23] also have AREs in their promoter regions and, thus, are also Nrf2-inducible.

ACTIVATION OF THE ANTI-OXIDANT RESPONSE

A brief explanation of the activation of the anti-oxidant response is given here, for more details please see Chapter 10 as well as recent reviews [24-28].

Role of Keap1

The protein Kelch-like ECH-Associated Protein-1 (Keap1), present in both the cytoplasm and nucleus, acts as a cellular redox sensor. Keap1 is present as a homodimer and it is the homodimer that binds Nrf2. Notably, Keap1 also acts as an adaptor protein for Cullin-3 (Cul3). Cul3 is a scaffold protein that assembles an E3-ubiquitin ligase complex [29]. The binding of Nrf2 by Keap1 allows the ubiquitin ligase complex to polyubiquinate Nrf2, thus tagging it for proteasomal degradation (Figure 1). The Keap1 homodimer-Cul3-ubiquitin ligase complex, thus, acts as a sink for Nrf2. Under normal redox conditions there is continual low-level synthesis of Nrf2 with the Nrf2 becoming bound to the Keap1 dimer allowing presentation to the ubiquitin ligase complex for polyubination followed by proteosomal degradation.

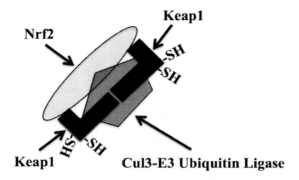

Figure 1. Diagram illustrating that under normal redox conditions Nrf2 is bound by a Keap1 dimer that presents Nrf2 to a Cul3-E3-Ubiquitin Ligase complex that polyubiquinates Nrf2, thus targeting it for proteasomal degradation.

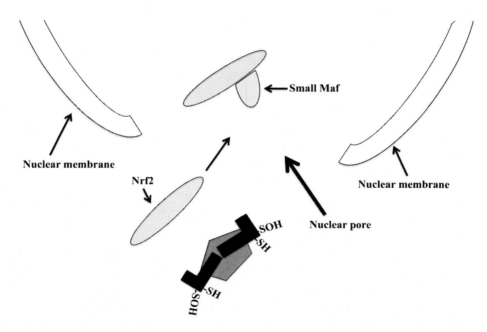

Figure 2. Diagram illustrating when Keap1 thiols are oxidized the Keap 1 dimer cannot bind Nrf2, allowing Nrf2 to translocate to the nucleus where it can heterodimerize with small Maf proteins, allowing binding to AREs.

Reduced cysteine residues present in Keap1 are required for binding of Nrf2. With oxidation of Keap1 cysteine residues Nrf2 no longer can bind to Keap1, thus allowing Nrf2 to translocate to the nucleus where it forms heterodimers with small Maf proteins, thereby promoting transcription of genes with AREs in their promoter regions (Figure 2). The ability of oxidants to oxidize Keap1 cysteine residues varies markedly and is likely due to their geometrical and electronic configurations. As can be seen in the next section, activation of the Nrf2 signalling system is not simply dependent upon oxidation of Keap1 thiols but is also influenced by phosphorylation of a number of amino acid residues on Nrf2.

The ability of molecules to oxidize Keap1 can vary by orders of magnitude. A measure of Nrf2 inducer ability is the Concentration of compound required to Double (CD) the activity of NAD(P)H quinone oxireductase activity in hepatoma cells grown in culture [30]. As an example of differences in CD activity is a comparison of dimethyl fumarate with sulforaphane. Dimethyl fumarate is an approved, but very expensive, treatment for multiple sclerosis [31]. Dimethyl fumarate has a CD of ~5 µM [32] whereas sulforaphane has a CD that is an order of magnitude less [33]. Since dimethyl fumarate as well as sulforaphane will oxidize many thiols in the cell, not just Keap1 thiols, this suggests that sulforaphane would do far less cellular damage than dimethyl fumarate at equal concentrations. This might be a consideration in carrying out a clinical trial with multiple sclerosis patients with sulforaphane.

Role of Amino Acid Residue Phosphorylation of Nrf2 Signalling Activity

This is still a relatively new area of research and only a few examples will be given of the ability of kinases to influence the anti-oxidant response. See Chapter 7 for more details. Phosphorylation of specific serine residues by glycogen synthase-3β inhibits the translocation of Nrf2 to the nucleus [34, 35], interferes with binding to Keap1 but allows it to be targeted for proteasomal degradation via another pathway where the phosphorylated Nrf2 binds to β-Transducing repeat-Containing Protein (β–TrCP) that is associated with a Cul1-ubiquitin ligase complex [36, 37]. Signalling pathways that influence glycogen synthase-3β activity will therefore influence Nrf2 signalling. Protein kinase C phosphorylates specific serine residues on Nrf2 inhibiting binding to Keap1, thus promoting translocation of Nrf2 to the nucleus [38]. The phosphorylation of amino acid residues within the transcriptional activation domain of Nrf2 by casein kinase-2 (serine/threonine kinase) also promotes nuclear translocation of Nrf2 as well as enhancement of transcription [39]. Phosphorylation of Nrf2 by c-Jun N-terminal Kinase (JNK) [40] as well as protein kinase C [41] also promotes nuclear translocation and enhancement of transcription.

It is clear that the regulation of the anti-oxidant response is complex and involves more than simply oxidizing Keap1 thiols. Polyphenolics in the diet influence a number of kinase pathways and can also have a major impact on the anti-oxidant response synergizing the effect of Keap1 oxidizers [42].

NON-CANONICAL ASPECTS OF NRF2 SIGNALLING

So far we have discussed the ability of Nrf2 to decrease oxidative stress. Nrf2 signalling also normalizes mitochondrial function as well as intermediary metabolism [28, 43, 44]. In part this is likely due to the more normal redox conditions since many of the critical enzymes in intermediary metabolism as well as electron carriers are susceptible to oxidative damage. Some of the effects of Nrf2 signalling may be indirect and due to increased expression of transcription factors with AREs in their gene promoter regions [45]. Examples of such involve lipid metabolism. Nrf2 signalling down-regulates lipid synthesis, in part by decreasing expression of sterol regulatory element-binding protein-1 (Sreb1), a main driver of expression of lipid synthesizing enzymes, while upregulating expression of enzymes involved in lipid oxidation [46]. AREs are also present in the Nuclear respiratory factor-1 (Nrf1) transcription factor gene [47]. Target genes of the Nrf1 transcription factor include mitochondrial biogenesis and mitochondrial function genes [48], likely accounting for much of the interaction between Nrf2 and intermediary metabolism.

CONCLUSION

Activation of the Nrf2 signalling pathway promotes normalization where homeostasis is disturbed. Much of the research attention has been paid to disturbances in redox homeostasis but recently attention has been paid to disturbances in mitochondrial homeostasis and metabolic homeostasis. Many of the positive effects of dietary small fruits and vegetables such as crucifers on our health are likely mediated through Nrf2 signalling.

In normal cells normalization of homeostasis is desired for better function; however, there are situations where one may not wish to activate the antioxidant response. A good example of this is cancer. Many cancer chemotherapeutic drugs increase oxidative stress and it is oxidant-induced DNA damage that activates apoptosis resulting in cancer cell death. Increasing the expression of phase 2 enzymes will increase the probability of drug inactivation and increasing the expression of phase 3 proteins will increase drug efflux [49], thus decreasing the effectiveness of the chemotherapeutics.

REFERENCES

[1] Itoh K, Mimura J, Yamamoto M. Discovery of the negative regulator of Nrf2, Keap1: a historical overview. *Antioxid. Redox Signal* 2010; 13: 1665-78.
[2] Jaiswal AK. Antioxidant response element. *Biochem. Pharmacol.* 1994; 48: 439-44.
[3] Nerland DE. The antioxidant/electrophile response element motif. *Drug Metab. Rev.* 2007; 39: 235-48.
[4] Itoh K, Chiba T, Takahashi S, et al. An Nrf2/small Maf heterodimer mediates the induction of phase II detoxifying enzyme genes through antioxidant response elements. *Biochem. Biophys. Res. Commun.* 1997; 236: 313-22.
[5] Pool-Zobel B, Veeriah S, Bohmer FD. Modulation of xenobiotic metabolising enzymes by anticarcinogens -- focus on glutathione S-transferases and their role as targets of dietary chemoprevention in colorectal carcinogenesis. *Mutat. Res.* 2005; 591: 74-92.
[6] Kwak MK, Itoh K, Yamamoto M, Sutter TR, Kensler TW. Role of transcription factor Nrf2 in the induction of hepatic phase 2 and antioxidative enzymes in vivo by the cancer chemoprotective agent, 3H-1, 2-dimethiole-3-thione. *Mol. Med.* 2001; 7: 135-45.

[7] Shen G, Kong AN. Nrf2 plays an important role in coordinated regulation of Phase II drug metabolism enzymes and Phase III drug transporters. *Biopharm. Drug Dispos.* 2009; 30: 345-55.

[8] Kalthoff S, Ehmer U, Freiberg N, Manns MP, Strassburg CP. Interaction between oxidative stress sensor Nrf2 and xenobiotic-activated aryl hydrocarbon receptor in the regulation of the human phase II detoxifying UDP-glucuronosyltransferase 1A10. *J. Biol. Chem.* 2010; 285: 5993-6002.

[9] Jaiswal AK. Regulation of genes encoding NAD(P)H:quinone oxidoreductases. *Free Radic. Biol. Med.* 2000; 29: 254-62.

[10] Thimmulappa RK, Mai KH, Srisuma S, Kensler TW, Yamamoto M, Biswal S. Identification of Nrf2-regulated genes induced by the chemopreventive agent sulforaphane by oligonucleotide microarray. *Cancer Res.* 2002; 62: 5196-203.

[11] Hayes JD, McMahon M, Chowdhry S, Dinkova-Kostova AT. Cancer chemoprevention mechanisms mediated through the Keap1-Nrf2 pathway. *Antioxid. Redox Signal* 2010; 13: 1713-48.

[12] Malhotra D, Portales-Casamar E, Singh A, et al. Global mapping of binding sites for Nrf2 identifies novel targets in cell survival response through ChIP-Seq profiling and network analysis. *Nucleic Acids Res.* 2010; 38: 5718-34.

[13] Shen G, Xu C, Hu R, et al. Comparison of (-)-epigallocatechin-3-gallate elicited liver and small intestine gene expression profiles between C57BL/6J mice and C57BL/6J/Nrf2 (-/-) mice. *Pharm. Res.* 2005; 22: 1805-20.

[14] Juurlink BH. Management of oxidative stress in the CNS: the many roles of glutathione. *Neurotox Res* 1999; 1: 119-40.

[15] Meister A. Glutathione. *Ann. Rev. Biochem.* 1983; 79: 711-60.

[16] Wild AC, Mulcahy RT. Regulation of gamma-glutamylcysteine synthetase subunit gene expression: insights into transcriptional control of antioxidant defenses. *Free Radic. Res.* 2000; 32: 281-301.

[17] Ishii T, Itoh K, Takahashi S, et al. Transcription factor Nrf2 coordinately regulates a group of oxidative stress-inducible genes in macrophages. *J. Biol. Chem.* 2000; 275: 16023-9.

[18] Kwak MK, Wakabayashi N, Itoh K, Motohashi H, Yamamoto M, Kensler TW. Modulation of gene expression by cancer chemopreventive dithiolethiones through the Keap1-Nrf2 pathway. Identification of novel gene clusters for cell survival. *J. Biol. Chem.* 2003; 278: 8135-45.

[19] Primiano T, Gastel JA, Kensler TW, Sutter TR. Isolation of cDNAs representing dithiolethione-responsive genes. *Carcinogenesis* 1996; 17: 2297-303.

[20] Campagne MV, Thibodeaux H, van Bruggen N, Cairns B, Lowe DG. Increased binding activity at an antioxidant-responsive element in the metallothionein-1 promoter and rapid induction of metallothionein-1 and -2 in response to cerebral ischemia and reperfusion. *J. Neurosci.* 2000; 20: 5200-7.

[21] Alayash AI, Patel RP, Cashon RE. Redox reactions of hemoglobin and myoglobin: biological and toxicological implications. *Antioxid. Redox Signal* 2001; 3: 313-27.

[22] Lee JM, Calkins MJ, Chan K, Kan YW, Johnson JA. Identification of the NF-E2-related factor-2-dependent genes conferring protection against oxidative stress in primary cortical astrocytes using oligonucleotide microarray analysis. *J. Biol. Chem.* 2003; 278: 12029-38.

[23] Katsuoka F, Motohashi H, Engel JD, Yamamoto M. Nrf2 transcriptionally activates the mafG gene through an antioxidant response element. *J. Biol. Chem.* 2005; 280: 4483-90.
[24] Keum YS, Choi BY. Molecular and chemical regulation of the Keap1-Nrf2 signalling pathway. *Molecules* 2014; 19: 10074-89.
[25] Canning P, Sorrell FJ, Bullock AN. Structural basis of KEAP1 interactions with Nrf2. *Free Radic. Biol. Med.* 2015.
[26] Niture SK, Khatri R, Jaiswal AK. Regulation of Nrf2-an update. *Free Radic. Biol. Med.* 2014; 66: 36-44.
[27] Suzuki T, Yamamoto M. Molecular basis of the Keap1-Nrf2 system. *Free Radic. Biol. Med.* 2015.
[28] Hayes JD, Dinkova-Kostova AT. The Nrf2 regulatory network provides an interface between redox and intermediary metabolism. *Trends Biochem. Sci.* 2014; 39: 199-218.
[29] Choo YY, Hagen T. Mechanism of cullin3 E3 ubiquitin ligase dimerization. *PLoS One* 2012; 7: e41350.
[30] Prochaska HJ, Santamaria AB, Talalay P. Rapid detection of inducers of enzymes that protect against carcinogens. *Proc. Natl. Acad. Sci. USA* 1992; 89: 2394-8.
[31] Sheremata W, Brown AD, Rammohan KW. Dimethyl fumarate for treating relapsing multiple sclerosis. *Expert Opin Drug Saf.* 2015; 14: 161-70.
[32] Spencer SR, Wilczak CA, Talalay P. Induction of glutathione transferases and NAD(P)H:quinone reductase by fumaric acid derivatives in rodent cells and tissues. *Cancer Res.* 1990; 50: 7871-5.
[33] Zhang Y, Talalay P, Cho CG, Posner GH. A major inducer of anticarcinogenic protective enzymes from broccoli: isolation and elucidation of structure. *Proc. Natl. Acad. Sci. USA* 1992; 89: 2399-403.
[34] Salazar M, Rojo AI, Velasco D, de Sagarra RM, Cuadrado A. Glycogen synthase kinase-3beta inhibits the xenobiotic and antioxidant cell response by direct phosphorylation and nuclear exclusion of the transcription factor Nrf2. *J. Biol. Chem.* 2006; 281: 14841-51.
[35] Rada P, Rojo AI, Evrard-Todeschi N, et al. Structural and functional characterization of Nrf2 degradation by the glycogen synthase kinase 3/beta-TrCP axis. *Mol. Cell Biol.* 2012; 32: 3486-99.
[36] Tebay LE, Robertson H, Durant ST, et al. Mechanisms of activation of the transcription factor Nrf2 by redox stressors, nutrient cues and energy status, and pathways through which it attenuates degenerative disease. *Free Radic. Biol. Med.* 2015.
[37] Chowdhry S, Zhang Y, McMahon M, Sutherland C, Cuadrado A, Hayes JD. Nrf2 is controlled by two distinct beta-TrCP recognition motifs in its Neh6 domain, one of which can be modulated by GSK-3 activity. *Oncogene* 2013; 32: 3765-81.
[38] Huang HC, Nguyen T, Pickett CB. Regulation of the antioxidant response element by protein kinase C-mediated phosphorylation of NF-E2-related factor 2. *Proc. Natl. Acad. Sci. USA* 2000; 97: 12475-80.
[39] Apopa PL, He X, Ma Q. Phosphorylation of Nrf2 in the transcription activation domain by casein kinase 2 (CK2) is critical for the nuclear translocation and transcription activation function of Nrf2 in IMR-32 neuroblastoma cells. *J. Biochem. Mol. Toxicol.* 2008; 22: 63-76.

[40] Vari R, D'Archivio M, Filesi C, et al. Protocatechuic acid induces antioxidant/detoxifying enzyme expression through JNK-mediated Nrf2 activation in murine macrophages. *J. Nutr. Biochem.* 2011; 22: 409-17.

[41] Buelna-Chontal M, Guevara-Chavez JG, Silva-Palacios A, Medina-Campos ON, Pedraza-Chaverri J, Zazueta C. Nrf2-regulated antioxidant response is activated by protein kinase C in postconditioned rat hearts. *Free Radic. Biol. Med.* 2014; 74: 145-56.

[42] Juurlink BH, Azouz HJ, Aldalati AM, AlTinawi BM, Ganguly P. Hydroxybenzoic acid isomers and the cardiovascular system. *Nutr. J.* 2014; 13: 63.

[43] Ludtmann MH, Angelova PR, Zhang Y, Abramov AY, Dinkova-Kostova AT. Nrf2 affects the efficiency of mitochondrial fatty acid oxidation. *Biochem. J.* 2014; 457: 415-24.

[44] Vomhof-Dekrey EE, Picklo MJ, Sr. The Nrf2-antioxidant response element pathway: a target for regulating energy metabolism. *J. Nutr. Biochem* 2012; 23: 1201-6.

[45] Chambel SS, Santos-Goncalves A, Duarte TL. The Dual Role of Nrf2 in Nonalcoholic Fatty Liver Disease: Regulation of Antioxidant Defenses and Hepatic Lipid Metabolism. *Biomed. Res. Int.* 2015; 2015: 597134.

[46] Yates MS, Tran QT, Dolan PM, et al. Genetic versus chemoprotective activation of Nrf2 signalling: overlapping yet distinct gene expression profiles between Keap1 knockout and triterpenoid-treated mice. *Carcinogenesis* 2009; 30: 1024-31.

[47] Piantadosi CA, Carraway MS, Babiker A, Suliman HB. Heme oxygenase-1 regulates cardiac mitochondrial biogenesis via Nrf2-mediated transcriptional control of nuclear respiratory factor-1. *Circ. Res.* 2008; 103: 1232-40.

[48] Satoh J, Kawana N, Yamamoto Y. Pathway Analysis of ChIP-Seq-Based NRF1 Target Genes Suggests a Logical Hypothesis of their Involvement in the Pathogenesis of Neurodegenerative Diseases. *Gene Regul. Syst. Bio.* 2013; 7: 139-52.

[49] Housman G, Byler S, Heerboth S, et al. Drug resistance in cancer: an overview. *Cancers (Basel)* 2014; 6: 1769-92.

In: Broccoli
Editor: Bernhard H. J. Juurlink

ISBN: 978-1-63484-313-3
© 2016 Nova Science Publishers, Inc.

Chapter 7

QUERCETIN AND KAEMPFEROL AMELIORATE INFLAMMATION THROUGH NRF2 AND OTHER SIGNALING PATHWAYS

Sarah E. Galinn and Petra A. Tsuji[*]
*Department of Biological Sciences,
Towson University, Towson, MD, US*

ABSTRACT

Quercetin and kaempferol are the dominant flavonoids in broccoli and many other vegetables and fruits. Both compounds have been implicated in the suppression of pro-inflammatory cytokine production. Because there is a strong link between inflammation and diseases, several signaling pathways have been investigated as potential strategies for therapeutic interventions using flavonoids. Quercetin and kaempferol are both strong antioxidants, and have been shown to target multiple of such signaling pathways, of which those involving Nf-κb, NRF2, MAPK, PI3K, and WNT/β-catenin are described within this chapter. The limited numbers of human clinical trials with flavonoids have yielded conflicting or inconclusive results thus far. However, the apparent pleiotropic functions of both kaempferol and quercetin, and their propensity for modulating NRF2 and other signaling pathways, continue to render them interesting therapeutics in inflammation and other diseases.

Keywords: quercetin, kaempferol, flavonoids, inflammation, cytokines, NRF2, Nf-κb, MAPK

INTRODUCTION

Flavonoids are phenolic secondary products isolated from a wide range of vascular plants, with over 8,000 individual compounds known thus far. Quercetin and kaempferol,

---

[*] Corresponding Author address: Email: ptsuji@towson.edu.

most frequently in their conjugated forms, count among the most regularly consumed flavonoids due to their widespread occurrence in plants [1].

Besides the family Brassicaceae, which includes broccoli and turnips, the families Amaryllidaceae (e.g., onions), Amaranthaceae (e.g., spinach), Fabaceae (e.g., green beans), Rosaceae (e.g., raspberry, strawberry, apple), and Solanaceae (e.g., tomoatoes) also contain significant amounts of these two and other flavonoids [2, 3]. The aglycone forms of kaempferol and quercetin are detectable in many edible plants with liquid chromatography–mass spectrometry. A large number of hydroxycinnamic acid esters of kaempferol and quercetin glucosides are also present, with the main acids detectable being sinapic, p-coumaric, caffeic and ferulic [4]. Some flavonoids have been suggested to be anti-histamines or to be protective against a variety of health conditions, including heart disease, cancer, high cholesterol, cystitis, prostatitis, brain ageing, and inflammation [5].

Oxidative stress, transition metal accumulation, and – importantly – inflammation are linked to endoplasmic reticulum stress and endothelial dysfunction, and are thought to influence the pathology of neurodegenerative diseases, such as Parkinson's disease and Alzheimer's disease [6, 7], the progression of cancer (e.g., [8]), and also contribute to metabolic abnormalities such as atherosclerosis, Type 2 diabetes, and obesity (e.g., [9]). Thus, there is a strong link between inflammation, dysfunction, and negative health outcomes. The inflammatory response is a highly regulated process and several signaling transduction pathways with significant overlap and crosstalk have been implicated in inducing inflammation, and this chapter focuses on the potential of the flavonoids quercetin and kaempferol in the regulation of inflammatory processes.

CHEMICAL STRUCTURE

Quercetin (3,3',4',5,7-pentahydroxyflavone) and kaempferol (3,4',5,7-tetrahydroxyflavone) are flavonols with minor different structural characteristics in their aglycone form (Figure 1). Kaempferol can be synthesized by hydroxylation of the flavanone naringenin, followed by insertion of a double-bond at the C2-C3 position by flavonol synthetase. Naringenin itself can be synthesized by chalcone synthase through condensation of 4-coumaroyl-CoA with three malonyol-CoA [10]. More commonly, kaempferol is often found as glycosidic forms, with various sugars (e.g., glucose, rutinose, rhamnose, galactose) bonded to the kaempferol skeleton (Figure 1).

Although quercetin is also a metabolite of kaempferol, quercetin can be similarly synthesized through conversion of naringenin into firstly eriodictyol using flavanoid 3'-hydroxylase, and then secondly into dihydroquercetin by flavanone 3-hydroxylase. This intermediate is then converted into quercetin using flavonol synthase. Quercitrin, also known as 3-rhamnosylquercetin, is a frequently encountered conjugated form of quercetin. Much like kaempferol, the aglycone quercetin is frequently found conjugated to sugar moieties such as glucose or rutinose. In the United States, quercetin's dietary intake is estimated to range from 6–18 mg/day [11-13].

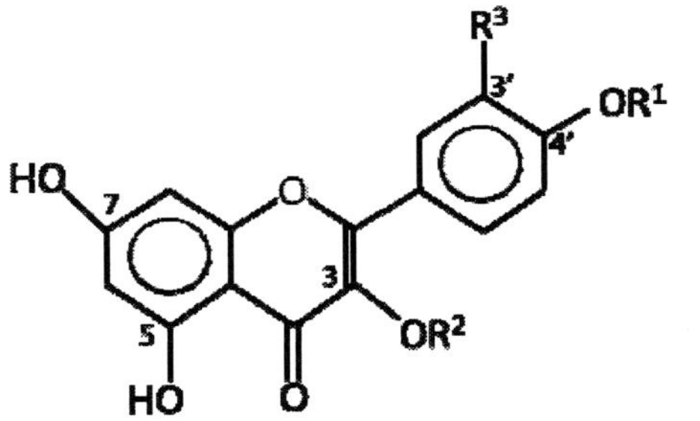

	R¹	R²	R³
Quercetin	H	H	OH
Quercetin 4'-monoglucoside	D-glucose	H	OH
Quercetin 3,4'-diglucoside	D-glucose	D-glucose	OH
Kaempferol	H	H	H
Kaempferol 3-glucoside	H	D-glucose	H

Figure 1. Basic chemical structure of quercetin and kaempferol. The aglycone form and some commonly consumed glucosides are indicated with their respective substitutions on R^1, R^2 and R^3.

BIOAVAILABILITY AND METABOLISM

The ability of biologically active (micro)nutrients to influence cellular function usually requires them to be bioavailable, including successful absorption from the gastrointestinal tract, and delivery to the peripheral blood system. Thus, bioavailability is traditionally correlated with the extent of absorption and subsequent serum level detection. However, if bioavailability of flavonoids is instead defined as reaching the intended target tissue [14], then for the tissues easily exposed to quercetin, kaempferol, and their metabolites, such as gastrointestinal epithelia, the bioavailability can often be considered much higher [15]. The quercetin glucosides are the major form of quercetin in foods. An early study in ileostomy patients suggested a 52% absorption of quercetin monoglucoside and diglucoside from an onion meal high in quercetin glucosides but with only trace amounts of quercetin taken up in its aglycone form [16]. However, in vitro studies with human intestinal Caco-2 cell monolayers demonstrated that the multidrug resistance-associated protein (MRP)-2 efficiently effluxed the 4'-β-glucoside across apical cell membranes [17], suggesting limited uptake and low serum concentrations of dietary quercetin glucosides. Subsequently, a study in the year 2000 with ileostomy patients, using a sophisticated analytical methodology for quantitating the intact glucosides and the quercetin aglycone, demonstrated that the dietary intake of 10.9 to 51.6 mg of quercetin mono- and diglucosides did not result in detectable amounts of quercetin glucosides in the ileostomy fluid. In stark contrast, 2.9 to 11.3 mg of the aglycone quercetin were detected, suggesting an absorption of 64.5 to 80.7% of total quercetin glucosides, followed by efficient hydrolysis in the small intestine by β-glucosidases to quercetin, most of which is then absorbed by the epithelium [18]. Variability in terms of absorption or uptake may depend on the plant source, and the type and linkage position of glucosides [15]. The oral intake of the aglycone quercetin results in poor absorption, which is attributed to the free hydroxyl groups allowing for rapid intestinal and hepatic conjugation and excretion [19, 20]. Accordingly, a daily supplementation of 1 g quercetin for 4 weeks increased plasma concentrations in humans only up to 1.5 µM, which may only provide limited health benefits [21]. Additionally, there appears to be a high interindividual variability in quercetin absorption, likely related to overall nutrient status and diet of the organism [22]. Once absorbed, quercetin is expected to undergo extensive first-pass metabolism in the liver by phase II enzymes, which includes glucuronidation, glycosylation, sulfation, isomeration, oxygenation, reduction or conjugation with glycine. Thus, low tissue and serum concentrations of the conjugated dietary forms of quercetin can be expected, but unconjugated forms may be produced by intestinal microflora or in-cell, resulting in relevant concentrations of quercetin in select tissues, with potentially beneficial effects on inflammation and oxidative stress. Intriguingly, recent studies using quercetin-loaded nanoparticles are pointing to increased membrane permeation and bioavailability [23], suggesting alternatives in therapeutic treatment strategies where quercetin has been shown to be of promise.

Although kaempferol is frequently consumed in substantial amounts, accounting for 25–33% of mean total flavonol intake in humans [11, 24], its oral bioavailability appears to be very low, and it demonstrates poor solubility [1, 25]. Co-administration with phytic acid appears to increase oral bioavailabltity in rats [26]; however, kaempferol is also a substrate for some ATP-binding cassette (ABC) transporters like the breast cancer resistance protein (BCRP, also known as ABCG2) and P-glycoprotein 1 (P-gp, also known as multidrug resistance protein 1 (MDR1) or ABCB1), thus regulating efflux of compounds such as kaempferol itself, and also quercetin [27, 28]. Additionally, in vitro studies have shown that any kaempferol taken up into the cell is readily conjugated by phase II enzymes, resulting primarily in uridine diphosphate glucuronic acid (UDGPA)-mediated formation of kaempferol-glucuronides [1]. Subsequently, *in vivo* experiments with rats indicated that neither orally nor intravenously administered kaempferol was detectable in serum after 24 hours, even at high doses of 25 mg/kg; however, both the parent compound as well as glucuronide metabolites were found in significant amounts in the urine following intravenous administration [1]. Much like quercetin, kaempferol is most frequently consumed as a conjucated form, such as kaempferol-3-glucuronide or kaempferol-3-glucoside (Figure 1). An earlier study reported on the total kaempferol concentrations in plasma or urine of human volunteers who had consumed tea (contained 49 mg quercetin and 27 mg kaempferol) and onions (contained 13 mg quercetin but no detectable kaempferol) for seven days [29]. However, it has remained unclear as to the extent the parent or conjugated forms of kaempferol contributed to the amounts detected in the clinical samples. In a small study completed in 2004, summer endives, which contained 8.65 mg kaempferol-equivalent as 79% kaempferol-3-glucuronide, 14% kaempferol-3-glucoside and 7% kaempferol-3-(6-malonyl)-glucoside, were fed to eight healthy human volunteers. Free kaempferol was detected in all plasma and urine samples, and 1.9% of the ingested amount were excreted [15]. Thus, it appears that the conjugated forms of kaempferol in the diet become un-conjugated at least to some extent, and are available for potential biological activity in the cells.

ANTI-OXIDATIVE AND RADICAL SCAVENGING ACTIVITIES

Whereas oxidation, which is the transfer of electrons from one atom to another, represents an essential part of aerobic life, the unbalanced condition between cellular oxidants and antioxidants leads to accumulation of free radicals or reactive oxygen and nitrogen species (reactive molecules with one or more unpaired electrons) in the cells, and subsequently results in oxidative stress [30, 31]. Generation of reactive oxygen and nitrogen species, especially in neutrophils and macrophages, can lead to lipid peroxidation, oxidative damage of nucleic acids and proteins, which frequently stimulates inflammatory mechanisms. Anti-oxidant mechanisms include suppressing reactive oxygen species formation or scavenging those free radicals in order to prevent the oxidation of other molecules by free radicals, and the potential for chelation of transition metals [32]. Humans have some endogenously produced anti-oxidative defenses, such as the enzymes glutathione peroxidase (GPX), thioredoxin reductase (TXNRD), catalase, and superoxide dismutase (SOD), which prevent formation of reactive oxygen species by metabolizing peroxides or by keeping non-enzymatic proteins important for this regulatory process, such as glutathione and thioredoxin, in their reduced states. Consumption of dietary anti-oxidants may also be helpful in attenuating the effects of oxidative damage, especially because humans are prone to excessively produced reactive oxygen and nitrogen levels (e.g., pollution, radiation, smoking) [5].

Among the flavonoids, the flavonols – which includes kaempferol and quercetin – appear to be the strongest anti-oxidants [33]. Both kaempferol and quercetin can help protect against lipid peroxidation through their anti-oxidative abilities, and thus free radicals can be prevented from removing electrons from the lipids in the cell membrane, which in turn can prevent cellular damage [34]. Direct evidence of anti-oxidative function has been demonstrated for both flavonoids in cell-free *in vitro* assays, where they were able to act as scavengers of superoxide anion, hypochlorous acid, chloramine, and nitric oxide, albeit not hydrogen peroxide [35]. Flavonoids can act as antioxidants by directly donating hydrogen to quench reactive oxygen species through the Michael acceptor function. Various investigations also reported anti-oxidative properties of kaempferol and/or quercetin using cell-based assays, including the protection of pancreatic beta cells from 2-deoxy-D-ribose-induced oxidative damage through the attenuation of ROS metabolism and lipid peroxidation by 10 µM kaempferol [36]. Treatment of human umbilical vein endothelial cells with kaempferol or quercetin at 5–50 µmol/L significantly decreased production of reactive oxygen and nitrogen species in a concentration-dependent manner [37]. There is increasing evidence for *in vivo* flavonoid anti-oxidant potential. Compared to untreated controls, animals treated with quercetin had significantly decreased levels of thiobarbituric acid reactive substances, which are byproducts of lipid peroxidation [38]. In a rat model of bladder injury, kaempferol was able to prevent formation of protamine sulfate-induced reactive oxygen species, which may likely have occurred though modulation of signaling pathways, including cyclooxygenase pathways [39]. Interestingly, kaempferol increased oxidative stress in glioblastoma cells, which in turn increased the production of reactive oxygen species accompanied by a decrease in the levels of the redox active proteins superoxide dismutase and thioredoxin, causing apoptosis to occur [40]. It also appears as if kaempferol may have a protective function in normal cells against oxidative stress, and induce oxidative stress in cancerous cells, pointing to an intriguing cell or tissue specificity in terms of the anti-oxidative nature of these flavonols [41].

Both kaempferol and quercetin have been shown to exert modulatory actions on endogenous anti-oxidative defense systems. Because the regulation of the redox state through oxidative stress is a key factor in the inflammatory process [42], quercetin and kaempferol may influence inflammation through regulation of intracellular signaling cascades and gene transcription. As a matter of fact, many of the biological effects of quercetin and kaempferol, and presumably other flavonoids, appear to be related to their ability to regulate cellular processes through modulation of cell-signaling pathways, rather than their direct anti-oxidant activity. These regulatory pathways include, but are not limited to, the NRF2 (nuclear factor (erythroid-derived 2)-like 2) pathway, nitric oxide synthase (NOS), cyclooxygenases (COX), mitogen-activated protein kinases (MAPK), redox-sensitive IκB kinase, and nuclear factor κ-light-chain-enhancer of activated B cells (NF-κB) pathways, which are further explained below. Importantly, substantial crosstalk among the various signaling pathways exists (Figure 2), suggesting a propensity for synergistic interactions kaempferol and quercetin may exert when activating or inhibiting a specific signaling pathway, and each only partially explains the pharmacological efficacy of flavonoids, such as quercetin and kaempferol as modulators of inflammation.

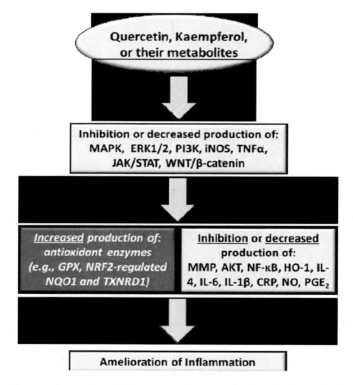

Figure 2. Inflammation can be ameliorated by quercetin, kaempferol or their metabolites through a wide array of signal transduction pathways. Substantial crosstalk among the signaling pathways exists. The various proteins may affect gene expression of anti-inflammatory pathways directly or indirectly, with tissue-specific targets, positive or negative feed-back mechanisms, and outcomes. For gene/protein abbreviations, please refer to the text.

REGULATION OF PRO-INFLAMMATORY PROSTAGLANDINS

Among the biomarkers affected by kaempferol and quercetin, prostaglandins and cytokines are important inflammatory mediators. Prostaglandins are a group of compounds enzymatically derived from fatty acids through arachidonic acid metabolism by cyclooxygenases, and are found in most tissues and organs. Whereas COX-1 (also known as prostaglandin-endoperoxide synthase 1, PTGS1) is constitutively expressed in many tissues, COX-2 (prostaglandin-endoperoxide synthase 2, PTGS2), which in most cells is usually not expressed under normal conditions, is inducible and produces prostaglandins in response to inflammation. Prostaglandin H2, the product of COX-2, is converted by prostaglandin E2 synthase (PGES) into prostaglandin E2 (PGE$_2$), which is increased during inflammation, and subsequently has been shown to promote cancer progression.

There have been many studies showing the effects of either quercetin or kaempferol on the expression of PGE$_2$-related inflammatory mediators. For example, unstimulated and IL-1β-induced proliferation of rheumatoid synovial fibroblast can be inhibited by quercetin, with subsequent inhibition of expression of matrix metalloproteinases (MMP), COX-2 and PGE$_2$ [43]. In another study, quercetin significantly suppressed COX-2 and PGE$_2$ production in human breast cancer cells, likely by inactivating the p300 signaling and blocking the binding of multiple transactivators, such as cAMP response element-binding protein (CREB)-2, C-JUN, and CCAAT/enhancer binding protein (C/EBP)-β, to the COX-2 promoter [44].

In a model of carrageenan induced rat air pouch, orally administered kaempferol at 50 and 100 mg/kg showed a significant inhibition of nitric oxide metabolite and PGE$_2$ production via modulation of the COX pathway [45]. Kaempferol also has been shown to suppress the release of nitric oxide and PGE$_2$ in histiocytic lymphoma/macrophage U937 cells, and the inhibition of gene expression for inducible nitric oxide synthase (iNOS), and COX-2 in lipopolysaccharide (LPS)- and sodium nitroprusside-treated mouse macrophage RAW264.7 cells and peritoneal macrophages [46].

iNOS is known to extend production of large amounts of nitric oxide, which likely results in a pro-inflammatory effect. Therefore, any compounds with the ability to suppress iNOS are considered to have anti-inflammatory effects, likely through inhibition of NF-κB and the signal transducer and activator of transcription 1 (STAT-1), two important transcription factors for iNOS [47].

Furthermore, in LPS-stimulated mouse microglial cells immortalized with a v-raf/v-myc recombinant retro-virus (macrophage-like BV2 cells), kaempferol significantly suppressed the expression of iNOS, COX-2, matrix metalloproteinase-3, attenuated LPS-induced nitric oxide, PGE$_2$, cytokine and reactive oxygen species production, and inhibited phagocytosis in a concentration-dependent manner, likely through the down-regulation of toll-like receptor-4, NF-κB, p38 MAPK, c-Jun N-terminal kinase (JNK) and the serine/threonine-specific kinase AKT [48], some of which are further discussed below. It should be noted that the suppression of PGE$_2$ production and inhibition of COX-2 expression is likely not unique to kaempferol and quercetin. Using activated macrophages, at least 10 other flavonoids, were shown to effectively inhibit LPS-induced PGE$_2$ production [47].

CYTOKINES AND NF-κB-MODULATED GENE EXPRESSION

Cytokines are a broad category of small, structurally-related, cell signaling proteins synthesized in the Golgi apparatus and produced by a range of cells, including immune cells such as macrophages, B lymphocytes, T lymphocytes and mast cells, as well as endothelial cells, fibroblasts, and various stromal cells. As such, cytokines include chemokines, interferons, interleukins (IL), lymphokines, and tumor necrosis factors (TNF), such as TNFα. There are various ways to classify cytokines: based on primary cell of origin, on structure, or their functional role in inflammatory responses. Several transcription factors, including NF-κB and activator protein-1 (AP-1), are crucial in the synthesis of cytokines such as TNFα [49]. In its inactivated state, the cytosolic NF-κB is complexed with the alpha inhibitory protein nuclear factor of κ light polypeptide gene enhancer in B-cells inhibitor, IκBα. Degradation of the ubiquitinated IκBα through the proteasome results in translocation of the activated NF-κB into the nucleus, where, either alone or in combination with other transcription factors such as AP-1 [50], it binds to response elements, eliciting gene expression. Particularly, IL-1, TNFα and IL-6 are cytokines known to drive the acute inflammatory response, and TNFα also regulates the growth, proliferation, differentiation, and viability of activated leukocytes. Downstream effects include production of hepatic C-reactive protein (CRP) in response to IL-6 (a cytokine with both pro- and anti-inflammatory effects [51]) secretion from macrophages and T-cells. The anti-inflammatory effects of flavonols, such as quercetin and kaempferol, can likely be explained by the correlation between inflammation and oxidative stress, and the involved regulation of NF-κB-modulated gene expression [52].

Quercetin has been shown to reduce oxidative stress and inflammatory biomarkers in a variety of models, both *in vitro* and *in vivo*, with studies spanning obesity, diabetes, cancer and other research. Quercetin has been shown to modulate NF-κB in human peripheral blood mononuclear cells, subsequently inhibiting both production as well as the gene expression of TNFα, which may possibly be mediated by the inhibition of the degradation of the inhibitory part (IκBα) of this transcription factor [53]. Primarily, the levels of pro-inflammatory cytokines, including IL-6, IL-1β, and TNFα, appear to be decreased in the presence of quercetin. Specifically, quercetin inhibited oxidative stress, reduced levels of pro-inflammatory cytokines, and increased activity of antioxidant enzymes, including SOD, catalase and GPX after traumatic brain injury in rats. This led to a reduced inflammatory response in the hippocampus, and the production of IL-6, IL-1β, and TNFα was decreased in the quercetin-treated groups compared to controls [38], whereas IL-10 was increased. LPS is a known trigger for inflammation-associated signal transduction, and in a model of LPS-induced acute lung injury through sepsis in mice, quercetin reduced expression of iNOS, COX-2 and NF-κB p65 phosphorylation, and inhibited IL-1β and IL-6, whereas secretion of IL-10 was increased [54]. Similarly, other groups were able to demonstrate that quercetin suppressed activation of the NF-κB pathway [55, 56], and thus inhibited inflammasome or nitric oxide production.

In a study by Zhang et al., using a rat brain intracerebral hemorrhage model, mRNA and protein expression of IL-1β, IL4, and TNFα (IL6: mRNA only) were downregulated with high doses (50mg/kg) of quercetin [57]. In another study, apple concentrate, which was composed of >90% quercetin or its glucosides/galactosides/rhamnoside/rutinosides, significantly reduced the LPS-induced serum inflammatory biomarkers IL-6 and CRP in rats, whereas IL-10 was elevated [58]. Takashima et al., reported that, in lung tissue, pro-inflammatory cytokines IL-6, IL-1β, and TNFα, secreted by macrophages, stimulated neutrophils, which, upon activation, released oxidants, proteases, leukotrienes and platelet activating factors, resulting in the development of respiratory distress. The authors used a model of chemically-induced acute respiratory distress syndrome in mice, and animals were intratracheally challenged with LPS in the absence and presence of quercetin pretreatment. A marked suppression in the mRNA expression and production of pro-inflammatory cytokines TNF-α, IL-1β, and IL-6 was observed with quercetin pretreatment [51]. Kumar et al., investigated the effects of quercetin in a diabetes model of retinal neurodegeneration, and found quercetin inhibited NF-κB and caspase-3 expression. Subsequently, levels of TNFα and IL-1β in retinas of quercetin-treated rats were significantly lower than untreated diabetic retinas [59]. In endothelial cells, quercetin, much like other flavonoids, such as luteolin and epigallocatechin gallate, reduced production of reactive oxygen species and inhibited endoplasmic reticulum stress-associated thioredoxin-interacting protein and nucleotide-binding oligomerization domain-like receptor pyrin domain containing-3 inflammasome activation, and led to down-regulation of IL-1β expression. Subsequently, endothelial cells were protected from inflammatory damage [60]. Interestingly, and contrary to much of the published literature, Kwon et al., reported that quercetin supplementation appeared to have no significant effect on inflammatory cytokine mRNA expression in skeletal muscle of mice [61], whereas in an earlier study, Le et al., reported that feeding mice a high fat diet for nine weeks resulted in obesity-induced skeletal muscle inflammation, which is closely associated with metabolic impairment. Dietary quercetin effectively reduced the protein levels of toll-like receptor 4, CD68 and monocyte chemoattractant protein-1, of the inflammatory cytokine TNFα, and as well as macrophage accumulation [62]. Furthermore, in a study to address the hepatoprotective effect of quercetin against cholestatic liver injury, quercetin affected superoxide dismutase and catalase mRNA expression, and attenuated recruitment/accumulation of inflammatory cells and bile duct ligation-induced oxidative stress [63]. Thus, quercetin has been shown to exert a wide range of anti-inflammatory effects in a variety of *in vitro* and *in vivo* models.

Various groups have investigated the effects of quercetin on inflammation in human clinical trials. The results, as they are for many nutritional intervention studies, are somewhat contradictory. Much of the controversy may be a result of the various forms of quercetin consumed, but may also depend on the population investigated, and the type of analyses (e.g., serum level cytokines *versus* tissue mRNA/protein expression). A number of groups have failed to find any links between quercetin supplementation and reduced inflammation in humans. For example, a double-blind, placebo-controlled, randomized clinical trial in community-dwelling adult females indicated that a 12-week supplementation with quercetin (500 or 1000 mg/day) had no influence on measures of innate immune function or inflammation biomarkers albeit significantly increased plasma quercetin levels [64]. A study in fifteen recreationally active, young adult men investigating the effect of quercetin consumption on performance of repeated sprints and inflammatory-marker response similarly found that quercetin supplementation in the form of quercetin-3-glucoside did not decrease IL-6 levels after sprint exercise. Furthermore, repeated-sprint performance was not improved by quercetin supplementation either, and was worse in the quercetin-treated group than in the placebo group when expressed as percent fatigue decrement [65]. However, as a study investigating the uptake of quercetin and quercetin glucuronide through the blood-brain barrier suggested, it appears that the non-conjugated quercetin and its methylated form isorhamnetin, but not quercetin-3-O-glucuronide, a major phase II metabolite of quercetin, are the bioactive forms. Thus, quercetin glucuronides may need to accumulate in specific types of cells, such as macrophages, and act as anti-inflammatory agents in the target tissue through deconjugation into the bioactive non-conjugated forms [66].

Contrary to the above mentioned negative trials, quercetin in combination with vitamin C reduced oxidative stress and inflammatory biomarkers c-reactive protein (CRP) and IL-6 in a small randomized double-blind clinical trial with healthy human subjects [67]. In another study, quercetin supplementation increased total plasma anti-oxidant capacity and reduced markers of oxidative stress and inflammation in the blood of sarcoidosis patients. The effects of quercetin supplementation appeared to be more pronounced in patients with higher baseline levels of oxidative stress and inflammation markers [68]. There are various clinical trials currently in process or recently completed (see: www.clinicaltrials.gov), where primary or secondary outcomes, for example, investigate effects of quercetin supplementation on the markers of oxidative stress, reactive oxygen species, and inflammation. Subjects have been or are being recruited from various populations, including (but not limited to) patients with chronic obstructive pulmonary disease, Fanconi anemia, or healthy volunteers. These studies will hopefully further elucidate the potential capacity of quercetin to function as an anti-oxidant or anti-inflammatory agent in humans.

Kaempferol has also been shown to modulate inflammation and oxidative stress in a variety of models, both *in vitro* and *in vivo*, and has been suggested to potentially temper effects of cardiovascular disease, diabetes, and cancer. Specifically, the expression of pro-inflammatory cytokines IL-1β, and TNFα appears to be affected, the two main cytokines that promote the activation of different enzymes in response to inflammation.

In an *in vitro* study using J744/2 macrophages, kaempferol substantially interfered with a number of different inflammation mechanisms. Treatment with kaempferol suppressed both IL-1β and TNFα mRNA levels, which inhibited their transcription and downstream effects. In addition, kaempferol has been demonstrated to be a disruptor of TNF-mediated operations [41]. A study using human embryonic kidney (HEK)-293 cells found that kaempferol was able to not only block TNF-induced IL-8 promotion but also IL-8 gene expression. Another inflammatory-signaling cytokine, IL-4, was inhibited by kaempferol, specifically targeting Janus kinase (JAK)-3 activity [41]. An *in vivo* study using female mice demonstrated that kaempferol suppressed UVB-induced COX-2 expression, likely by blocking Src kinase activity [36]. In a four-group mouse study, male C57BL/6 mice were used to determine the effect of kaempferol pretreatment on inflammation and oxidative stress following hemorrhagic shock. Compared to the hemorrhagic shock only group and the group that received kaempferol after the shock, the group pretreated with kaempferol had significantly decreased levels of the pro-inflammatory cytokines TNF-α and IL-6 [69]. Kaempferol and its glycosylated derivative, kaempferol-3-O-rhamnoside, inhibited the increase of Th2 cytokines (IL-4, IL-5, IL-13) and TNFα in a mouse model of allergic asthma. Total immunoglobulin E levels in serum were also blocked [70].

Human clinical trials with kaempferol appear to be lacking. However, several studies investigated total flavonol intake, which is, of course, mostly comprised of quercetin and kaempferol, and whose metabolites are detectable in serum. For example, in a four-year randomized, multi-center, nutritional intervention study, intake of low-fat, high-fiber, and high fruit/vegetable was correlated with a reduced serum level of IL-6. Furthermore, a decrease in IL-6 concentration was inversely associated with high-risk adenoma recurrence. The results are likely a combined effect of the flavonols, primarily kaempferol, quercetin and isorhamnetin, that are present in such a diet, but not of kaempferol by itself [71]. Any synergistic effects among flavonoids remain to be elucidated.

MODULATION OF NRF2/KEAP1/ARE PATHWAY EXPRESSION

The transcription factor nuclear factor (erythroid-derived 2)-like 2 (NFE2L2 or NRF2) is a basic leucine zipper protein with essential functions in the upregulation of anti-oxidant response element-mediated phase 2 enzymes in response to oxidative stress, injury and inflammation. Under normal or unstressed conditions, NRF2 is kept in the cytoplasm by Kelch like-ECH-associated protein 1 (KEAP1) and Cullin 3, which degrade NRF2 by ubiquitination. Much of NRF2 and KEAP1, is discussed in other chapters, because the isothiocyanate sulforaphane interacts with KEAP1 [72]. However, NRF2 also can be activated by various flavonoids, including kaempferol and quercetin, and activation of NRF2 occurs through protein kinase signaling pathways involved in inflammation, and is linked to several other signaling pathways that are further explained below. Thus we will briefly discuss NRF2-pathway function here, and its relation to kaempferol and quercetin in inflammation.

Under conditions of oxidative stress, NRF2-degradation is inhibited, and NRF2 is instead translocated to the nucleus, where it binds to the antioxidant response element (ARE), and transcription of anti-oxidative and anti-inflammatory genes is initiated. Subsequently, expression of phase II detoxifying enzymes and intracellular redox balancing proteins is enhanced. The prototypical NRF2-target is the phase II enzyme NAD(P)H quinone oxidoreductase 1 (NQO1), which prevents the one electron reduction of quinone as a detoxification reaction, and also stabilizes p53 [72-74]. It should be noted that the expression of redox balancing proteins are important for anti-oxidative and anti-inflammatory activities of other proteins, including thioredoxin (TRX), heme oxygenase (HO), and the NRF2-regulated selenoprotein TXNRD1, thus preventing oxidative and electrophilic insults [75].

There are many reports of quercetin and other flavonoids directly or indirectly modulating NRF2 in cell culture and animal models, subsequently inducing expression of NQO1 (e.g., [76-78]). Quercetin not only induces the nuclear translocation of NRF2, but also results in increased expression of the anti-oxidant responsive element (ARE)-dependent genes like heme oxygenase-1 (HO-1). This has been shown, for example, in human normal liver L-02 cells, possibly through inducing or activating p62 and JNK [79], in BV2 microglial cells [55], in trabecular meshwork cells [80], in rat dorsal root ganglion neurons [81], in human lung carcinoma A549 cells [82], and in mycotoxin-induced human hepatocarcinoma HepG2 cells, with subsequent down-regulation of COX2 [83]. NRF2-dependent modulation of the glutathione redox system also appears to be an important effect of quercetin's ability to modulate inflammation [84], because glutathione is important as an antioxidant and also as a signaling molecule in the regulation of innate immunity [85]. Animal models further support quercetin's action on NRF2. Zhang et al., [86] as well as Domitrović et al., [87] showed that quercetin increased the expression of NRF2 and HO-1 in carbon tetrachloride-induced acute liver injury in mice. The former also demonstrated up-regulation of peroxiredoxins and Txnrd1 mRNA upon intraperitoneally administered quercetin.

Although not as intensively studied as quercetin, similarly, kaempferol has also been shown to activate the NRF2 pathway in modified HepG2 cells [88], and to induce HO-1 expression by the aid of NRF2 translocation, as Gao et al., demonstrated using House Ear Institute-Organ of Corti 1 (HEI-OC1) cells [89]. Animal models supporting these observations unfortunately appear to be lacking for kaempferol thus far.

MODULATION OF PI3K/AKT PATHWAYS

The serine/threonine-specific kinase AKT (also known as protein kinase B, PKB) is involved in the phosphatidylinositol 3-kinase (PI3K)/AKT/mTOR and other signaling pathways, thus regulating a wide array of cellular functions relating to metabolism, proliferation, cell survival, mRNA and protein synthesis.

Phosphorylation of AKT is an indicator of the activation of PI3Ks, and PI3Ks are important targets in inflammation and immune diseases [90]. In mouse models, selective inhibition of PI3Ks has been shown to reduce the severity of inflammation [91]. It should be repeated, that the activation of protein kinase signaling pathways, including PI3K, can also mediate NRF2-translocation to the nucleus, thus suggesting the aforementioned cross talk between signaling cascades, and the importance of the NRF2-pathway in PI3K-mediated effects on inflammation.

Using human breast cancer cell lines lacking the tumor suppressor phosphatase and tensin homolog (PTEN), which as a result constitutively activates the AKT pathway, Gulati et al., were able to demonstrate that quercetin effectively inhibited cell proliferation by suppressing AKT activity [92]. Many other studies demonstrated similar inhibitory effects on PI3K-AKT signaling, such as reported in UVB-irradiated murine skin melanoma B16F10 cells [93], in cervical carcinoma HeLa cells [94], in human glioma cells in a time- and dose-dependent manner [95], as well as in mouse models of diet-induced nonalcoholic fatty liver disease [96] and Dalton's lymphoma [97]. In a similar fashion, kaempferol has also been shown to decrease PI3K/Akt pathways in human bladder cancer cells [98], in human HT-29 colon cancer cells likely though inhibiting insulin-like growth factor receptor and ERBB3 signaling [99], and in chronic myelogenous leukemia cell line K562 and in promyelocitic human leukemia U937 cells [100]. In mouse epidermal JB6 P+ cells, kaempferol competes with ATP binding to PI3K, neutralizing PI3K, and inhibits subsequent downstream activity of AKT and its transcription factors [41]. In a mouse model of allergic asthma, kaempferol and its glycosylated derivative, kaempferol-3-O-rhamnoside, inhibited increase of Th2 cytokines and TNFα through inhibition of AKT phosphorylation [70].

MODULATION OF MAPK/ERK/MEK/RAF/JNK PATHWAYS

The highly conserved family of mitogen-activated protein kinases (MAPK), which includes protein kinases with various isoforms, regulates gene expression, physiological and pathological cell proliferation, and apoptosis in response to stimuli, such as mitogens, osmotic stress, heat shock and pro-inflammatory cytokines. Increased activity of MAPK regulates synthesis of inflammation mediators at the level of transcription and translation, make the MAPK proteins potential targets for anti-inflammatory compounds. Important MAPK include the c-Jun N-terminal kinases (JNK) and the extracellular signal-regulated kinase (ERK) 1/2 pathway, which has the RAF (rapidly accelerated fibrosarcoma) proteins as upstream regulators [101, 102]. RAF proteins are not only essential connectors between RAS and the MAPK-kinase (MEK)/ERK pathway, but also play a role in the regulation of apoptosis and cell migration. It should be noted, that there are many different signaling proteins interacting with the proteins of the MAPK, ERK, MEK pathways [103], providing many angles for flavonoids to influence cell signaling as it relates to inflammation. Quercetin and kaempferol appear to modulate MAPK and its associated signaling proteins in various cell culture models. For example, Lee et al., showed that quercetin inhibited MEK-1 and RAF1 kinase activities in mouse skin epidermal (JB6 P+) cells [104], and Cho et al., demonstrated quercetin's inhibitory effects on MAPK and NF-κB and subsequent suppression of pro-inflammatory cytokine production in LPS-stimulated macrophages [105]. Quercetin also markedly reduced activation of ERK, p38 MAPK, and NF-κB in co-cultured mouse myotubes/macrophages [62], and suppressed the RAS/MAPK/ERK and PI3K/AKT signaling pathways in glioma cells, thus promoting senescence and apoptosis in a model of the most common and malignant primary brain tumors [106].

Kaempferol impacts the MAPK pathway at various points, and, depending on the cell type or conditions, appears to have both inhibitory as well as activating effects. In adherent PC12 cells maintained under low serum conditions for 16 hours, 60 μM kaempferol caused a prolonged ERK activation, preventing oxidative damage in these cells [107], and 70 μM kaempferol induced MAPK activation in human lung cancer A549 cells while inhibiting AKT and phosphorylated AKT [108]. In contrast, Huang et al., demonstrated that kaempferol suppressed LPS-induced MAPK pathways in human monocyte THP-1 cells, including inhibiting the phosphorylation of the upstream regulators c-raf and MEK1/2. Subsequently, the production of monocyte-derived chemokines, such as IL-8, was inhibited [109]. Similarly, intragastrical administration of large amounts of kaempferol (100mg/kg) prior to intranasal instillation of LPS attenuated pulmonary edema in mice with acute lung injury by significantly inhibiting MAPK and NF-κB signaling pathways [110], and kaempferol also inhibited IL-1β-stimulated phosphorylation of ERK 1/2, p38 and JNK MAP kinases in osteoclasts from 6-week old mice [111] and in human U-2 OS osteosarcoma cells [112].

MODULATION OF WNT/ β-CATENIN SIGNALING PATHWAYS

The WNT/β-catenin signaling pathway can play a regulatory role in the inflammatory response to infections caused by pathogenic bacteria. As an intracellular signal transducer in the WNT signaling pathway, β-catenin regulates the coordination of cell–cell adhesion and gene transcription, and is itself controlled through its ubiquitination and proteosomal degradation by the β-catenin destruction complex. In the absence of a WNT stimulus, β-catenin is constantly phosphorylated by the casein kinase Iα (CKIα) and the serine/threonine protein kinase glycogen synthase kinase (GSK) 3β [113]. It has been reported that the phosphorylation of a protein by GSK3β to promote or suppress an inflammatory response is tissue-specific. Furthermore, there appears to be considerable crosstalk to other signaling pathways. Pro-inflammatory stimuli, including TNFα, IFNγ, and NO, are able to increase the expression proteins within the WNT/β-catenin signaling pathway [113]. Recent data also suggest crosstalk with NRF2 through its participation in a protein complex with AXIN1, which is regulated by the canonical WNT pathway [114], and also through GSK3β, which in the active state prepares NFR2 as well as β-catenin for proteasomal degradation [40].

Quercetin, in models of human colon cancer SW480 cells and human embryonal kidney HEK293 cells, inhibited the transcriptional activity of β-catenin by decreasing the nuclear concentration of β-catenin and the transcriptional coactivator of transcription factors [115]. In other studies, the metabolism of β-catenin was modified by quercetin both directly and through activated endocannabinoids receptor in colon cancer cells [116], and quercetin also inhibited the WNT/β-catenin signaling pathway and subsequent nuclear translocation of β-catenin in B-1 lymphocytes [117] and in human teratocarcinoma NT2/D1 cells [118].

Kaempferol, on the other hand, has been less described in relation to WNT/β-catenin signaling. One study reported that kaempferol inhibited WNT signaling in β-catenin-activated human embryonal kidney HEK293 cells [119], and another study showed that a kaempferol derivative, kaempferol-3-methyl ether, inhibited β-catenin in a cell-based luciferase assay [120].

CONCLUSION

Kaempferol and quercetin are two of the most common flavonoids and widely distributed in fruits, herbs, and vegetables including Brassicaceae (broccoli). Numerous scientific reports have linked either or both flavonoids to beneficial anti-oxidative and anti-inflammatory regulation. Not surprisingly, many diseases have been linked to acute or chronic inflammation, including cancer, obesity, and allergies. This chapter described some of the diverse mechanisms through which the flavonoids kaempferol and quercetin are thought to regulate the expression of pro-inflammatory cytokines, which includes direct and indirect modulation of a wide range of signaling kinases (Figure 2), including, but not limited to, NRF2/KEAP1, IκB Kinases α and β [53], AKT/PKB, PI3K [92], MAPK [105], JAK/STAT, and also cell cycle-regulatory molecules, such as cyclins, and cyclin dependent kinases [121]. Many of these signaling pathways are involved in a number of cellular processes, including those related to the inflammatory response, and significant crosstalk points to involvement of NRF2-signaling pathways at various levels.

The idea of kaempferol and/or quercetin ameliorating diseases by suppressing the inflammatory response may be constrained due to limited bioavailability of quercetin and kaempferol beyond tissues of the gastrointestinal tract because of efflux and extensive metabolism. However, bioavailability depends on the other foods consumed (e.g., dietary fat has been shown to improve quercetin bioavailability by increasing its absorption [122]), and de-conjugation of glucuronidated flavonoids is possible in tissues or by intestinal microbes. Data from food-based clinical trials or those with quercetin thus far have yielded conflicting or inconclusive results, and trials with kaempferol as the sole compound appear to be lacking. However, the apparent pleiotropic functions of both kaempferol and quercetin and their propensity for synergistic interactions, including those related to the NRF2-signaling pathway, continue to render them intriguing compounds for therapeutic efforts in inflammation and other diseases.

REFERENCES

[1] Barve A, Chen C, Hebbar V, Desiderio J, Saw C, Kong A. Metabolism, oral bioavailability and pharmacokinetics of chemopreventive kaempferol in rats. *Biopharm. Drug Dispos.* 2013;30(7):356-65.
[2] Kelly G. Quercetin. Monograph. Altern Med Rev. 2011;16(2):172-94.
[3] Nishimuro H, Ohnishi H, Sato M, Ohnishi-Kameyama M, Matsunaga I, Naito S, et al., Estimated daily intake and seasonal food sources of quercetin in Japan. 7. 2015;4(45-58).
[4] Vallejo F, Tomas-Barberan F, Ferreres F. Characterisation of flavonols in broccoli (Brassica oleracea L. var. italica) by liquid chromatograpghy-UV diode-array detection-electrospray ionisation mass spectrometry. *Journal of Chromatography.* 2004;1054(1-2):181-93.
[5] Pietta PG. Flavonoids as antioxidants. *J. Natur Prod.* 2000;63(7):1035-42.
[6] Guo H, Callaway J, Ting J. Inflammasomes:mechanism of action, role in disease, and therapeutics. *Nature Medicine.* 2015;21(7).
[7] Ramassamy C. Emerging role of polyphenolic compounds in the treatment of neurodegenerative diseases: a review of their intracellular targets. *European Journal of Pharmacology.* 2006;545(1):51-64.
[8] Fichtner-Feigl S, Kesselring R, Strober W. Chronic inflammation and the development of malignancy in the GI tract. Trends Immunol. 2015.
[9] Strowig T, Henao-Mejia J, Elinav E, Flavell R. Inflammasomes in health and disease. *Nature* 2012;481(7381):278-86.
[10] Kim BG, Joe EJ, Ahn JH. Molecular characterization of flavonol synthase from poplar and its application to the synthesis of 3-O-methylkaempferol. *Biotechnol. Lett.* 2010;32(4):579-84.
[11] Sampson L, Rimm E, Hollman P, de Vries J, Katan M. Flavonol and Flavone Intakes in US Health Professionals. *Journal of the American Dietetic Association.* 2002;102(10):1414-20.
[12] Wang L, Lee I, Zhang S, Blumberg J, Buring J, Sesso H. Dietary intake of selected flavonols, flavones, and flavonoid-rich foods and risk of cancer in middle-aged and older women. *The American Journal of Clinical Nutrition.* 2009;89(3):905-12.
[13] Winkel-Shirley B. Flavonoid Biosynthesis. A Colorful Model for Genetics, Biochemistry, Cell Biology, and Biotechnology. *Plant Physiol.* 2001;126(2):485-93.
[14] Walle T. Absorption and metabolism of flavonoids. *Free Radic. Biol. Med.* 2004;36(7):829-37.
[15] DuPont M, Day A, Bennett R, Mellon F, Kroon P. Absorption of kaempferol from endive, a source of kaempferol-3-glucuronide, in humans. *European Journal of Clinical Nutrition.* 2004;58:947-54.

[16] Hollman P, de Vries J, van Leeuwen S, Mengelers M, Katan M. Absorption of dietary quercetin glycosides and quercetin in healthy ileostomy volunteers. *J. Clin. Nutr.* 1995;62(6):1276-82.

[17] Walgren RA, Karnaky KJ, Lindenmayer GE, Walle T. Efflux of dietary flavonoid quercetin 4'-b-glucoside across human intestinal Caco-2 cell monolayers by apical multidrug resistance-associated protein2. *J. Pharmacol. Exp. Ther.* 2000;294(3):830-6.

[18] Walle T, Otake Y, Walle U, Wilson F. Quercetin glucosides are completely hydrolyzed in ileostomy patients before absorption. *Journal of Nutrition.* 2000;130(11):2658-61.

[19] Otake Y, Hsieh F, Walle T. Glucuronidation versus oxidation of the flavonoid galangin by human liver microsomes and hepatocytes. *Drug Metab. Dispos.* 2002;30:576-81.

[20] Walle T, Ta N, Kawamori T, Wen X, Tsuji PA, Walle UK. Cancer chemopreventive properties of orally bioavailable flavonoids - methylated versus unmethylated flavones. *Biochem. Pharmacol.* 2007;79(9):1288-96.

[21] Conquer J, Maiani G, Azzini E, Raquzzini A, Holub B. Supplementation with quercetin markedly increases plasma quercetin concentration without effect on selected risk factors for heart disease in healthy subjects. *Journal of Nutrition* 1998;128(3):593-7.

[22] Guo Y, Mah E, Bruno R. Quercetin bioavailability is associated with inadequate plasma vitamin C status and greater plasma endotoxin in adults. *Nutrition.* 2014;30(11-12):1279-86.

[23] Testa G, Gamba P, Badilli U, Gargiulo S, Maina M, Guina T, et al., Loading into nanoparticles improves quercetin's efficacy in preventing neuroinflammation induced by oxysterols. *PLoS One.* 2014;9(5):e96795.

[24] Hertog M, Hollman P, Katan M, Kromhout D. Intake of potentially anticarcinogenic flavonoids and their determinants in adults in The Netherlands. *Nutr. Cancer.* 1993;20(1):21-9.

[25] Chen Z, Sun J, Chen H, Xiao Y, Liu D, Chen J, et al., Comparative pharmacokinetics and bioavailability studeis of quercetin, kaempferol and isorhamnetin after oral administration of Ginkgo biloba extracts, Ginkgo biloba extract phospholipid complexes and Ginkgo biloba extract solid dispersions in rats. *Fitoterapia.* 2010;81(8):1045-52.

[26] Xie Y, Luo H, Duan J, Hong C, Ma P, Li G, et al., Phytic acid enhances the oral absorption of isorhamnetin, quercetin, and kaempferol in total flavones of Hippophae rhamnoides L. *Fitoterapia.* 2014;93:216-65.

[27] An G, Gallegos J, Morris M. The bioflavonoid kaempferol is an Abcg2 substrate and inhibits Abcg2-mediated quercetin efflux. *Drug Metab. Dispos.* 2011;39(3):426-32.

[28] Zhang S, Yang X, Coburn R, Morris M. Structure activity relationships and quantitative structure activity relationships for the flavonoid-mediated inhibition of breast cancer resistance protein. *Biochem. Pharmacol.* 2005;70(4):627-39.

[29] De Vries J, Hollman P, Meyboom S, Buysman M, Zock P, van Staveren W, et al., Plasma concentrations and urinary excretion of the antioxidant flavonols quercetin and kaempferol as biomarkers for dietary intake. *Am. J. Clin. Nutr.* 1998;68(1):60-5.

[30] Chiavaroli V, Giannini C, De Marco S, Chiarelli F, Mohn A. Unbalanced oxidant-antioxidant status and its effect in pediatric diseases. *Redox Rep.* 2011;16(3):101-7.

[31] Boots A, Haenen G, Bast A. Health effects of quercetin: from antioxidant to nutraceutical. *Eur. J. Pharmacol.* 2008;585(2-3):325-37.

[32] Rice-Evans CA. Flavonoid antioxidants. *Curr. Med. Chem.* 2001;8:797-807.

[33] Burda S, Oleszek W. Antioxidant and antiradical activities of flavonoids. *J. Agric. Food Chem.* 2001;49(6):2774-9.

[34] Galinn SE, Hartman J, Tsuji PA. Diet and Cancer. In: Caballero B, Finglas, Toldra, editors. Encylopedia of Food and Health. Oxford, U.K.: Elsevier; (in press).

[35] Vellosa J, Regasini III L, Khalil IV N, Bolzani III V, Khalil V O, Manente I F, et al., Antioxidant and cytotoxic studies for kaempferol, quercetin and isoquercitrin. *Ecletica Quimica.* 2011;36(2).

[36] Lee K, Lee K, Junh S, Lee E, Heo Y, Bode A, et al., Kaempferol inhibits UVB-induced COX-2 expression by suppressing Src kinase activity. *Biochem. Pharmacol.* 2010;80(12):2042-9.

[37] Crespo I, Garcia-Mediavilla M, Gutierrez B, Sanchez-Campos S, Tunon M, Gonzalez-Gallego J. A comparison of the effects of kaempferol and quercetin on cytokine-induced pro-inflammatory status of cultured human endothelial celss. *Br. J. Nutr.* 2008;100(5):968-76.

[38] Yang T, Kong B, Gu J-W, Kuang Y-Q, Cheng L, Yang W-T, et al., Anti-apoptotic and Anti-oxidative Roles in Quercetin After Traumatic Brain Injury. *Cell Mol. Neurobiol.* 2014;34:797-804.

[39] Huang Y, Lin M, Chao Y, Huang C, Tsai Y, Wu P. Anti-oxidant activity and attenuation of bladder hyperactivity by the flavonoid compound kaempferol. *International Journal of Urology.* 2013;21(1):94-8.

[40] Jiang Y, Bao H, Ge Y, Tang W, Cheng D, Luo K, et al., Therapeutic targeting of GSK3β enhances the Nrf2 antioxidant response and confers hepatic cytoprotection in hepatitis C. *Gut.* 2013;64(1):168-79.

[41] Chen A, Chen Y. A review of the dietary flavonoid, kaempferol on human health and cancer chemoprevention. *Food Chemistry.* 2013;138:2009-107.

[42] Fernandez V, Tapia G, Varela P, Romanque P, Cartier-Ugarte D, Videla L. *Comparative Biochemistry and Physiology Part C: Toxicology and Pharmacology.* 142. 2006;3-4(231-239).

[43] Sung M, Lee E, Jeon H, Chae H, Park S, Lee Y, et al., Quercetin inhibits IL-1b-induced proliferation and production of MMPs, COX-2, and PGE2 by rheumatoid synovial fibroblast. *Inflammation* 2012;35(4):1585-94.

[44] Xiao X, Shi D, Liu L, Wang J, Xie X, Kang T, et al., Quercetin suppresses cyclooxygenase-2 expression and angiogenesis through inactivation of P300 signaling. *PLoS One.* 2011;6(8):e22934.

[45] Mahat MY, Kulkarni NM, Vishwakarma SL, Khan FR, Thippeswamy BS, Hebballi V, et al., Modulation of the cyclooxygenase pathway via inhibition of nitric oxide production contributes to the anti-inflammatory activity of kaempferol. *Eur. J. Pharmacol.* 2010;642(1-3):169-76.

[46] Kim S, Park J, Sung G, Yang S, Yan W, Kim E, et al., Kaempferol, a dietary flavonoid, ameliorates acute inflammatory and nociceptive symptoms in gastrisis pancreatitis, and abdominal pain. *Molecular Nutrition & Food Research* 2015.

[47] Hämäläinen M, Nieminen R, Vuorela P, Heinonen M, Moilanen E. Anti-inflammatory effects of flavonoids: genistein, kaempferol, quercetin, and daidzein inhibit STAT-1 and NF-kB activations, whereas flavone, isorhamnetin, naringenin, and pelargonidin inhibit NF-kB activation along with their inhibitory effect on iNOS expression and NO production in activated macrophages. *Mediators of Inflammation.* 2007;2007:1-10.

[48] Park S, Sapkota K, Kim S, Kim H, Kim S. Kaempferol acts through mitogen-activated protein kinases and protein kinase B/AKT to elicit protection in a model of nueroinflammation in BV2 microglial cells. *Br. J. Pharmacol.* 2011;164(3):1008-25.

[49] McInnes IB, Schett G. Cytokines in the pathogenesis of rheumatoid arthritis. *Nat. Rev. Immunol.* 2007;4(6):429-42.

[50] Rahman I, Gilmour P, Jimenez L, MacNee W. Oxidative stress and TNF-alpha induce histone acetylation and N-kappaB/AP-1 activation in alveolar epithelial cells: potential mechanism in gene transcription in lung inflammation. *Mol. Cell Biochem.* 2002;234-235(1-2):239-48.

[51] Takashima K, Matsushima M, Hashimoto K, Nose H, Sato M, Hashimoto N, et al., Protective effects of intratracheally administered quercetin on lipopolysaccharide-induced acute lung injury. *Respiratory Research.* 2014;15(150).

[52] Nair MP, Mahajan S, Reynolds J, Aalinkeel R, Nair H, Schwartz S, et al., The flavonoid quercetin inhibits proinflammatory cytokine (tumor necrosis factor alpha) gene expression in normal peripheral blood mononuclear cells via modulation of the NF-kappa beta system. *Clin. Vaccine Immunol.* 2006;13(3):319-28.

[53] Peet G, Li J. IkappaB kinases alpha and beta show a random sequential kinetic mechanism and are inhibited by staurosporine and quercetin. *J. Biol Chem.* 1999;274(46):32655-61.

[54] Wang L, Chen J, Wang B, Wu D, Li H, Lu H, et al., Protective effect of quercetin on lipopolysaccharide-induced acute lung injury in mice by inhibiting inflammatory cell influx. *Exp. Biol. Med. (Maywood).* 2014;239(12):1653-62.

[55] Kang C, Choi Y, Moon S, Kim W, Kim G. Quercetin inhibits lipopolysaccharide-induced nitric oxide production in BV2 microglial cells by suppressing the NF-kB pathway and activating the Nrf2-dependent HO-1 pathway. *Int. Immunopharmacol.* 2013;17(3):808-13.

[56] Zhang Q, Pan Y, Wang R, Kang L, Xue Q, Wang X, et al., Quercetin inhibits AMPK.TXNIP activation and reduces inflammatory lesions to improve insulin signaling defect in the hypothalamus of high fructose-fed rats. *J. Nutr. Biochem.* 2014;25(4):420-8.

[57] Zhang Y, Yi B, Ma J, Zhang L, Zhang H, Yang Y, et al., Quercetin promotes neuronal and behavioral recovery by suppressing inflammatory response and apoptosis in a rat model of intracerebral hemorrhage. *Neurochem. Res.* 2015;40(1):195-203.

[58] Sekhon-Loodu S, Catalli A, Kulka M, Wang Y, Shahidi F, Rupasinghe H. Apple flavonols and n-3 polyunsaturated fatty acid-rich fish oil lowers blood C-reactive protein in rats with hypercholesterolemia and acute inflammation. *Nutr. Res.* 2014;36(6):535-43.

[59] Kumar N, Gupta S, Naq T, Srivastava S, Saxena R, Jha K, et al., Retinal neuroprotective effects of quercetin in streptozotocin-induced diabetic rats. *Exp. Eye Res.* 2014;125:193-202.

[60] Wu J, Xu X, Li Y, Kou J, Huang F, Liu B, et al., Quercetin, luteolin and apigallocatechin gallate alleviate TXNIP and NLRP3-mediated inflammation and apoptosis with regulation of AMPK in endothelial cells. *European Journal of Pharmacology.* 2014;745:59-68.

[61] Kwon S, Park H, Jun J, Lee W. Exercise, but not quercetin, ameliorates inflammation, mitochondrial biogenesis, and lipid metabolism in skeletal msucle after strenuous exercise by high-fat diet mice. *J. Exerc. Nutrition Biochem.* 2014;18(1):51-60.

[62] Le N, Kim C, Park T, Park J, Sung M, Lee D, et al., Quercetin protects against obesity-induced skeletal muscle inflammation and atrophy. *Mediators Inflamm.* 2014.

[63] Lin S, Wang Y, Chen W, Chuang Y, Pan P, Chen C. Beneficial effect of quercetin on cholestatic liver injury. *J. Nutr. Biochem.* 2014;25(11):1183-95.

[64] Heinz S, Henson D, Nieman D, Austin M, Jin F. A 12-week supplementation with quercetin does not affect natural killer cell activity, granulocyte oxidative burst activity or granulocyte phagocytosis in female human subjects. *Br. J. Nutr.* 2010;104(6):849-57.

[65] Abbey E, Rankin J. Effect of quercetin supplementation on repeated-sprint performance, xanthine oxidase activity, and inflammation. *Int. J. Sport Nutr. Exerc. Metab.* 2011;21(2):91-6.

[66] Ishisaka A, Mukai R, Terao J, Shibata N, Kawai Y. Specific localization of quercetin-3-O-glucuronide in human brain. *Archives of Biochemistry and Biophysics.* 2014;557:11-7.

[67] Askari G, Ghiasvand R, Feizi A, Ghanadian S, Karimian J. The effect of quercetin supplementation on selected markers of inflammation and oxidative stress. *J. Res. Med. Sci.* 2012;17(7):637-41.

[68] Boots A, Drent M, de Boer V, Bast A, Haenen G. Quercetin reduces markers of oxidative stress and inflammation in sarcoidosis. *Clin. Nutr.* 2011;30(4):506-12.

[69] Yang Q, He L, Zhou X, Zhao Y, Shen J, Xu P, et al., Kaempferol pretreatment modulates systemic inflammation and oxidative stress following hemorrhagic shock in mice. *Chinese Medicine.* 2015;10(6):1-7.

[70] Chung M, Pandey R, Choi J, Sohng J, Choi D, Park Y. Inhibitory effects of kaempferol-3-O-rhmnoside on ovalbumin-induced lung inflammation in a mouse model of allergic asthma. 25. 2015(302-310).

[71] Bobe G, Albert P, Sansbury L, Lanza E, Schatzkin A, Colburn N, et al., Interleukin-6 as a Potential Indicator for Prevention of High Risk Adenoma Recurrence by Dietary Flavonols in the Polyp Prevention Trial. *Cancer Prev. Res.* 2010;3(6):764-75.

[72] Kensler TW, Egner PA, Agyeman AS, Visvanathan K, Groopman JD, CHen TY, et al., Keap1-nrf2 signaling: a target for cancer prevention by sulforaphane. *Top. Curr. Chem.* 2013;329:163-77.

[73] Nioi P, McMahon M, Itoh K, Yamamoto M, Hayes JD. Identification of a novel Nrf2-regulated antioxidant response element (ARE) in the mouse NAD(P)H;quinone oxidoreductase 1 gene: reassessment of the ARE consensus sequence. *Biochem. J.* 2003;374:337-48.

[74] Talalay P, Fahey JW, Holtzclaw WD, Prestera T, Zhang Y. Chemoprotection against by phase 2 enzyme induction. *Toxicol. Lett.* 1995;82-83:173-9.

[75] Kou X, Kirberger M, Yang Y, Chen N. Natural prodcuts for cancer prevention associated with Nrf2-ARE pathway. *Food Science and Human Wellness* 2013;2:22-8.

[76] Dinkova-Kostova AT, Fahey JW, Talalay P. Chemical structures of inducers of nicotinamide quinone oxidoreductase 1 (NQO1). *Methods in Enzymology.* 2004;382:423-49.

[77] Fahey JW, Stephenson KK. Pinostrobin from honey and Thai ginger (Boesenbergia pandurata): a potent flavonoid inducer of mammalian phase 2 chemoprotective and antioxidant enzymes. *J. Agric. Food Chem.* 2002;50:7472-6.

[78] Tsuji PA, Stephenson KK, Wade KL, Liu H, Fahey JW. Structure-activity analysis of flavonoids: direct and indirect antioxidant, and anti-inflammatory potencies and toxicities. *Nutrition and Cancer: An international journal.* 2013;65(7):1014-25.

[79] Ji LL, Sheng YC, Zheng ZY, Shi L, Wang ZT. The involvement of p62-Keap1-Nrf2 antioxidative signaling pathway and JNK in the protextion of natural flavonoid quercetin against hepatotoxicity. *Free Radic. Biol. Med.* 2015;85:12-23.

[80] Miyamoto N, Izumi H, Miyamoto R, Kondo H, Tawara A, Sasaguri Y, et al., Quercetin induces the expression of peroxiredoxins 3 and 5 via the Nrf2/NRF1 transcription pathway. *Invest Ophtalmol. Vis. Sci.* 2011;52(2):1055-63.

[81] Shi Y, Liang X, Zhang H, Wu Q, Qu L, Sun Q. Quercetin protects rat dorsal root ganglion neurons against high glucose-induced injury in vitro through Nrf-2/HO-1 activation and NF-kB inhibition. *Acta Pharmacol. Sin.* 2013;34(9):1140-8.

[82] Zerin T, Kim YS, Hong SY, Song HY. Quercetin reduces oxidative damage induced by paraquat via modulating expression of antioxidant genes in A549 cells. *J. Appl. Toxicol.* 2013;33(12):1460-7.

[83] Ramyaa P, Krishnaswamy R, Padma VV. Quercetin modulates OTA-induced oxidative stress and redox signalling in HepG2 cells - up regulation of Nrf2 expression and down regulation of NF-κB and COX-2. *Biochim. Biophys. Acta.* 2014;1840(1):681-92.

[84] Arredondo F, Echeverry C, Abin-Carriquiry JA, Blasina F, Antúnez K, Jones DP, et al., After cellular internalization, quercetin causes Nrf2 nuclear translocation, increases glutathione levels, and prevents neuronal death against an oxidative insult. *Free Radic. Biol. Med.* 2010;49(5):738-47.

[85] Ghezzi P. Role of glutathione in immunity and inflammation in the lung. *Int. J. Gen. Med.* 2011;4:105-13.

[86] Zhang JQ, Shi L, Xu XN, Huang SC, Lu B, Ji LL, et al., Therapeutic detoxificatin of quercetin against carbon tetrachloride-induced acute liver injury in mice and its mechanism. *J. Zheijang Univ Sci B.* 2014;15(12):1039-47.

[87] Domitrović R, Jakovac H, Vasiljev Marchesi V, Vladimir-Knežević S, Cvijanović O, Tadić Z, et al., Differential hepatoprotective mechanisms of rutin and quercetin in CCl(4)-intoxicated BALB/cN mice. *Acta Pharmacol. Sin.* 2012;33(10):1260-70.

[88] Saw C, Guo Y, Yang AY, Paredes-Gonzalez X, Ramirez C, Pung D, et al., The berry constituents quercetin, kaempferol, and pterostilbene synergistically attenuate reactive oxygen species: involvement of the Nrf2-ARE signaling pathway. *Food Chem. Toxicol.* 2014;72(303-311).

[89] Gao SS, Choi BM, Chen XY, Zhu RZ, Kim Y, So H, et al., Kaempferol suppresses cisplatin-induced apoptosis via inductions of heme oxygenase-1 and glutamate-cysteine ligase catalytic subunit HEI-OC1 cell. *Pharm Res.* 2010;27(2):235-45.

[90] Ghigo A, Damilano F, Braccini L, Hirsch E. PI3K inhibition in inflammation: Toward tailored therapies for specific diseases. *Bioessays.* 2010;32(2):185-96.

[91] Hawkins PT, Stephens LR. PI3K signalling in inflammation. *Biochim. Biophys. Acta.* 2015;1851(6):882-97.

[92] Gulati N, Laudet B, Zohrabian V, Murali R, Jhanwar-Uniyal M. The antiproliferative effect of Quercetin in cancer cells is mediated via inhibition of the PI3K-Akt/PKB pathway. *Anticancer Res.* 2006;26(2A):1177-81.

[93] Rafiq RA, Quadri A, Nazir LA, Peerzada K, Ganai BA, Tasduz SA. A Potent Inhibitor of Phosphoinositide 3-Kinase (PI3K) and Mitogen Activated Protein (MAP) Kinase Signalling, Quercetin (3, 3', 4', 5, 7-Pentahydroxyflavone) Promotes Cell Death in Ultraviolet (UV)-B-Irradiated B16F10 Melanoma Cells. *PLoS One.* 2015;10(7):e0131253.

[94] Xiang T, Fang Y, Wang SX. Quercetin suppresses HeLa cells by blocking PI3K/Akt pathway. *J. Huazhong Univ. Sci. Technolog. Med. Sci.* 2014;34(5):740-4.

[95] Endale M, Parkm S, Kim S, Kim S, Yang Y, Cho J, et al., Quercetin disrupts tyrosine-phosphorylated phosphatidylinositol 3-kinase and myeloid differentiation factor-88 associatio, and inhibits MAPK/AP-1 and IKK/NF-kB-induced inflammatory mediators production in RAW 264.7 cells. *Immunobiology.* 2013;218(12):1452-67.

[96] Pisonero-Vaquero S, Martínez-Ferreras Á, García-Mediavilla MV, Martínez-Flórez S, Fernández A, Benet M, et al., Quercetin ameliorates dysregulation of lipid metabolism genes via the PI3K/AKT pathway in a diet-induced mouse model of nonalcoholic fatty liver disease. *Mol. Nutr. Food Res.* 2015;59(5):879-93.

[97] Maurya AK, Vinayak M. Quercetin regresses Dalton's lymphoma growth via suppression of PI3K/AKT signaling leading to upregulation of p53 and decrease in energy metabolism. *Nutr Cancer.* 2015;67(2):354-63.

[98] Xie F, Su M, Qiu W, Zhang M, Guo Z, Su B, et al., Kaempferol promotes apoptosis in human bladder cancer cells by inducing the tumor suppressor, PTEN. *Int. J. Mol. Sci.* 2013;14(11):21215-26.

[99] Lee HS, Cho HJ, Kwon GT, Park JH. Kaempferol Downregulates Insulin-like Growth Factor-I Receptor and ErbB3 Signaling in HT-29 Human Colon Cancer Cells. *J. Cancer Prev.* 2014;19(3):161-9.

[100] Marfe G, Tafani M, Indelicato M, Sinibaldi-Salimei P, Reali V, Pucci B, et al., Kaempferol induces apoptosis in two different cell lines via Akt inactivation, Bax and SIRT3 activation, and mitochondrial dysfunction. *J. Cell Biochem.* 2009;106(4):643-50.

[101] Kaminska B. MAPK signalling pathways as molecular targets for anti-inflammatory therapy--from molecular mechanisms to therapeutic benefits. *Biochim. Biophys. Acta.* 2005;1754(1-2):253-62.

[102] Kyriakis JM, Avruch J. Mammalian MAPK signal transduction pathways activated by stress and inflammation: a 10-year update. *Physiol. Rev.* 2012;92(2):689-737.

[103] Matallanas D, Birtwistle M, Romano D, Zebisch A, Rauch J, von Kriegsheim A, et al., Raf family kinases: old dogs have learned new tricks. *Genes Cancer.* 2011;2(3):232-60.

[104] Lee K, Kang N, Heo Y, Rogozin E, Pugliese A, Hwang M, et al., Raf and MEK protein kinases are direct molecular targets for chemopreventive effect of quercetin, a major flavonol in red wine. *Cancer Res.* 2008;68(3):946-55.

[105] Cho S, Park S, Kwon M, Jeong T, Bok S, Choi W, et al., Quercetin suppresses proinflammatory cytokines production through MAP kinases and NF-kappaB pathway in lipopolysaccharide-stimulated macrophage. *Mol. Cell Biochem.* 2003;243(1-2):153-60.

[106] Pan HC, Jiang Q, Yu Y, Mei JP, Cui YK, Zhao WJ. Quercetin promotes cell apoptosis and inhibits the expression of MMP-9 and fibronectin via the AKT and ERK signalling pathways in human glioma cells. *Neurochem. Int.* 2015;80:60-71.

[107] Hong JT, Yen JH, Wang L, Lo YH, Chen ZT, Wu MJ. Regulation of heme oxygenase-1 expression and MAPK pathways in response to kaempferol and rhamnocitrin in PC12 cells. *Toxicol. Appl. Pharmacol.* 2009;237(1):59-68.

[108] Nguyen TT, Tran E, Ong CK, Lee SK, Do PT, Huynh TT, et al., Kaempferol-induced growth inhibition and apoptosis in A549 lung cancer cells is mediated by activation of MEK-MAPK. *J. Cell Physiol.* 2003;197(1):110-21.

[109] Huang CH, Jan RL, Kuo CH, Chu YT, Wang WL, Lee MS, et al., Natural flavone kaempferol suppresses chemokines expression in human monocyte THP-1 cells through MAPK pathways. *J. Food Sci.* 2010;75(8):H254-9.

[110] Chen X, Yang X, Liu T, Guan M, Feng X, Dong W, et al., Kaempferol regulates MAPKs and NF-κB signaling pathways to attenuate LPS-induced acute lung injury in mice. *Int. Immunopharmacol.* 2012;14(2):209-16.

[111] Lee WS, Lee EG, Sung MS, Yoo W. Kaempferol inhibits IL-1β-stimulated, RANKL-mediated osteoclastogenesis via downregulation of MAPKs, c-Fos, and NFATc1. *Inflammation.* 2014;37(4):1221-30.

[112] Chen HJ, Lin CM, Lee CY, Shih NC, Peng SF, Tsuzuki M, et al., Kaempferol suppresses cell metastasis via inhibition of the ERK-p38-JNK and AP-1 signaling pathways in U-2 OS human osteosarcoma cells. *Oncol. Rep.* 2013;30(2):925-32.

[113] Silva-Garcia O, Valdez-Alarcon J, Baizabal-Aguirre V. The Wnt/b-catenin Signaling Pathway Controls the Inflammatory Response in Infections Caused by Pathogenic Bacteria. *Mediators of Inflammation.* 2014.

[114] Rada P, Rojo AI, Offergeld A, Feng GJ, Velasco-Martín JP, González-Sancho JM, et al., WNT-3A regulates an Axin1/NRF2 complex that regulates antioxidant metabolism in hepatocytes. *Antioxid. Redox Signal.* 2015;22(7):555-71.

[115] Park C, Chang J, Hahm E, Park S, Kim H, Yang C. Quercetin, a potent inhibitor against B-catenin/Tcf signaling in SW480 colon cancer cells. *Biochemical and Biophysical Research Communications.* 2005; 328(1):227-34.

[116] Refolo MG, D'Alessandro R, Malerba N, Laezza C, Bifulco M, Messa C, et al., Anti Proliferative and Pro Apoptotic Effects of Flavonoid Quercetin Are Mediated by CB1 Receptor in Human Colon Cancer Cell Lines. *J. Cell Physiol.* 2015;(in press).

[117] Novo MC, Osugui L, dos Reis VO, Longo-Maugéri IM, Mariano M, Popi AF. Blockage of Wnt/β-catenin signaling by quercetin reduces survival and proliferation of B-1 cells in vitro. *Immunobiology.* 2015;220(1):60-7.

[118] Mojsin M, Vicentic JM, Schwirtlich M, Topalovic V, Stevanovic M. Quercetin reduces pluripotency, migration and adhesion of human teratocarcinoma cell line NT2/D1 by inhibiting Wnt/β-catenin signaling. *Food Funct.* 2014;5(10):2564-73.

[119] Park S, Choi J. Inhibition of beta-catenin/Tcf signaling by flavonoids. *J. Cell Biochem.* 2010;110(6):1376-85.

[120] Park HY, Toume K, Arai MA, Koyano T, Kowithayakorn T, Ishibashi M. β-Sitosterol and flavonoids isolated from Bauhinia malabarica found during screening for Wnt signaling inhibitory activity. *J. Nat. Med.* 2014;68(1):242-5.

[121] Casagrande F, Darbon J. Effects of structurally related flavonoids on cell cycle progression of human melanoma cells: regulation of cyclin-dependent kinases CDK2 and CDK1. *Biochem. Pharmacol.* 2001;61(10):1205-15.

[122] Guo Y, Mah E, Davis C, Jalili T, Ferruzzi M, Chun O, et al., Dietary fat increases quercetin bioavailability in overweight adults. *Mol. Nutr. Food Res.* 2013;57(5):896-905.

In: Broccoli
Editor: Bernhard H. J. Juurlink

ISBN: 978-1-63484-313-3
© 2016 Nova Science Publishers, Inc.

Chapter 8

RADIOMITIGATING POTENTIAL OF SULFORAPHANE, A CONSTITUENT OF BROCCOLI

Paban K. Agrawala[∗] *and Omika Katoch*

Department of Radiation Genetics and Epigenetics,
Institute of Nuclear Medicine and Allied Sciences, Delhi, India

ABSTRACT

Broccoli, a cole crop belonging to the cruciferae family, originated in Italy. Broccoli is a nutrient powerhouse with phytochemicals such as dithiolthiones, s-methyl cysteine sulfoxide, indole-3-carbinol, glucosinolates such as glucoraphanin, isothiocyanates, indoles, etc. Broccoli is an excellent source of vitamins A (in the form of carotenoids), B1, B3, B5, B6, B9, C, E, and K. It is also a very good source of calcium, chromium, copper, iron, magnesium, manganese, phosphorus, potassium, selenium, zinc as well as choline, omega-3 fatty acids and dietary fiber. Besides its nutritional properties, broccoli also shows health benefits including cancer prevention, cholesterol reduction, detoxification, anti-inflammatory effects and improved digestion. The isothiocyanate sulphoraphane significantly suppresses oxidative stress and inflammation. Sulforaphane and indole-3-carbinol present in broccoli have protective effects against cancer. These phytochemicals boost detoxifying enzymes and promote expression of antioxidant enzymes, thereby reducing oxidative stress. They also may affect estrogen levels which may help reduce breast cancer risk. Recently we have shown that sulforaphane mitigates radiation-induced DNA damage as studied in terms of micronuclei formation in human lymphocytes following radiation administration. Sulforaphane also inhibited the rise in histone deacetylase activity that normally is a consequence of irradiation. In this chapter we discuss the ability of sulforaphane to increase the viability, using MTT, XTT and CyQuant methods, of several cell types following radiation exposure. Estimation of reactive oxygen species (ROS) formation using H_2-DCF-DA fluorescent dye showed a reduction in radiation-induced ROS levels in sulforaphane-treated group.

[∗] Corresponding author: Paban K. Agrawala. Institute of Nuclear Medicine and Allied Sciences, Division of Radiation Biosciences, Brig SK Mazumdar Marg, Timarpur, Delhi 110054, India. E: mail: paban@inmas.drdo.in, tel: 91-11-23905187, fax: 91-11-23919509.

Sulforaphane also increased the acetylation status of histone H4. H4 acetylation has a role in DNA damage repair. Overall, reduction of ROS and increased histone acetylation may be important mechanisms responsible for radiation damage mitigation.

INTRODUCTION

Broccoli (*Brassica oleracea*), a member of the cruciferae family is a cool season cole crop. Originally, broccoli was cultivated in Italy under the name of "*Broccolo.*" The name is derived from the Latin word 'brachium' meaning 'branch' or 'arm' and describes broccoli's branching pattern. Broccoli is closely related to cauliflower, requires a sandy type of soil, with a temperature as low as 40°F, whose pH range from slight acidic to neutral for its cultivation. The colour of this vegetable can range from deep sage to dark green to purplish-green depending upon the variety.

Nutritional Value

Broccoli contains important phytochemicals like glucosinolates, dithiolthiones, indoles, glucoraphanin, s-methyl cysteine sulfoxide, isothiocyanates and indole-3-carbinol. Cruciferous vegetables including broccoli are the dietary source of glucosinolates, a large group of sulfur-containing glucosides. The enzyme myrosinase (EC 3.2.1.147, thioglucoside glucohydrolase) is a member of the family of enzymes involved in plant defense against herbivores and converts glucosinolates into isothiocyanates. In intact tissue myrosinase remains physically separated from glucosinolates; upon chewing that allows the plant myrosinase to come into contact with glucosinolates, glucosinolates are converted to isothiocyanates and other metabolites.

Intact glucosinolates that reach the intestine can be converted to isothiocyanates and other metabolites by intestinal microbes. Isothiocyanates are absorbed from the small bowel and colon, and metabolites are detectable in human urine two to three hours after consumption of brassica vegetables [1]. Isothiocyanates are further metabolized by glutathione-S-transferases (GSTs) to mercapturic acid. The urine isothiocyanate metabolites concentrations are directly related to the dietary intake of cruciferous vegetables [2].

Cooking modifies the glucosinolate-myrosinase system by partial or complete inactivation of myrosinase, loss of enzymic cofactors such as epithiospecifier protein, thermal breakdown and/or leaching of glucosinolates and their metabolites or volatilisation of metabolites. Consumption of raw brassica (containing active plant myrosinase) leads to the release of glucosinolate breakdown products in the upper gastrointestinal tract while the consumption of cooked brassica (devoid of plant myrosinase) results in glucosinolate hydrolysis in the colon by gut microflora [3].

The anti-cancer property of broccoli is due to its isothiocyanates (e.g., sulforaphane) and indole -3- carbinol (I3C) a hydrolysis product of glucobrassicin. The I3C molecules undergo acid condensation in the acidic environment of the stomach to form biologically active compounds such as 3, 3'-diindolylmethane (DIM) [4]. Broccoli is an excellent source of micronutrients. For example it is a good source of vitamins A (in the form of carotenoids), B1, B3, B5, B6, B9, C, E, and K.

It is also a very good source of calcium, chromium, copper, iron, magnesium, manganese, phosphorus, potassium, selenium, zinc as well as choline, omega-3 fatty acids and dietary fibre.

Health Benefits of Sulforaphane

Sulforaphane (SFN), a metabolite of glucoraphanin, is the most widely studied isothiocyanate derived from glucosinolates found in broccoli.

Sulforphane and cancer: Cancer is induced by genetic and epigenetic changes leading to the uncontrolled proliferation, apoptosis, differentiation and migration. Inadequate detoxification of carcinogens in the body, chronic inflammation and oxidative stress increase the risk of cancer development. SFN can inhibit the development and proliferation of cancer cells by targeting various signaling pathway, inhibiting Phase I enzymes and inducing Phase II enzymes [5] (See Chapter 4 for phase I and II enzymes).

SFN is reported to inhibit growth, activate apoptosis in cancer cells, upregulate HDAC activity and suppress expression of key proteins involved in breast cancer progression. SFN treatment results in the generation of ROS and induction of ROS-mediated signaling may contribute to at least some of its chemopreventive properties [6-8].

SFN inhibits the proliferation and progression of cancer by arresting the cell cycle through inhibition of cyclins that together with cyclin-dependent kinases (CDKs) drive the cell from one phase of the cycle to the next. SFN also inhibits angiogenesis and microtubule formation, thereby inhibiting metastasis. SFN down-regulates inflammation markers such as TNF-α, IL-1, NO and PGE2 [9] through decreasing NF-κB signalling.

Sulforaphane in kidney diseases and diabetes: Nrf2-mediated upregulation of phase II enzymes by SFN and reduction in ROS results in the protection from cytotoxicity induced by hypoxia-reoxygenation [10] and renal damage including glomerular, tubulointerstatial and endothelial alteration [11].

Pretreatment of streptozotocin-treated mice with SFN resulted in maintenance of normal insulin secretion and prevents the development of Type 1 diabetes [12]. This protective effect of SFN is mediated by activation of the Nrf2 signaling pathway. Activation of Nrf2 signaling by SFN reduces oxidative stress, prevents hyperglycemia-induced activation of hexosamine and protein kinase C (PKC) and prevents increased cellular accumulation of the glycating agent methylglyoxal [13].

Sulforaphane and genotoxicity: Recently, we have shown that SFN ameliorated radiation-induced genotoxicity in lymphocytes of people accidentally exposed to radiation. Of significance is that SFN was used at low concentrations following exposure to radiation.

Specifically, we have shown the ability of SFN to protect $CD34^+$ cells in peripheral blood against radiation induced lethality [14]. SFN was shown to increase the acetylation status of histones that normally are reduced following radiation exposure.

In the current study we show the increased viability of several cell types by SFN using various methods of cell viability assay. Levels of cellular and mitochondrial reactive oxygen species (ROS) were measured fluorometrically and the global acetylation status of individual histones were determined by ELISA.

MATERIAL AND METHODS

Lymphocyte Isolation and Culture

Blood from healthy volunteers were collected by trained personals in BD vacutainers and lymphocytes were isolated using Histopaque 1077 (Sigma) and cultured using RPMI as described earlier [14].

Culture of HUVEC and MRC-5 Cells

HUVEC cells were purchased from PromoCells, Germany and cultured in endothelial cell growth medium with growth factor supplements (PromoCells GmbH, Germany). MRC-5 cells were cultured in DMEM supplemented with 10% FBS and antibiotics.

Irradiation and SFN Treatment

A Co^{60} gamma source (Teletharapy unit, Bhabatron, Panacea) was used to irradiate the cells with desired dose (5 Gy) of radiation at a dose rate of 1 Gy per min. Dosimetry of the irradiator was performed using ion chamber dosimetry and Fricke's method.

A stock solution of sulforaphane (Sigma) was prepared in dimethyl sulfoxide (DMSO) and further dilutions were made in Hank's Balanced Salt Solution (HBSS) as per requirement and added to culture medium.

Ethical Statement

All the experiments were carried out in strict accordance with the guidelines laid down by the institutional ethical committee. Collection and use of human lymphocyte for the experiments was duly approved by the Institutional Regulatory Board (IRB approval letter INM/TS/IEC/01/2012) and all blood samples were collected with proper consents by trained medical technicians of the institute.

Metabolic Viability Assays

3-(4,5-Dimethylthiazol-2-yl)-2,5-Diphenyltetrazolium Bromide (MTT) and 2,3-bis (2-methoxy-4-nitro-5-sulfophenyl)-5-[(phenylamino) carbonyl]-2H-tetrazolium hydroxide (XTT) viability assays were performed using HUVEC, MRC-5 and human lymphocytes. MTT assay was performed essentially as described earlier [15]. Briefly, 10000 cells were seeded per well of a 96 well plate. These were administered 5 Gy radiation and/or the desired concentrations of sulforaphane before adding 20 µl of MTT (5 mg/ml stock in PBS) for 2 h at 24 or 48 h post-irradiation time. The formazan developed was dissolved in 200 µl DMSO after carefully removing the medium (for lymphocyte cultures a centrifugation for 10 min was done before removing medium) and optical density (OD) recorded at 570 nm on a SpectraMax M2 multimodal plate reader (Molecular Devices, US).

XTT assay was performed using cell proliferation assay kit (Roche Diagnostics GmbH, Germany) as per the instructions provided by the manufacturer.

Briefly, 10000 cells/well in Broccoli, a cole crop belonging to the cruciferae family treatments administered. At the end of 24 or 48 h of treatment 50 µl XTT solution and electron coupling reagent mixture was added to the wells. After 4 h of incubation at 37°C absorbance was read at 450 nm with a reference wavelength of 650 nm.

Cell Proliferation Assay

CyQuant cell proliferation assay (Invitrogen, UK) was followed as per instructions and DNA content measured [16]. Briefly, 0.5×10^3 cells were seeded per well of a black cell culture plate compatible for flourimetry. 24 and 48 h after various treatments cells were processed as per the manufacturer's instructions and fluorescence was recorded with Ex/Em 480/520 nm using a multimodal plate reader (SpectraMax M2, Molecular Devices, US).

Determination of Free Radicals

2',7'-Dichlorodihydroflurescein diacetate (H_2-DCFDA) fluorescent probe (Invitrogen, UK) was used for the fluorometric detection of reactive oxygen species (ROS) in cells [15]. Briefly cells were plated and treated as described earlier. Cells were treated with 10 µM H_2-DCFDA at desired time intervals for 30 min and fluorescence was recorded using a multimodal plate reader (SpectraMax M2, Molecular Devices, US).

Acetylation Status of Histones

Acetylation status of H2A, H2B, H3 and H4 histones were studied using PathScan® Sandwich ELISA kit from Cell Signaling Technology, US as per the manufacturer's instructions. Briefly, cell lysates were prepared with cell lysis buffer provided with the kit and stored at -80°C until analysis. 100 µl of diluted (1:1) cell lysate from each treatment groups were added to the wells of respective histone antibody coated plates, incubated overnight at 4°C and the instructions for detection were followed. The OD values were read within 30 min of adding 100 µl of stop solution at 450 nm spectophotometrically.

Statistics

Data are presented as mean ± SD of three independent experiments. Students' *t*-test was employed to determine the level of significance and $P < 0.05$ was considered significant.

RESULTS

MTT Assay

Metabolic viability, determined using MTT assay, showed a significant time-dependent reduction in viability of all cell types (HUVEC, MRC-5 and lymphocytes) following exposure to 5 Gy γ-radiation. SFN treatment alone rendered no toxic effects at any time point (24 or 48 h) or doses (40 nM or 400 nM) in all cell types. SFN (400 nM) treatment given 2 h post-irradiation caused a significant increase in metabolic viability in all cell types compared to irradiated group alone and was comparable to untreated control values.

For HUVEC, SFN (400 nM) administered 2 h after irradiation resulted in a significant increase ($P < 0.05$) in MTT reduction at 48 h time point compared to irradiation group: this increase in MTT reduction was not seen at 24 h time point.

40 nM SFN had no significant impact on metabolic viability of HUVECs at either of the time points studied. It should be pointed out that neither of the SFN concentrations alone had any toxic effect on HUVECs at any of the two time points (Figure 1a). With MRC-5 (Figure 1b), 40 nM SFN was observed to be more effective in countering radiation induced reduction of metabolic viability at both time points, however the values were not statistically different from the 400 nM SFN dose.

For lymphocytes collected from healthy volunteers both concentration of SFN were equally effective in protecting against radiation damage at both time points examined (Figure 1c). SFN alone showed no toxicity for any of the cell types examined.

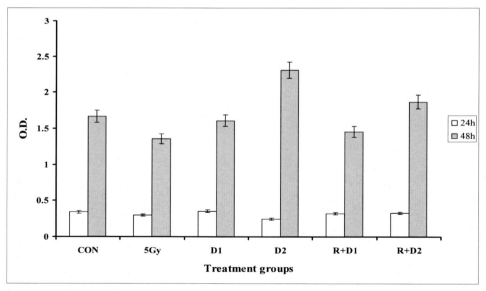

a

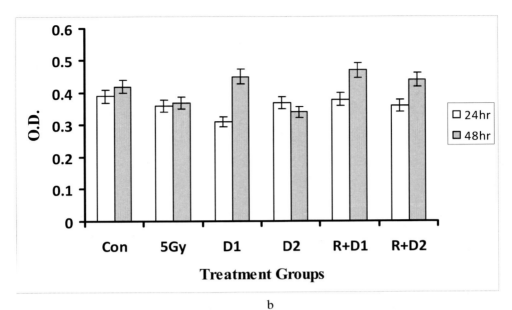

b

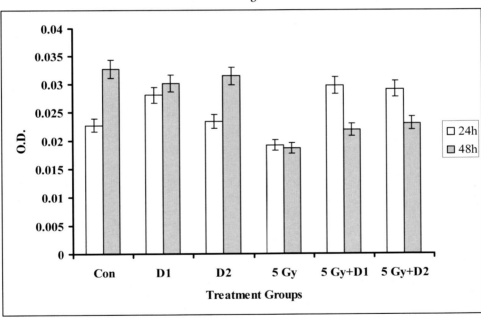

c

Data represents mean ± SD of three independent experiments.

Figure 1. Effect of sulforaphane on metabolic viability of irradiated a) HUVEC, b) MRC-5 and c) human lymphocytes using MTT assay. Cells were exposed to 5 Gy γ-radiation, (D1) 40 or (D2) 400 nM SFN or radiation along with SFN. MTT reduction was measured at 24 and 48 h.

XTT Assay

The XTT assay has the advantageous over the MTT assay in that there is no need to dissolve the formazan product developed in DMSO or acid-alcohol since the formazan developed in XTT assay is water soluble and can be read directly. The results obtained with XTT assay (Figure 2a-c) correlated well with the MTT assay for all the three cell types studied.

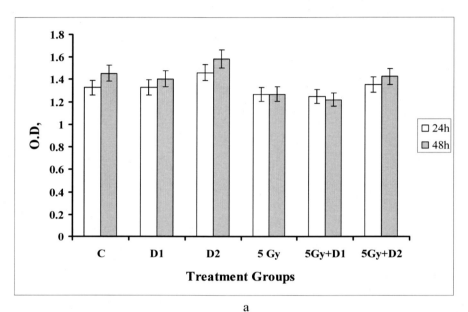

a

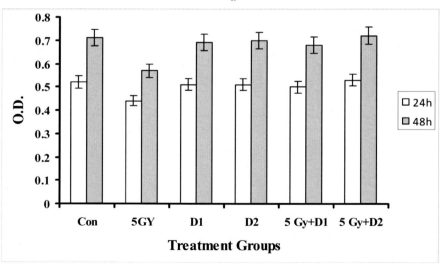

b

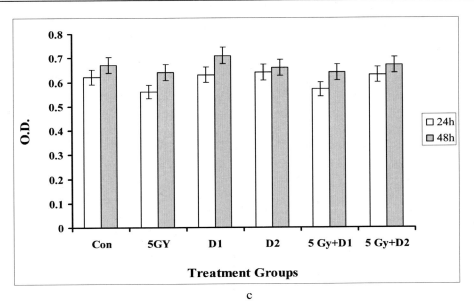

c

Data represents mean ± SD of three independent experiments.

Figure 2. Effect of sulforaphane on cell proliferation assay using XTT cell proliferation assay kit of irradiated a) HUVEC, b) MRC-5 and c) human lymphocytes. Cells were exposed to 5 Gy γ-radiation, (D1) 40 or (D2) 400 nM SFN or radiation along with SFN. XTT was added at 24 and 48 h and the water soluble formazan was measured spectrophotometrically.

CyQuant Cell Proliferation Assay

The CyQuant assay for cell proliferation was performed only with cultured lymphocytes. Both the concentration of SFN (40 nM and 400 nM) alone were shown to have no effect on cell proliferation as the fluorescence intensity remained comparable to that of untreated control at both 24 and 48 h time points. 5 Gy exposure showed significant ($P < 0.05$) decrease in fluorescence (478.32 ± 43.34 vs 728.32 ± 17.29 and 730.77 ± 31.82 vs 1224.48 ± 30.71 at 24 and 48 h respectively) intensity. SFN plus radiation showed comparable fluorescence intensity to the control group at both drug concentrations and at both the time points (Figure 3).

Determination of ROS

ROS was measured in human lymphocyte cultures 30 min post-SFN treatment time. Note that SFN was administered at 2 h post-irradiation time.

Untreated control, 40 nM and 400 nM SFN treatment were observed to have no significant difference in fluorescence intensity (Figure 4) indicating that SFN treatment had no effect on cellular free radical generation.

Irradiation (5 Gy) however showed a significant ($P < 0.05$) increase in DCF-DA fluorescence (217.49 ± 13.97) compared to control (165.97 ± 12.44) at 30 min time point.

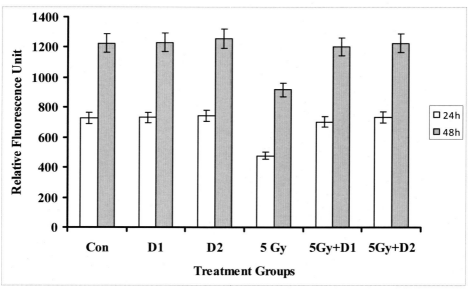

Data represents mean ± SD of three independent experiments.

Figure 3. CyQuant cell proliferation assay in human lymphocytes depicting the effect of radiation and sulforaphane. Cells were exposed to 5 Gy γ-radiation, (D1) 40 or (D2) 400 nM SFN or radiation along with SFN. Lymphocyte cultures in 96-well plates were centrifuged and plates were kept at -80°C at 24 or 48 h of various treatments. After repeated freeze-thaw, CyQuant nucleic acid staining was performed and fluorescence was measured.

SFN at both concentrations led to significant reductions in radiation-induced free radical generation with the values being comparable to untreated control values.

ELISA Assay for Histone Acetylation Status

Sandwich ELISAs with antibodies against H2A, H2B, H3 and H4 were performed with human lymphocytes at different time points (1, 2, 4 and 24 h post-treatment) using PathScan ELISA kit (Figure 5a-d). A 5 Gy irradiation led to a temporary but significant ($P < 0.05$) increase in H2A acetylation status compared to untreated control cells up to the 2 h post-irradiation time and then tended to revert back to control levels from 4 h onwards (Figure 5a).

SFN administration (400 nM) caused a steady increase in H2A acetylation from 4 h to 24 h in the control cells and further increased in the cells also exposed to radiation (note that SFN was administered 2 h following irradiation). H2B histone acetylation was increased significantly only at 2 h post-irradiation time in case of 5 Gy group. SFN treatment increased acetylation only at the 24 h point and SFN increased the acetylation status of the irradiated cells at the 24 h point.

A 5 Gy exposure led to significant decrease in H3 acetylation compared to control at 1 h, 2 h and 4 h but increased at 24 h where the values were comparable to control value. SFN alone induced a temporary significant increase in H3 acetylation at 4 h and the values became comparable to control value at 24 h. SFN further decreased H3 acetylation at 4 h but at 24 h it was comparable to control values.

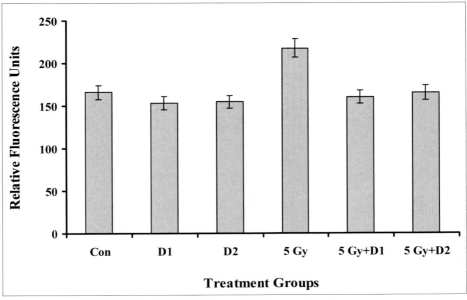

Data represents mean ± SD of three independent experiments.

Figure 4. ROS determination using H_2-DCFDA in human lymphocytes irradiated with 5 Gy and its modification by sulforaphane post-irradiation administration. Lymphocyte cultures in 35 mm culture dishes were exposed to 5 Gy, SFN 400 nM or both. 30 min after SFN administration time, DCF-DA was added and after 30 min of incubation at 37°C fluorescence was recorded.

In case of H4 acetylation status, a 5 Gy exposure led to a significant decrease at 1 h and reverted back to control values from 2 h onwards. SFN alone induced an increase in acetylation from 4 h onwards which was similar in the case of SFN plus radiation group.

DISCUSSION

SFN has been studied extensively as a potent activator of Nrf2 [17], Nrf2 regulates a broad network of more than 500 genes with versatile cytoprotective functions [18]. Besides its ability to reduce oxidative stress induced by UV radiation, Kantko et al. have shown SFN to reduce the levels of proinflammatory cytokines such IL-6, IL-1β and COX-2 [18].

Recently SFN's ability to inhibit histone deacetylases has been reported by several researchers [14, 19-20]. Senanayake et al. have shown the ability of SFN to modulate renal methylation in hypertensive stroke-prone rats and to normalize methylated deoxycytosine levels. The normalized methyl deoxycytidine was related to improved blood pressure in these rats [21]. Katoch et al. have shown that nanomolar concentrations of SFN administered hours after radiation exposure of human lymphocytes reduces radiation-induced cytogenetic damage without affecting the nuclear division index [14]. SFN was also found effective in reducing micronuclei in lymphocyte cultures of accidentally exposed individuals where the blood was collected several days after radiation exposure.

Under post-irradiation treatment scenarios where radiation-induced DNA damage has already taken place any antioxidant treatment is less likely to have any ameliorating effect on

DNA damage like strand breaks, micronuclei or chromosomal aberration, etc., unlike in pre-irradiation treatment scenario where manifestation of damage to DNA can be reduced by the scavenging of free radicals.

The observed reduction of DNA damage in post-irradiation administration scenario therefore could be due to enhancement of DNA repair or accelerated removal of cells harbouring DNA damage.

The current study aimed at evaluating the potential of SFN post-irradiation treatment in enhancing cell viability in different cell types such as HUVEC, MRC-5 and human lymphocytes and studying the acetylation pattern of H2A, H2B, H3 and H4 histones.

MTT and XTT assays performed over 48 h time periods clearly demonstrated that SFN post-irradiation administration at nano-molar concentrations (40 nM and 400 nM) enhanced cell viability (Figure 1 and 2). The cell proliferation assay with CyQuant dye showed enhanced proliferation compared to irradiated group (Figure 3).

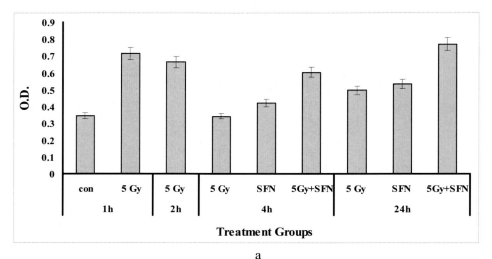

a

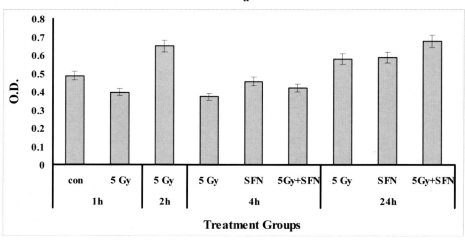

b

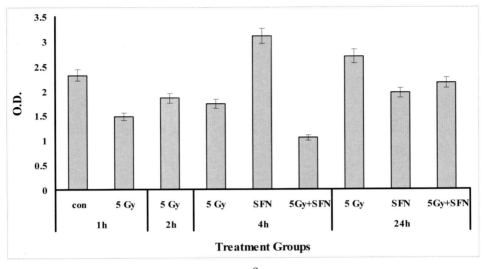

c

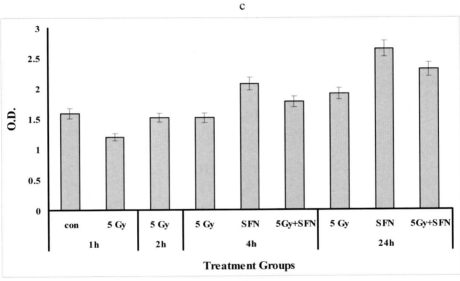

d

Data represents mean ± SD of three independent experiments.

Figure 5. Histone acetylation pattern in human lymphocytes a) H2A, b) H2B, c) H3 and d) H4 at various time points following exposure to 5 Gy γ-radiation and its modification by sulforaphane (400 nM). Cultures were terminated at 1, 2, 4 and 24 h of various treatments and processed for ELISA.

In both studies the concentrations of SFN used (40 nM and 400 nM) were observed to be beneficial, 400 nM being marginally more effective except in the case of human lung fibroblast MRC-5 where the 40 nM concentration was observed to be more effective. In our earlier report on reduction in radiation-induced cytogenetic damage by SFN, we showed that the 400 nM SFN concentration was more effective. However, it should be noted that the earlier study was based on a lower radiation dose (2 Gy) with the thought that the cohort of people accidentally exposed to radiation might have accumulated a similar radiation dose.

The current study is based on exposure of 5 Gy radiation to the cells. Radiation exposure is known to induce cell cycle delay, particularly G2/M arrest, as a result of radiation-induced DNA damage and cell death mainly through apoptosis. Increased cell viability and increased cell proliferation by 2 h post-irradiation SFN treatment suggests a reduction in DNA damage and other death signals induced by radiation.

SFN administration 2 h after 5 Gy irradiation effectively countered radiation-induced free radical generation in lymphocytes (Figure 4) at both concentrations. However, the cells were under high oxidative stress for at least 2 h before SFN administration and during this time the cells should have accumulated biomolecular damage.

We have postulated earlier that HDAC inhibition after induction of radiation damage might help repair and recovery and thus ameliorate radiation injury [22]. We have shown that a 2 Gy exposure led to enhanced HDAC activity in human lymphocytes that was inhibited by SFN post-irradiation treatment leading to a reduction in genotoxicity [14].

It has been observed that SFN post-irradiation treatment led a continuous increase in H4 acetylation status in 2 Gy-exposed lymphocytes. H4 acetylation status plays a significant role in DNA repair process [23] which might have helped reduce micronuclei frequency in irradiated lymphocytes.

In the current study we also observed a continuous prolonged enhanced H4 acetylation level in 5 Gy radiation-exposed human lymphocytes. An enhanced acetylation status was observed at different time points post-SFN treatment for the other histones. It is important to note that despite increased HDAC activity observed at 2 h post-irradiation in the earlier study, the current study showed an increase in acetylation status of H2B and H3 and a reduced acetylation status of H4 in irradiated lymphocytes.

CONCLUSION

The current study shows the changes in global acetylation patterns of various histones as a result of sulforaphane administration and irradiation. The contribution of increased H2B and H3 acetylation in various cellular functions following radiation exposure needs to be investigated further. In contrast, the role of increased H4 acetylation status has been extensively studied with respect to DNA damage repair.

The contribution of such changes in global acetylation status on chromatin dynamics and subsequent functional alterations needs to be studied in more details. Promotor specific acetylation levels and gene expression studies may help in better understanding the mechanism of amelioration of radiation injury by HDAC inhibitors.

ACKNOWLEDGMENTS

The work was supported by DRDO, Government of India. Support and encouragements provided by Director INMAS is sincerely acknowledged.

Conflict of Interest: No conflict of interest exists.

REFERENCES

[1] Johnson, I. T. (2002) Glucosinolates: bioavailability and importance to health. *Int. J. Vitam. Nutr. Res.*, 72: 26-31.

[2] Seow, A., Shi, C. Y., Chung, F. L. et al. (1998). Urinary total isothiocyanate (ITC) in a population-based sample of middle-aged and older Chinese in Singapore: relationship with dietary total ITC and glutathione S-transferase M1/T1/P1 genotypes. *Cancer Epidemiol. Biomarkers Prev.*, 7: 775-781.

[3] Rungapamestry, V., Duncan, A. J., Fuller, Z., Ratcliffe, B. (2007). Effect of cooking brassica vegetables on the subsequent hydrolysis and metabolic fate of glucosinolates. *Proc. Nutr. Soc.*, 66: 69-81.

[4] Shertzer, H. G., Senft, A. P. (2000). The micronutrient indole-3-carbinol: implications for disease and chemoprevention. *Drug Metabol. Drug Interact.*, 17: 159-188.

[5] Lenzi, M. et al. (2014), Sulforaphane as a promising molecule for fighting cancer. *Advances in Nutrition and Cancer* Eds. Vincenzo Zappia et al. Springer publisher.

[6] Simon, H. U., Haj-Yehia, A., Levi-Schaffer, F. (2000). Role of reactive oxygen species (ROS) in apoptosis induction. *Apoptosis*, 5: 415-418.

[7] Pham, N. A., Jacobberger, J. W., Schimmer, A. D., Cao, P., Gronda, M., Hedley, D. W. (2004). The dietary isothiocyanate sulforaphane targets pathways of apoptosis, cell cycle arrest, and oxidative stress in human pancreatic cancer cells and inhibits tumor growth in severe combined immunodeficient mice. *Mol. Cancer Ther.*, 3: 1239-1248.

[8] Singh, S. V., Srivastava, S. K., Choi, S., Lew, K. L., Antosiewicz, J., Xiao, D., Zeng, Y., Watkins, S. C., Johnson, C. S., Trump, D. L., Lee, Y. J., Xiao, H., Herman-Antosiewicz, A. (2005). Sulforaphane-induced cell death in human prostate cancer cells is initiated by reactive oxygen species. *J. Biol. Chem.*, 280: 19911-19924.

[9] Cheung, K. L., Khor, T. O., Kong, A. N. (2009). Synergistic effect of combination of phenethyl isothiocyanate and sulforaphane or curcumin and sulforaphane in the inhibition of inflammation. *Pharm. Res.*, 26: 224-231.

[10] Yoon, H. Y., Kang, N. I., Lee, H. K., Jang, K. Y., Park, J. W., Park, B. H. (2008). Sulforaphane protects kidneys against ischemia-reperfusion injury through induction of the Nrf2-dependent phase 2 enzyme. *Biochem. Pharmacol.*, 75: 2214-2223.

[11] Ragheb, A., Attia, A., Eldin, W. S., Elbarbry, F., Gazarin, S., Shoker, A. (2009). The protective effect of thymoquinone, an anti-oxidant and antiinflammatory agent, against renal injury: A review. *Saudi J. Kidney Dis. Transpl.*, 20: 741-752.

[12] Song, M. Y., Kim, E. K., Moon, W. S., Park, J. W., Kim, H. J., So, H. S., Park, R., Kwon, K. B., Park, B. H. (2009). Sulforaphane protects against cytokine- and streptozotocin-induced beta-cell damage by suppressing the NFkappaB pathway. *Toxicol. Appl. Pharmacol.*, 235: 57-67.

[13] Xue, M., Qian, Q., Adaikalakoteswari, A., Rabbani, N., Babaei-Jadidi, R., Thornalley, P. J. (2008). Activation of NF-E2-related factor-2 reverses biochemical dysfunction of endothelial cells induced by hyperglycemia linked to vascular disease. *Diabetes*, 57: 2809-2817.

[14] Katoch, O., Kumar, A., Adhikari, J. S., Dwarakanath, B. S., Agrawala, P. K. (2013b). Sulforaphane mitigates genotoxicity induced by radiation and anticancer drugs in human lymphocytes. *Mutat. Res.*, 758: 29-34.

[15] Agrawala, P. K. and Adhikari, J. S. (2009). Modulation of raidiation-induced cytotoxicity in U 87 cells by RH-3 (a preparation of Hippophae rhamnoides). *Indian J. Med. Res.*, 130: 542-549.

[16] Agrawala, P. K., Adhikari, J. S., Malhotra, N., Goel, H. C. (2005). Modulation of radiation induced cell cycle perturbations by RH-3, a preparation from Hippophae Rhamnoides. *Indian J. Rad. Res.*, 2: 33-40.

[17] He, C., Li, B., Song, W., Ding, Z., Wang, S., Shan, Y. (2014). Sulforaphane attenuates homocysteine-induced endoplasmic reticulum stress through Nrf-2-driven enzymes in immortalized human hepatocytes. *J. Agric. Food Chem.*, 62: 7477-85.

[18] Knatko, E. V., Ibbotson, S. H., Zhang, Y., Higgins, M., Fahey, J. W., Talalay, P., Dawa, R., Ferguson, J., Huang, J. T., Clarke, R., Zheng, S., Saito, A., Kalra, S., Benedict, A. L., Honda, T., Proby, C. M., Dinkova-Kostova, A. T. (2015) Nrf2 activation protects against solar-simulated ultraviolet radiation in mice and humans. *Cancer Prev. Res.* (Phila.) pii: canprevres.0362.2014.

[19] Qu, X., Pröll, M., Neuhoff, C., Zhang, R., Cinar, M. U., Hossain, M. M., Tesfaye, D., Große-Brinkhaus, C., Salilew-Wondim, D., Tholen, E., Looft, C., Hölker, M., Schellander, K., Uddin, M. J. (2015) Sulforaphane epigenetically regulates innate immune responses of porcine monocyte-derived dendritic cells induced with lipopolysaccharide. *PLoS One.*, 20; 10(3):e0121574.

[20] Royston, K. J. and Tollefsbol, T. O. (2015) he Epigenetic Impact of Cruciferous Vegetables on Cancer Prevention. *Curr. Pharmacol. Rep.*, 1;1(1):46-51.

[21] Senanayake, G. V. K., Banigesh Ali, Wu Lingyun, Lee Paul and Juurlink, B. H. J. (2012) The dietary phase 2 protein inducer sulforaphane can normalize the kidney epigenome and improve blood pressure in hypertensive rats. Am. J. Hypertens. 25(2): 229-235.

[22] Katoch, O., Dwarakanath, B. S., Agrawala, P. K. (2013a). HDAC inhibitors: applications in oncology and beyond. *HOAJ Biol.* DOI: http://dx.doi.org/10.7243/2050-0874-2-2.

[23] Sharma, G. G., So, S., Gupta, A., Kumar, R., Cayrou, C., Avvakumov, N., Bhadra, U., Pandita, R. K., Porteus, M. H., Chen, D. J., Cote, J., Pandita, T. K. (2010). MOF and histone H4 acetylation at lysine 16 are critical for DNA damage response and double-strand break repair. *Mol. Cell. Biol.*, 30: 3582-3595.

In: Broccoli
Editor: Bernhard H. J. Juurlink

ISBN: 978-1-63484-313-3
© 2016 Nova Science Publishers, Inc.

Chapter 9

BROCCOLI SPROUT SUPPLEMENTATION AS A NOVEL METHOD FOR PREVENTING PERINATAL BRAIN INJURY

Jerome Y. Yager[*], MD, Antoinette T. Nguyen, BSc, Jennifer Corrigan, MD, Ashley M. A. Bahry, Ann-Marie Przyslupski, BSc and Edward A. Armstrong, MSc

Department of Pediatrics, University of Alberta, Edmonton, Canada

ABSTRACT

Cerebral palsy is the *sine quo non* phenotypical outcome measure of perinatal brain injury. It continues to occur with an incidence of 2-3/1000 live births in term infants. The incidence increases 10-fold in infants born prematurely, and yet another 10-fold in developing countries. Risk factors causative for the development of cerebral palsy in childhood predominantly occur during gestation, prior to the onset of labor and delivery, whereas only 10-20% of causes occur as a result of a traumatic birth.

Despite these epidemiologic findings, efforts regarding the treatment of perinatal brain injury are focused on rescue and/or rehabilitation. To address the majority of causes, however, *preventive* therapies, provided during gestation, must be developed in order to treat the 'at risk' fetus. Natural health products such as broccoli sprouts and its active metabolite, sulforaphane, as potent phase-II enzyme inducers, show excellent promise, given their safety and efficacy profile. In this chapter, we describe a host of pre-clinical studies in rodent models of the human risk factors responsible for the majority of causes of cerebral palsy in children. In this regard, we have utilized Broccoli Sprouts as a dietary supplement during pregnancy, and shown it to prevent the behavioural and pathological characteristics typical of perinatal brain damage. Our findings suggest this to be a viable avenue for further exploration, and a potential safe and efficacious approach for the prevention of perinatal brain injury and cerebral palsy.

---

[*] Correspondence to: Jerome Y. Yager, Department of Pediatrics, University of Alberta, Room 4-020D, Katz Group Centre for Pharmacy and Health Research, 114 St, Edmonton AB, T6G 2E1, Email: jyager@ualberta.ca.

Keywords: broccoli sprouts, cerebral palsy, developmental disability, fetal growth restriction, fetal inflammation, natural health products, neonatal stroke, oxidative stress, placental insufficiency, prematurity

INTRODUCTION

Children with developmental disabilities (DDs) face lifelong challenges that prevent them from fully participating in education, work, and family roles [1, 2]. Families experience tremendously increased stress and health problems [3, 4]. According to the National Foundation for Brain Research (USA), a spectrum of disorders related to white matter injury in the immature brain -including cerebral palsy (CP), mental retardation (MR), vision and hearing loss, and learning difficulties - account for 27% of all childhood disabilities.

Cerebral palsy is the *sine quo non* outcome measure regarding perinatal brain injury. However, numerous co-morbidities occur in children with CP and perinatal brain injury, inclusive of cognitive impairment, attention deficit disorder, autism spectrum disorder, learning disabilities, and seizures [5-11]. Despite countless advances in neonatal medicine, the prevalence of neurodevelopmental disabilities such as Cerebral Palsy (CP) has not declined. Over the last three decades the incidence of CP has remained constant at 2-4 per 1000 live term births; rendering it the most common physical disability of childhood [12]. In prematurely born infants, the incidence rises 10-fold to 22/1000 infants born before 37 weeks gestation [13]; and in developing countries CP reportedly occurs at an incidence 10 times higher.

Cerebral palsy is a heterogeneous disease consisting of non-progressive motor disorders that result from injury to the developing fetal or infant brain. It was first described in the early 19th century by Dr. William John Little, who referred to the lower limb hypertonia and spasticity he observed as "Little's disease." This entity is now known as spastic diplegia and represents the most common form of CP. Little attributed the condition to difficult delivery resulting in intra-partum asphyxia [14]. The notion that CP occurs primarily as a result of birth asphyxia has persisted into the 21st century and is still present today. However, new research suggests that less than 10% of children with CP has suffered an asphyxial event at the time of birth [15, 16], and that 80-90% of those children who are ultimately diagnosed with CP, have an inciting event or risk factor that occurs during the ante-partum time frame, most likely during the 3rd trimester of pregnancy.

In 1888, Sir William Osler coined the term Cerebral Palsy. He divided CP into different subtypes based on clinically apparent motor disorder phenotypes, and then correlated these phenotypes with neuroanatomical pathology [15, 16]. The four major subtypes of CP are spastic, dyskinetic, ataxic and mixed. Spastic CP is characterized by hypertonia and affects greater than 80% of patients with CP. It can be further described as diplegic, hemiplegic or quadriplegic, depending on the topographical distribution [17]. The vast majority of patients with CP (>60%) have mild to moderate motor impairment [18]. In addition to constituting the majority of patients with CP, these children are also the most likely to benefit from therapeutic intervention [19]. Yet, all therapeutic interventions to date have addressed perinatal asphyxia after the injury has already occurred, as a rescue therapy, and therefore targeting only 10% of the children at risk for the later development of CP. Indeed, there are few pre-clinical models designed to mimic the human condition and those risk factors that occur during gestation, and associated with the later onset of CP in childhood. Developing animal models reminiscent of all stages of CP, inclusive of the most significant risk factors, is crucial to the introduction, testing and translation of novel therapeutic agents.

In addition to motor dysfunction, cognitive and behavioural co-morbidities are prominent among patients with CP and contribute considerably to the disease's morbidity [19a]. According to the 2008 Centers for Disease Control (CDC) report, greater than 60% of children with CP have at least one associated neurodevelopmental disorder including, but not limited to, intellectual disability (40%), epilepsy (35%) and vision impairment (15%). Recent studies have demonstrated that executive dysfunction is present in approximately half the children with CP [20-22]. The prevalence increases with prematurity and bilateral brain lesions [23]. In this regard, the Executive Committee for the Definition and Classification of CP released an updated definition in 2006 to more accurately reflect these associated neurodevelopmental disabilities. CP is now defined as "*a group of permanent disorders of the development of movement and posture, causing activity limitations, attributed to non-progressive disturbances ...often accompanied by disturbances of sensation, perception, cognition, communication, and behaviour—epilepsy and musculoskeletal problem* [5].

Cerebral palsy (CP) is a heterogeneous and complex disease, predisposed to by a host of risk factors [24, 25]. Until recently, the neurological disturbances observed in CP had been primarily attributed to acute intra-partum asphyxia that resulted in a hypoxic ischemic encephalopathy (HIE). Acute oxygen and glucose deprivation undoubtedly results in neuronal cell death and varying degrees of neurological sequelae. Low APGAR scores, which are indicative of intra-partum hypoxia, are a risk factor for the development of CP [26]. The majority of children with CP, however, do not have low APGAR scores at the time of birth, nor a neonatal encephalopathy [27]. One explanation for this is that the majority of risk factors leading to perinatal brain injury and CP actually occur prior to birth.

ETIOLOGIC RISK FACTORS FOR CEREBRAL PALSY

Several independent risk factors have been identified for the development of CP, and while these have included genetic anomalies and exposure to toxins, the following discussion will focus on those risk factors that phenotypically account for over 80% of all forms of cerebral palsy and are at the basis for the development of relevant animal models in our laboratory [11, 28]. Infants later diagnosed with CP and other developmental disabilities (DD), may experience a range of hypoxic/asphyxic ante-partum events that lead to brain injury and aberrant development. Of those causes that may be preventable, a late prenatal or perinatal hypoxic-hemodynamic insult is the dominating final common pathway in the pathogenesis of the static encephalopathies during development [29]. In this regard, hypoxia-ischemia can occur through the ante-partum -- intra-partum continuum, resulting in the birth of a neurologically impaired newborn [30]. Hence, while some intra-partum factors may occur in isolation, other factors may be on a causal pathway that starts before birth, but which includes intra-partum hypoxia-ischemia as a contributor (so-called 'double-hit' theory).

Ante-Partum Period	Intra-Partum Period	Newborn Outcome
1	Insult	Encephalopathy
2 Insult	Further Insult	Encephalopathy
3 Insult		Encephalopathy

From Badawi, 1998.

As indicated above, the most significant of these is low birth weight, commonly associated with premature birth, and associated with a 10-fold rise in the incidence of CP. Preterm birth is responsible for 5–11% of all births but is the root cause of 70% of neonatal deaths. Moreover, preterm survivors account for 75% of neonatal morbidity [31, 32] resulting from the brain damage that often occurs. The most common lesion affecting premature infants is cerebrovascular in nature, and results in damage to the subcortical periventricular white matter [33]. *Damage to this region is known as periventricular leukomalacia (PVL), and is a distinct pathologic entity of the human newborn brain.* The peak gestational age for the development of PVL is between 24 and 32 weeks. *PVL is the anatomical substrate for the development of cerebral palsy (CP).* Of infants with PVL, 25% develop cerebral palsy, and upwards of 50% develop cognitive and learning disabilities by school age [34-36]. With more severe lesions [37], the incidence of accompanying mental retardation rises from 14% to 54%.

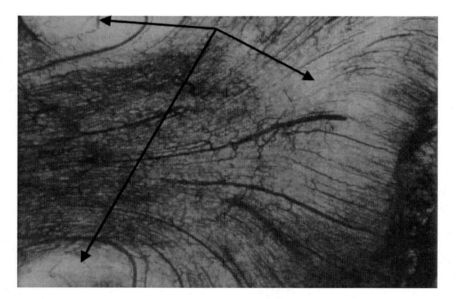

Figure 1. Coronal Section of 28-week gestation fetus with blood vessels perfused with red dye. Arrows depict areas of topographically vulnerable regions due to lack of blood vessel development between penetrating arteries. The areas depicted are in the periventricular region.

PVL lesions "interrupt" fibres descending from the motor cortex (in the corticospinal tract) that normally control the upper and lower extremities, as well as muscles controlling the face, speech, and the swallowing reflex. Pathologically, PVL occurs in an area of the brain adjacent to the lateral ventricles [33, 38]. These sites are considered 'border' or 'watershed' zones between penetrating branches of the anterior, middle and posterior cerebral arteries in the premature infant. Oligodendroglial deficiency, myelin loss and astrogliosis are dominant features, microscopically. Two main factors contribute to PVL in the immature newborn infant. First, the degree of vascular immaturity plays a major role in the selective distribution of PVL. Vessels in the region of PVL are derived largely from the middle cerebral artery and penetrate the cerebral wall from the pial (outer) surface. These long penetrators are *end arteries* and therefore do not anastomose with surrounding vessels. As a result, the region is vulnerable to a reduction in perfusion pressure. This vulnerability accounts for the prevalence of PVL in neonates of 24–32 weeks gestation (Figure 1 & 2) [39, 40].

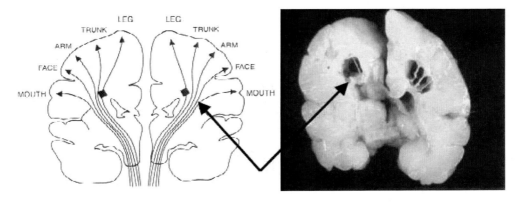

Figure 2. Pictorial cartoon on left and coronal section of fetal brain on right. Arrows point to periventricular area involved in white matter injury in premature infant due to hypoxia-ischemia. Cartoon depiction on left indicates descending fibres, which when interrupted, results in spastic diplegic or quadriplegic cerebral palsy. Pathological specimen on the right indicates the area of cystic formation that are seen with the evolution of white matter injury.

Second, the intrinsic vulnerability of the oligodendrocyte contributes to the pathogenesis of PVL. A series of elegant studies by Back et al., [41-44] has demonstrated the maturation-dependent nature of white matter injury. Hence, the stage of development that best coincides with vulnerability is that of the pre-oligodendrocyte (preOL), prominent in the 24–32 week gestation fetus. The decline in risk for white matter injury occurs with the onset of oligodendroglial maturation, and gestational age, both of which coincide with increasing myelination. The remarkable sensitivity of oligodendroglial precursors to excitotoxic injury has also been demonstrated by Oka et al. [45] Relevant to the mechanism of broccoli sprout neuroprotection, the cell death, in their series of experiments, was not due to a receptor-mediated mechanism but rather to a depletion of intracellular cysteine and a subsequent reduction in the concentration of glutathione (an important endogenous free-radical scavenger [symbolized as GSH when in the reduced redox state]) [46, 47] [see Chapter 5 for review] Juurlink and colleagues [48-51] found that the specific sensitivity of the oligodendroglial cells to damage by free radicals is also related, in part to the low GSH content of these cells [52]. Studies of astrocytes revealed that they have a 3-fold greater GSH content than oligodendroglial cells, and that oligodendrocytes displayed less than 10% of the glutathione peroxidase activity seen in astrocytes [53]. Finally and most recently, the Back group of investigators has further delineated that, not only are oligodendroglia exquisitely sensitive to neurotoxicity, they also display aberrant maturation and growth as a result of impaired dendritic arborization and synaptogenesis [54, 55].

Intrauterine growth restriction (IUGR) refers to a fetus that is small for gestational age (weight <10th percentile) as a result of a pathological process that prevents it from meeting its genetic growth potential [56]. IUGR is attributed to one or more fetal, placental, or maternal factors. With the exception of intrinsic fetal factors such as a genetic anomaly, the most common cause of IUGR, in the western hemisphere, is placental insufficiency (PI). Placental insufficiency, also known as utero-placental vascular insufficiency, precludes adequate delivery of blood to the fetus resulting in an inadequate supply of oxygen and substrate supply, or fetal ischemia. The relationship between placental blood flow, IUGR and neurological outcomes has been demonstrated clinically and in animal models. Doppler studies consistently reveal high placental vascular resistance in IUGR human fetuses. If umbilical artery resistance increases to the point of impairment, loss or ultimately reversal of end diastolic flow; the rates of poor neurological outcome and neonatal death increase exponentially [38, 57].

Based on epidemiologic data, IUGR increases the likelihood of neonatal encephalopathy by 40-fold (an adjusted odds ratio of 38.23) [58, 59]. The National Collaborative Perinatal Project [60] found that children with IUGR were more likely than controls to have cerebral palsy or mental retardation at 7 years of age. Others [61] have shown a relationship between IUGR and *(i)* learning deficits or behavioural problems of inattention and anxiety in 48% of children assessed between 9 and 11 years of age, and *(ii)* poor school performance at 12 and 18 years of age [62-64]. In addition, malnutrition of the fetus (including placental insufficiency) is a principal cause of abnormal development of the fetal brain, contributing to cognitive impairment, autism [64a], schizophrenia and possibly other issues of mental health [65, 66].

Fetal Inflammation: A further important recognized antepartum risk factor for cerebral palsy is the systemic fetal inflammatory response (FI) [67]; reportedly associated with a four-fold increase in the risk of developing CP [24, 25]. Both clinical and experimental studies have provided strong evidence supporting the association between FI and brain injury leading to CP [68-71]. And others have shown that inflammation/infection of the prematurely newborn infant also increases the risk for CP [72].

Fetal inflammation can arise following maternal infection and inflammation, such as chorioamnionitis, and is characterized by inflammation of the chorion and amniotic membranes. Pregnant mothers may have no symptoms, biochemical or histologic findings alone, or systemic findings consistent with infection. All are significant risk factors for CP and premature birth. Chorioamnionitis can occur from ascending bacteria, normally localized in the vaginal flora, where it gains access to the decidua, initiating a maternal inflammatory response. Both bacterial products and maternal inflammatory mediators can gain access to the fetus causing the FI. Overall, chorioamnionitis, FI, and prematurity, can act in conjunction or independently, leading to CP. These different factors reflect the complexity and interplay of risk factors resulting in the clinical phenotype of CP.

Once FI has commenced, inflammatory mediators cause injury to the developing brain, particularly targeting the pre-oligodendrocytes. Thus, exposure to the FI during this period can result in cell death and/or blockage of maturation to mature myelin producing oligodendrocytes, leading to white matter injury in the developing brain [43, 44, 73, 74]. In addition to oligodendrocytes, neuronal injury such as those in the hippocampus, involved in learning and memory, can also be negatively affected by the FI [75, 76]. Furthermore, intrauterine inflammation has been shown to interact with additional risk factors, by either sensitizing or exaggerating brain injury when given prior to a sub-threshold insults such as hypoxia [77, 78].

Unfortunately, current therapeutic strategies for predisposed and injured newborns are limited. The only regime available is post-ischemic hypothermia, a form of rescue therapy available for term infants diagnosed with intrapartum asphyxia. As indicated earlier, even under the best of circumstances, this therapy will only address 10-20% of all newborns at risk for cerebral palsy. Moreover, the beneficial effects of hypothermia are only partial; having no effect on those infants most severely injured, and only a moderate benefit to those presenting at birth with a mild to moderate encephalopathy. Indeed, clinical trials indicate a 'need to treat' benefit of 8 patients in order to derive improved outcome in 1 [79-83].

Several years ago our laboratory recognized the need to address the issue of cerebral palsy, its co-morbidities, and the risk factors associated with them from a different perspective. Particularly as it relates to our knowledge that the majority of these causative risk factors occurred during gestation, and the damage was 'already done' at the time of birth, continued pursuit of our current pre-clinical models [84] (Rice-Vannucci Model – see reference) were clearly inadequate, as therapeutically they addressed only a small percentage of infants affected, and was rescue in nature. In this regard, we worked with two additional models that reflected the intra-uterine environments of placental insufficiency, fetal inflammation, and fetal growth restriction.

The adaptation of models which reflect the intrauterine environment allows for the introduction of preventive therapies, as opposed to those that are 'rescue.' However, such an approach requires treatment of the mother, in order to address the concerns of the fetus. In this regard, significant fear continues to be present with respect to the application of traditional pharmaco-therapeutics during pregnancy, dating back to the unfortunate events linked to the use of thalidomide [85]. Furthermore, conventional medicines used to treat adult injured brains can cause significant harm to the developing brain [86, 87], emphasizing the need to identify safe interventions to protect both the mother and fetus.

Natural health products offer an innovative, safe, and effective approach to protect the developing brain. Beginning with investigations in the field of cancer research (see Chapter 1) interest in broccoli sprouts (BrSps) over the last number of years has exploded. BrSps contain the precursor of sulforaphane, glucoraphanin; sulforaphane is a powerful antioxidant and anti-inflammatory agent [88-90]. Sulforaphane, which is produced with chewing of the sprouts, has now been extensively studied in the fields of oncology, cardiovascular disease, and stroke and has shown very promising results. These studies demonstrate that sulforaphane induces a significant reduction in both inflammation and oxidative stress, mechanisms involved in the evolution of perinatal brain injury [91, 92]. Juurlink and colleagues have determined the effects of phase 2 enzyme inducers on up-regulating the glutathione system, a powerful endogenous group of enzymes that reduce oxidative stress (Chapter 5) [93-97]. The impetus for this work came from literature, which indicated that many types of chemoprotectors against malignancy caused the induction of phase 2 enzymes, which in turn increased glutathione levels. Epidemiologic data suggested that diets rich in fruits and vegetables were associated with a dose-related reduction in the risk of developing cancer. Sulforaphane was identified as the potent phase-2 enzyme inducer within the crucifers (i.e., plants of the genus *Brassica*). A critical result was that 3-day-old broccoli sprouts were found to contain 10–100 times the concentration of glucoraphanin (the precursor to sulforaphane) than that found in more mature broccoli or other crucifers [88, 90, 98].

Wu et al., used broccoli sprouts in pharmacologic doses as an anti-oxidant in a model of the spontaneously hypertensive (SH) stroke-prone rat. They showed that feeding 200 mg/day of dried broccoli sprouts for 14 weeks, lowered blood pressure and decreased markers of oxidative stress, as indicated by increased glutathione content, decreased oxidized-glutathione, and a reduction in the concentration of infiltrating macrophages in the tissues of the treated animals [92]. More recent studies have indicated that feeding broccoli sprouts to pregnant SH rats during gestation lowered blood pressure in their offspring and reduced their markers of oxidative stress and inflammation [93, 95, 99, 100]. Others have found potent beneficial effects on the reduction of stroke in adult rodent models [101].

Preventing perinatal brain injury offers up several challenges. The pregnant woman and fetus, though clearly a vulnerable population, have largely been neglected by pharma due to the complexity of maternal fetal interactions, risk to the rapidly developing fetus, the difficulties that arise regarding the identification of a fetus at risk, and of course the consequent threat of litigation. Yet, the importance of developing strategies that address the ·80% of infants and children who develop cerebral palsy as a result of ante-partum risk factors remains.

It was for these reasons that our laboratory determined that an approach to this issue might be through the use of natural health products, and particularly broccoli sprouts. Our aims are to develop the scientific evidence for the efficacy of this therapy during pregnancy, demonstrate its safety profile, and determine the dose/responsiveness for a beneficial effect. In so doing, we have completed a number of experiments, which will be outlined briefly below.

EXPERIMENTAL MODELS

Placental Insufficiency

Placental insufficiency is perhaps the most common underlying risk factor for premature delivery and intra-uterine growth restriction. It accounts for between 6 and 11% of deliveries. We developed a model of bilateral uterine artery ligation (BUAL) [102], following that described by Lane et al., [103, 104] In brief, pregnant Long-Evans rats were utilized for all studies. On E20, a longitudinal abdominal incision was made and the uterine horns were exposed. The latter were ligated bilaterally, proximal to the chain of fetal sacs. Visual confirmation assured the interruption of blood flow. Following closure of the abdomen, the Dams were allowed to deliver vaginally on E23. The model produces an IUGR newborn, which at birth is age equivalent to a 24-28 week gestation prematurely newborn human infant.

Our results indicated a mortality rate of approximately 50%. Birth weights were uniformly below the 3%ile compared to control. Growth restriction occurred in an asymmetrical fashion, meaning that there was relatively greater loss of growth in length and weight of the offspring, compared to brain weight, identical to that which occurs in human newborns with placental insufficiency in the 3rd trimester. Four groups of animals were analyzed: 1) Control Sham, 2) Sham plus BrSp supplementation, 3) BUAL, and 4) BUAL plus BrSp supplementation. Control animals received a normal diet of rat chow provided *ad libitum,* and sham surgery in which the abdominal incision was performed, without uterine artery ligation. Pregnant dams in the experimental groups received BrSp dietary supplementation in the 3rd trimester of pregnancy, beginning on E15. Dried broccoli sprouts, at a dose of 200 mg/day were provided in a petri dish. Rat dams were observed to eat the sprouts completely. Those Dams that did not feed on the sprouts were excluded from the study. Supplementation to the Dams was provided from E15 to PD14. Rat pups were weaned from their Dams on day 21 after which they were sacrificed for neuropathologic assessment. From PD3 to PD21, rat pups underwent a series of early developmental behavioural tests [102].

All growth restricted rat pups that did not receive BrSp supplementation did significantly more poorly on all developmental reflex behaviours, compared to all other groups. Most importantly, those pups receiving BrSp supplementation through feeding of their Dam, showed normal performance of their developmental reflexes, indicating the BrSp supplementation prevented the behavioural alterations. Pathologically, IUGR pups displayed reduced corpus callosum thickness and myelination, compared to controls. In addition, hippocampal cell counting revealed a reduced number of cells in CA$_1$ and CA$_3$ in the IUGR pups compared to the controls. Once again, BrSp supplementation prevented these changes from occurring. (Figure 3 and 4) Studies validating the long term and behavioural affects of these findings have recently been supported in our laboratory. In this regard, behavioural abnormalities on PD80 involving cognitive, motor and anxiety in the IUGR rats, were normalized in those pups exposed to BrSp supplementation of their Dams.

Table 1.

Test	Group	Means			Main	Effects	(p-value)
	SHAM	SHAM+B	IUGR	IUGR+B	Treatment	Diet	Interaction
n	16	20	27	25			
Righting PD7 (s)	1.3 ± 0.4	1.3 ± 0.3	5.2 ± 4.8	4.6 ± 4.8	0.000	0.715	0.708
Forelimb grasp (PD)	2.9 ± 0.3	3.0 ± 0.3	4.6 ± 1.0	3.3 ± 0.9	0.000	0.000	0.000
Hind limb grasp	4.3 ± 0.9	3.8 ± 0.8	6.8 ± 2.2	6.1 ± 2.1	0.000	0.124	0.848
Hind limb placing	5.5 ± 1.2	5.1 ± 0.9	8.1 ± 1.4	6.8 ± 1.5	0.000	0.002	0.118
Cliff Aversion	6.6 ± 0.7	5.0 ± 1.0	7.7 ± 1.5	5.5 ± 0.9	0.002	0.000	0.291
Gait	7.8 ± 1.1	7.1 ± 1.0	8.9 ± 1.3	8.8 ± 1.1	0.000	0.121	0.229
Posture	14.3 ± 0.6	14.4 ± 0.6	16.5 ± 1.3	15.7 ± 0.9	0.000	0.067	0.024
Eye Opening	16.2 ± 0.5	16.4 ± 0.6	16.6 ± 0.9	16.7 ± 0.6	0.028	0.360	0.903
Auditory	11.9 ± 0.7	12.4 ± 0.8	13.7 ± 1.2	14.0 ± 0.7	0.000	0.094	0.547
Acceleration-righting	15.3 ± 1.0	15.6 ± 0.9	18.0 ± 2.1	17.2 ± 1.0	0.000	0.413	0.085

Legend: Table 1 shows means ± SD as well as p-values by two-way ANOVA for early reflex, behaviour and maturation tests. Two-way ANOVA of the data clearly show a main effect of treatment in all tests. There is an effect of diet in forelimb grasp, hind limb placing and cliff aversion and an interaction in forelimb grasp and posture tests. All tests with the exception of gait resulted in a significant Levine test (p ≤ 0.043; data not shown).

Table 2.

Test	Group				Main Effects		(p-value)
	Means				Treatment	Diet	Interaction
	SHAM	SHAM+B	IUGR	IUGR+B			
n	16	20	26	24			
Ambulation (squares)	67.6 ± 23.8	87.1 ± 21.6	115 ± 24.1	86.0 ± 29.5	0.000	0.390	0.000
Head lifts	13.9 ± 4.4	13.5 ± 3.8	24.0 ± 6.8	18.5 ± 7.2	0.000	0.022	0.045
Rearing	35.3 ± 9.6	38.4 ± 8.8	36.8 ± 9.6	33.0 ± 12.2	0.393	0.850	0.127
Grooming	1.7 ± 1.4	0.9 ± 0.8	1.0 ± 0.8	1.3 ± 0.8	0.519	0.182	0.010
Defecation	2.3 ± 1.0	1.7 ± 1.1	1.3 ± 1.4	1.2 ± 1.6	0.011	0.268	0.447

Legend: Table 2 shows results from the open field behavioural test. Data are reported as mean ± SD. Two-way ANOVA shows a main effect of treatment for ambulation, head lifts and defecation. A main effect of diet is observed in head lifts and an interaction in ambulation, head lifts and grooming. The Levine statistic was significant for head lifts and grooming (p ≤ 0.02; data not shown).

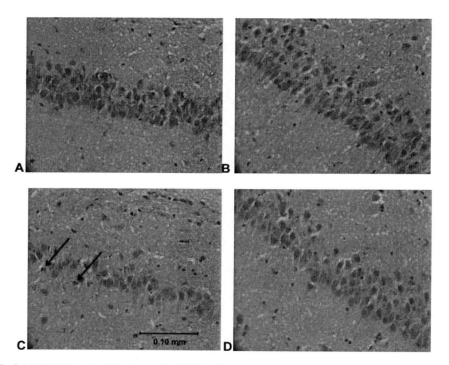

Figure 3. CA1 SHAM (A); SHAM+B (B); IUGR (C); IUGR+B (D). The images illustrate the observable reduction in pyramidal cells in the CA1 area of the IUGR section (slide C) compared with the other groups at PD21. Pyknotic cells are still visible in IUGR sections, indicated by the black arrows.

Figure 5 shows an example of these findings, providing evidence of the long-term beneficial effect of BrSp provided during pregnancy. Interestingly, pathologic assessment of this more senior group of animals did not show any differences between groups, suggesting that there was some compensation or adaptation to earlier pathologic alterations. Ongoing research in the area of connectivity continues in our laboratory.

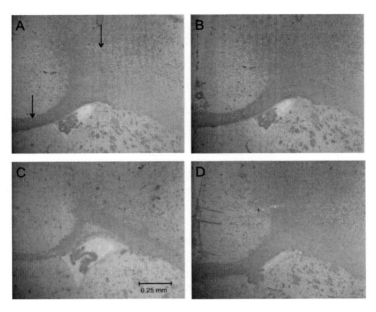

Figure 4. Photomicrographs show myelin basic protein (MBP) stained images, A. SHAM, B. SHAM+B, C. IUGR, D. IUGR+B. Close-up anterior brain images were taken at a vantage point to include the right hemisphere ventricle, corpus callosum (cc) and cingular projections. In SHAM animals (A), white matter is densely stained, portraying thick myelinated bundles of the cc and long axonal projections of the cingulum (black arrows). The weak MBP signal observable in the same areas of the IUGR image (C) is typical of our findings and reveals a thinning of the cc and shorter cingular projections. Ventricular dilation typical of the IUGR animals is also visible. The IUGR+B image shows clear improvement over IUGR in all these aforementioned areas.

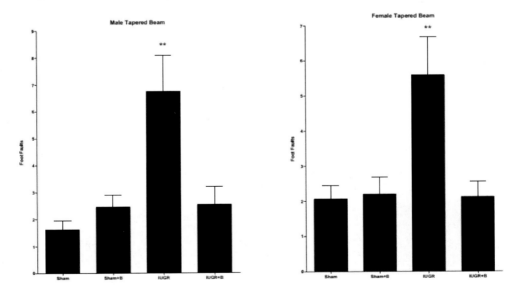

Figure 5. Male and Female tapered beam test. ** $p < 0.0001$ significantly different between IUGR pups at PD 80 compared to all other groups. Importantly, those pups whose Dams received BrSp supplementation during the last trimester and prior to weaning, suggesting a prevention in motor disability, as a result of placental insufficiency.

Fetal Inflammation

Our model of fetal inflammation utilized LPS as a stimulant. Pregnant Long Evans Dams were injected with 200 µg/kg of LPS (*Escherichia* coli serotype 0127:B8; Sigma Biochemical, Oakville, ON, Canada) diluted in 100 µl of saline, every 12 hours on E19 and 20, for a total of 4 injections [105]. Dams temperature actually reduced in the first 12 hours after which it normalized. Dams were randomly divided into four groups to receive the following treatments: 1) Saline, 2) Saline plus BrSp, 3) LPS, and 4) LPS + BrSp. Developmental reflex testing was again accomplished from PD3 to PD21, followed by pathologic assessment. In these groups of animals, BrSp supplementation again prevented abnormalities in a number of reflexes tested (Table 3). Pathologically, there were no differences amongst the groups tested. Although our findings were positive with respect to reflex testing, they were not as robust as those findings in our model of placental insufficiency. We conclude from this that was the case because the model itself was not as severe an injury model as that displayed by placental insufficiency. Nonetheless, it's relevance is important, given that the majority of children with cerebral palsy have mild to moderate disability, as opposed to those in the severe group. Hence providing benefit to this group of children is clearly important.

Table 3.

	Saline	Saline + BrSp	LPS	LPS + BrSp
Birth Weights*#	6.3 ± 0.1	6.2 ± 0.1	5.1 ± 0.1	5.8 ± 0.1
Neurodevelopmental Reflexes				
Forelimb Grasp	3.0 ± 0.0	3.0 ± 0.0	3.0 ± 0.0	3.0 ± 0.0
Hindlimb Grasp*#	3.6 ± 0.1	3.4 ± 0.1	4.7 ± 0.4	3.3 ± 0.1
Hindlimb Placing	4.3 ± 0.1	4.3 ± 0.1	4.6 ± 0.1	4.5 ± 0.1
Righting*#	4.4 ± 0.3	4.8 ± 0.3	6.6 ± 0.6	4.0 ± 0.3
Cliff Avoidance*#	4.4 ± 0.1	4.6 ± 0.1	5.8 ± 0.2	5.0 ± 0.2
Gait*#	7.5 ± 0.2	7.4 ± 0.2	9.6 ± 0.3	7.6 ± 0.2
Auditory Startle	11.4 ± 0.2	11.5 ± 0.1	11.9 ± 0.3	12.0 ± 0.0
Posture*#	15.6 ± 0.3	15.5 ± 0.2	16.9 ± 0.3	14.7 ± 0.2
Eye Openings	16.3 ± 0.1	16.0 ± 0.0	16.0 ± 0.0	15.3 ± 0.1
Accelerated Righting*	16.0 ± 0.3	16.4 ± 0.2	17.0 ± 0.3	17.0 ± 0.2
Behaviour				
Headlifts	30.6 ± 2.1	27.7 ± 1.7	26.7 ± 1.0	29.3 ± 1.7
Rearing	34.3 ± 2.4	35.7 ± 2.3	30.1 ± 2.6	33.1 ± 2.1
Grooming*#	1.3 ± 0.2	1.0 ± 0.0	2.1 ± 0.2	1.1 ± 0.2
Urination	0.3 ± 0.1	0.3 ± 0.1	0.6 ± 0.1	0.3 ± 0.1
Defecation	3.1 ± 0.3	2.4 ± 0.2	2.3 ± 0.3	2.7 ± 0.2
Center*	21.4 ± 2.0	21.5 ± 2.2	14.1 ± 1.2	21.0 ± 1.8
Ambulation	86.0 ± 4.1	91.4 ± 7.0	66.3 ± 2.5	76.4 ± 4.3

The data is represented as mean ± SEM.
*Significant difference between Saline and LPS.
#Significant difference between LPS and LPS + BrSp.

Interestingly, as opposed to supplementation in our placental insufficiency model, in our FI model, birth weights were restored with the feeding of BrSp. These findings suggest that the effect of BrSp may be acting at several levels, including the vaso-responsiveness of the umbilical artery blood flow, as was shown by Wu et al., [95, 100] in their model of the spontaneously hypertensive rat.

Perinatal Asphyxia

The model of perinatal asphyxia has been utilized for many years, and continues to act as the most commonly used. Briefly, this model, described by Rica and Vannucci [84] utilizes 7-day old rat (or mice) pups as being near term equivalent. Under anesthesia, pups have their common carotid artery ligated unilaterally. After a period of recovery, the pups are placed into thermo and humidity controlled jars, through which 8% oxygen is piped in through inlet and outlet portals, for periods between 60 and 180 minutes, depending on the extent of injury required.

Pathologically, this insult, though utilized as a model of perinatal asphyxia, more likely reflects a model of perinatal stroke and hemiplegic CP, given that the brain damage is largely unilateral in nature, reflects that of a porencephalic cyst of the newborn, and results in unilateral behavioural abnormalities, on testing [106]. Nonetheless, neonatal stroke accounts for upwards of 30% of the children with CP, and as such is a valid model to utilize as a therapeutic target. In this regard however, therapy would, in fact be rescue in nature. In other words, rather than preventive, treatment would be provided after the injury occurs and the infant is born.

For this experimental paradigm, we utilized the classic PD7, Rice-Vannucci model of unilateral carotid artery ligation. In an attempt to determine whether pre-treatment would be effective in reducing injury vs. post-injury treatment, Dams were fed the 200mg/kg BrSp, as noted above. Groups were divided into those Dams who were fed prior to conception, at conception, and at the time of birth, until the date of the induced injury at PD7 days. Another group of Dams was fed BrSp from the time of the injury at PD7 until the date of weaning at PD21. Rat pups, of course, received the active constituent of the broccoli, sulforaphane, through mothers milk during feeding. As seen in Figure 6, the only group of rat pups that obtained significant beneficial effect from the supplemental BrSp, were those that received concentrations of the sulforaphane following the injury, and during the course of its evolution. Remember that those in the other groups, because their supplementation ended on the date of injury, would not have had any in their system during the evolution of the injury (i.e., During the inflammatory and/or period of free radical production).

Given that the current standard of care involves the utilization of post-ischemic hypothermia, we conducted further studies to determine if the addition of sulforaphane, as a complement to hypothermia, would improve overall outcome. In this set of studies, pregnant Dams delivered their rat pups vaginally. On PD7, the pups underwent unilateral common carotid artery ligation and exposure to 8% oxygen for 90 minutes.

Following exposure to the HI insult, pups were divided into the following groups: 1) Recovery in normothermia (37^0C), 2) Receiving either 1 mg/kg, 5mg/kg, or 10 mg/kg sub-cutaneously for 7 days, or 3) Hypothermia for 24 hours in 28^0C (environmental temperature) plus either 1 mg/kg, 5mg/kg, or 10 mg/kg sub-cutaneously for 7 days. Interestingly, sulforaphane at 1 and 5 mg/kg alone significantly reduced brain damage, compared to control, but 10 mg/kg dosing had no effect.

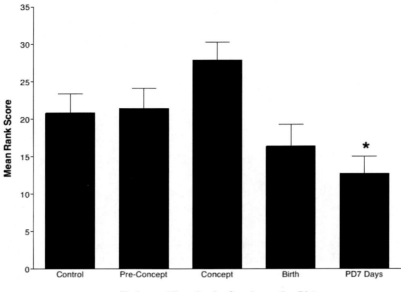

Figure 6. Bar graph depicting mean rank score damage of rat pup brains examined at 30 days of age following a hypoxic-ischemic insult at 7 days of post-natal age. * $p < 0.05$ compared to controls.

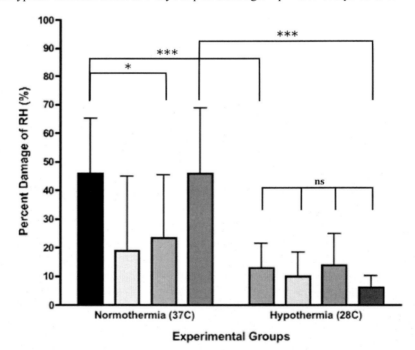

Figure 7. Bar graphs depicting the effects of hypothermia, SFN, and the combination of both therapies compared to control. The findings indicate an overall protective effect of hypothermia, a protective effect of 1 and 5 mg/kg of SFN compared to control, but no effect of combined treatment over hypothermia alone.

Likewise hypothermia was effective in significantly reducing injury. However, the combination of hypothermia plus sulforaphane had no additive effect on reducing injury (Figure 7), compared to hypothermia alone. The findings are important as it relates, not only the effect of sulforaphane on perinatal hypoxic-ischemic brain damage but the interaction of hypothermia and other medications, as they relate to perinatal brain injury.

DISCUSSION

Natural health products have always held medicinal potential. Recent years has brought a greater understanding of the underlying mechanisms by which these beneficial effects occur. Broccoli sprouts and their active metabolite, sulforaphane, are potent phase-II enzyme inducers and effective anti-inflammatories and anti-oxidants. Their effect has been increasingly clear in adult disease, with good evidence for its effect in pre-clinical animal models for cancer, hypertension, and stroke. The work we have outlined in this chapter, however, is the first application of broccoli sprouts as a preventive approach during pregnancy against causes associated with cerebral palsy and its co-morbidities.

To date, our lab has also completed a systematic review of the safe medicinal use of cruciferous vegetables [107]. The review found that, when used medicinally, cruciferous vegetables are safe. Caution should be used in those individuals who are also utilizing anticoagulants, as it may exacerbate the effects. Ongoing investigations within our laboratory include discussions with focus groups of pregnant woman, to determine their willingness to alter or supplement their diets with broccoli sprouts or a similar vitamin, during their diet, for the health of their fetus. In addition, we are looking at dosing concentrations and its effects on multi-organ systems as a phase one trial. Preliminary data show absolutely no adverse effects across all systems.

Given the association of fetal growth restriction with later onset adult disease, the 'Barker' hypothesis, there is every possibility that treating 'at risk' pregnancies may reduce the risk for later onset disorders, and even the potential for mental health issues, known to have an increased incidence in children with cerebral palsy [108-113]. Moving forward for the treatment of pregnancy related risks requires the utmost of care, the ensuring of safety and efficacy and the development of a product that retains its bioavailability over time. Nonetheless, this approach may be the most efficacious and safe, in the therapy of this vulnerable population.

REFERENCES

[1] Clark A, Hirst M. Disability in adulthood: ten year follow-up of young people with disabilities. *Disability, Handicap and Society*. 1989;4:271-83.

[2] Fuhrer MJ. Subjective well-being: Implications for medical rehabilitation outcomes and models of disablement. *Am J Phys Med Rehab.* 1994;73:358-64.

[3] Cadman D, Boyle, M., Szatmari, P., Offord, D. R. Chronic illness, disability, and mental and social well-being: Findings of the Ontario Child Health Study. *Pediatrics.* 1987;79:805-13.

[4] Cadman D, Rosenbaum, P., Boyle, M., Offord, D. R. Children with chronic illness: Family and parent demographic characteristics and psycho-social adjustment. *Pediatrics.* 1991;87:884-9.

[5] Rosenbaum P, Paneth N, Leviton A, Goldstein M, Bax M, Damiano D, et al., A report: the definition and classification of cerebral palsy April 2006. *Dev. Med. Child Neurol. Suppl.* 2007 Feb;109:8-14. PubMed PMID: 17370477. Epub 2007/03/21. eng.

[6] Webster RI, Majnemer A, Platt RW, Shevell MI. Motor function at school age in children with a preschool diagnosis of developmental language impairment. *The Journal of pediatrics.* 2005 Jan;146 (1):80-5. PubMed PMID: 15644827.

[7] Simard-Tremblay E, Shevell M, Dagenais L. Determinants of ambulation in children with spastic quadriplegic cerebral palsy: a population-based study. *Journal of child neurology.* 2010 Jun;25 (6):669-73. PubMed PMID: 19794101. Epub 2009/10/02. eng.

[8] Shikako-Thomas K, Lach L, Majnemer A, Nimigon J, Cameron K, Shevell M. Quality of life from the perspective of adolescents with cerebral palsy: "I just think I'm a normal kid, I just happen to have a disability." *Quality of life research: an international journal of quality of life aspects of treatment, care and rehabilitation.* 2009 Sep;18 (7):825-32. PubMed PMID: 19548117. Epub 2009/06/24. eng.

[9] Shevell MI, Majnemer A, Miller SP. Neonatal neurologic prognostication: the asphyxiated term newborn. *Pediatric neurology.* 1999 Nov;21 (5):776-84. PubMed PMID: 10593666.

[10] Shevell MI, Dagenais L, Hall N. The relationship of cerebral palsy subtype and functional motor impairment: a population-based study. *Developmental medicine and child neurology.* 2009 Nov;51 (11):872-7. PubMed PMID: 19416339. Epub 2009/05/07. eng.

[11] Shevell MI, Dagenais L, Hall N. Comorbidities in cerebral palsy and their relationship to neurologic subtype and GMFCS level. *Neurology.* 2009 Jun 16;72 (24):2090-6. PubMed PMID: 19528515. Epub 2009/06/17. eng.

[12] Paneth N, Hong T, Korzeniewski S. The descriptive epidemiology of cerebral palsy. *Clinics in perinatology.* 2006 Jun;33 (2):251-67. PubMed PMID: 16765723.

[13] Robertson CM, Watt MJ, Yasui Y. Changes in the prevalence of cerebral palsy for children born very prematurely within a population-based program over 30 years. *JAMA: the journal of the American Medical Association.* 2007 Jun 27;297 (24):2733-40. PubMed PMID: 17595274. Epub 2007/06/28. eng.

[14] Panteliadis C, Panteliadis P, Vassilyadi F. Hallmarks in the history of cerebral palsy: from antiquity to mid-20th century. *Brain & development.* 2013 Apr;35 (4):285-92. PubMed PMID: 22658818.

[15] McIntyre S, Taitz D, Keogh J, Goldsmith S, Badawi N, Blair E. A systematic review of risk factors for cerebral palsy in children born at term in developed countries. *Developmental medicine and child neurology.* 2013 Jun;55 (6):499-508. PubMed PMID: 23181910.

[16] McIntyre S, Blair E, Badawi N, Keogh J, Nelson KB. Antecedents of cerebral palsy and perinatal death in term and late preterm singletons. *Obstetrics and gynecology.* 2013 Oct;122 (4):869-77. PubMed PMID: 24084547.

[17] Mandaleson A, Lee Y, Kerr C, Graham HK. Classifying cerebral palsy: are we nearly there? *Journal of pediatric orthopedics.* 2015 Mar;35 (2):162-6. PubMed PMID: 24919134.

[18] Reid SM, Carlin JB, Reddihough DS. Classification of topographical pattern of spasticity in cerebral palsy: a registry perspective. *Research in developmental disabilities*. 2011 Nov-Dec;32 (6):2909-15. PubMed PMID: 21624819.

[19] Chen YN, Liao SF, Su LF, Huang HY, Lin CC, Wei TS. The effect of long-term conventional physical therapy and independent predictive factors analysis in children with cerebral palsy. *Developmental neurorehabilitation.* 2013 Oct;16 (5):357-62. PubMed PMID: 23477591.

[19a] Hou M, Sun DR, Shan RB, Wang K, Yu R, Zhao JH, et al. [Comorbidities in patients with cerebral palsy and their relationship with neurologic subtypes and Gross Motor Function Classification System levels]. Zhonghua er ke za zhi Chinese journal of pediatrics. 2010 May;48(5):351-4. PubMed PMID: 20654035.

[20] Bodimeade HL, Whittingham K, Lloyd O, Boyd RN. Executive function in children and adolescents with unilateral cerebral palsy. *Developmental medicine and child neurology*. 2013 Oct;55 (10):926-33. PubMed PMID: 23809003.

[21] Bottcher L, Flachs EM, Uldall P. Attentional and executive impairments in children with spastic cerebral palsy. *Developmental medicine and child neurology*. 2010 Feb;52 (2):e42-7. PubMed PMID: 20002117.

[22] Hakkarainen E, Pirila S, Kaartinen J, Meere JJ. Stimulus evaluation, event preparation, and motor action planning in young patients with mild spastic cerebral palsy: an event-related brain potential study. *Journal of child neurology.* 2012 Apr;27 (4):465-70. PubMed PMID: 21940693.

[23] Pirila S, van der Meere JJ, Rantanen K, Jokiluoma M, Eriksson K. Executive functions in youth with spastic cerebral palsy. *Journal of child neurology.* 2011 Jul;26 (7):817-21. PubMed PMID: 21398561.

[24] Wu YW, Colford JM, Jr. Chorioamnionitis as a risk factor for cerebral palsy: A meta-analysis. *JAMA: the journal of the American Medical Association*. 2000 Sep 20;284 (11):1417-24. PubMed PMID: 10989405.

[25] Wu YW, Escobar GJ, Grether JK, Croen LA, Greene JD, Newman TB. Chorioamnionitis and cerebral palsy in term and near-term infants. *JAMA: the journal of the American Medical Association*. 2003 Nov 26;290 (20):2677-84. PubMed PMID: 14645309.

[26] Nelson KB, Ellenberg JH. Apgar scores as predictors of chronic neurologic disability. *Pediatrics*. 1981 Jul;68 (1):36-44. PubMed PMID: 7243507.

[27] Lie KK, Groholt EK, Eskild A. Association of cerebral palsy with Apgar score in low and normal birthweight infants: population based cohort study. *Bmj.* 2010;341:c4990. PubMed PMID: 20929920. Pubmed Central PMCID: 2952090.

[28] Shevell MI, Dagenais L, Hall N. The relationship of cerebral palsy subtype and functional motor impairment: a population-based study. *Developmental medicine and child neurology*. 2009 Nov;51 (11):872-7. PubMed PMID: 19416339. Epub 2009/05/07. eng.

[29] Lou HC. Hypoxic-hemodynamic pathogenesis of brain lesions in the newborn. *Brain & Development*. 1994;16:423-31.

[30] Badawi N, Watson, L., Petterson, B., Blair, E., Slee, J., et al., What constitutes cerebral palsy? *Dev. Med. Child Neurol*. 1998;40:520-7.

[31] Wen SW, Smith G, Yang Q, Walker M. Epidemiology of preterm birth and neonatal outcome. *Seminars in fetal & neonatal medicine.* 2004 Dec;9 (6):429-35. PubMed PMID: 15691780.

[32] Joseph KS, Huang L, Liu S, Ananth CV, Allen AC, Sauve R, et al., Reconciling the high rates of preterm and postterm birth in the United States. *Obstetrics and gynecology.* 2007 Apr;109 (4):813-22. PubMed PMID: 17400841.

[33] Volpe JJ. Neurology of the Newborn, 4th Ed. Philadelphia: WB Saunders; 2001.

[34] Hack M, Taylor HG, Drotar D, Schluchter M, Cartar L, Andreias L, et al., Chronic conditions, functional limitations, and special health care needs of school-aged children born with extremely low-birth-weight in the 1990s. *Jama.* 2005 Jul 20;294 (3):318-25. PubMed PMID: 16030276.

[35] Litt J, Taylor HG, Klein N, Hack M. Learning disabilities in children with very low birthweight: prevalence, neuropsychological correlates, and educational interventions. *Journal of learning disabilities.* 2005 Mar-Apr;38 (2):130-41. PubMed PMID: 15813595.

[36] Taylor HG, Klein N, Drotar D, Schluchter M, Hack M. Consequences and risks of <1000-g birth weight for neuropsychological skills, achievement, and adaptive functioning. *Journal of developmental and behavioral pediatrics: JDBP.* 2006 Dec;27 (6):459-69. PubMed PMID: 17164618.

[37] Pharoah PO, Cooke T, Rosenbloom L, Cooke RW. Effects of birth weight, gestational age, and maternal obstetric history on birth prevalence of cerebral palsy. *Archives of disease in childhood.* 1987 Oct;62 (10):1035-40. PubMed PMID: 3674922.

[38] Volpe JJ. Brain injury in premature infants: a complex amalgam of destructive and developmental disturbances. *The Lancet Neurology.* 2009 Jan;8 (1):110-24. PubMed PMID: 19081519. Pubmed Central PMCID: 2707149. Epub 2008/12/17. eng.

[39] Inage YW, Itoh M, Takashima S. Correlation between cerebrovascular maturity and periventricular leukomalacia. *Pediatric neurology.* 2000 Mar;22 (3):204-8. PubMed PMID: 10734251.

[40] Miyawaki T, Matsui K, Takashima S. Developmental characteristics of vessel density in the human fetal and infant brains. *Early human development.* 1998 Nov;53 (1):65-72. PubMed PMID: 10193927.

[41] Back SA, Riddle A, McClure MM. Maturation-dependent vulnerability of perinatal white matter in premature birth. *Stroke; a journal of cerebral circulation.* 2007 Feb;38 (2 Suppl):724-30. PubMed PMID: 17261726.

[42] Back SA, Luo NL, Mallinson RA, O'Malley JP, Wallen LD, Frei B, et al., Selective vulnerability of preterm white matter to oxidative damage defined by F2-isoprostanes. *Annals of neurology.* 2005 Jul;58 (1):108-20. PubMed PMID: 15984031.

[43] Back SA, Luo NL, Borenstein NS, Volpe JJ, Kinney HC. Arrested oligodendrocyte lineage progression during human cerebral white matter development: dissociation between the timing of progenitor differentiation and myelinogenesis. *Journal of neuropathology and experimental neurology.* 2002 Feb;61 (2):197-211. PubMed PMID: 11853021.

[44] Back SA, Luo NL, Borenstein NS, Levine JM, Volpe JJ, Kinney HC. Late oligodendrocyte progenitors coincide with the developmental window of vulnerability for human perinatal white matter injury. *The Journal of neuroscience: the official*

journal of the Society for Neuroscience. 2001 Feb 15;21 (4):1302-12. PubMed PMID: 11160401.

[45] Oka A, Belliveau MJ, Rosenberg PA, Volpe JJ. Vulnerability of oligodendroglia to glutamate: pharmacology, mechanisms, and prevention. *The Journal of neuroscience: the official journal of the Society for Neuroscience.* 1993 Apr;13 (4):1441-53. PubMed PMID: 8096541.

[46] Yonezawa M, Back SA, Gan X, Rosenberg PA, Volpe JJ. Cystine deprivation induces oligodendroglial death: rescue by free radical scavengers and by a diffusible glial factor. *Journal of neurochemistry.* 1996 Aug;67 (2):566-73. PubMed PMID: 8764581.

[47] Back SA, Gan X, Li Y, Rosenberg PA, Volpe JJ. Maturation-dependent vulnerability of oligodendrocytes to oxidative stress-induced death caused by glutathione depletion. *The Journal of neuroscience: the official journal of the Society for Neuroscience.* 1998 Aug 15;18 (16):6241-53. PubMed PMID: 9698317.

[48] Husain J, Juurlink BH. Oligodendroglial precursor cell susceptibility to hypoxia is related to poor ability to cope with reactive oxygen species. *Brain research.* 1995 Nov 6;698 (1-2):86-94. PubMed PMID: 8581507.

[49] Jelinski SE, Yager JY, Juurlink BH. Preferential injury of oligodendroblasts by a short hypoxic-ischemic insult. *Brain research.* 1999 Jan 2;815 (1):150-3. PubMed PMID: 9974135.

[50] Juurlink BH, Thorburne SK, Hertz L. Peroxide-scavenging deficit underlies oligodendrocyte susceptibility to oxidative stress. *Glia.* 1998 Apr;22 (4):371-8. PubMed PMID: 9517569.

[51] Juurlink BH. Management of oxidative stress in the CNS: the many roles of glutathione. *Neurotox Res.* 1999 Dec;1 (2):119-40. PubMed PMID: 12835108.

[52] Thorburne SK, Juurlink BH. Low glutathione and high iron govern the susceptibility of oligodendroglial precursors to oxidative stress. *Journal of neurochemistry.* 1996 Sep;67 (3):1014-22. PubMed PMID: 8752107.

[53] Nanda D, Tolputt J, Collard KJ. Changes in brain glutathione levels during postnatal development in the rat. *Brain research Developmental brain research.* 1996 Jul 20;94 (2):238-41. PubMed PMID: 8836583.

[54] Back SA. Brain Injury in the Preterm Infant: New Horizons for Pathogenesis and Prevention. *Pediatric neurology.* 2015 Sep;53 (3):185-92. PubMed PMID: 26302698. Pubmed Central PMCID: 4550810.

[55] McClendon E, Chen K, Gong X, Sharifnia E, Hagen M, Cai V, et al., Prenatal cerebral ischemia triggers dysmaturation of caudate projection neurons. *Annals of neurology.* 2014 Apr;75 (4):508-24. PubMed PMID: 24395459. Pubmed Central PMCID: 4013245.

[56] Sehested LT, Pedersen P. Prognosis and risk factors for intrauterine growth retardation. *Danish medical journal.* 2014 Apr;61 (4):A4826. PubMed PMID: 24814595.

[57] Volpe JJ. The encephalopathy of prematurity--brain injury and impaired brain development inextricably intertwined. Seminars in pediatric neurology. 2009 Dec;16 (4):167-78. PubMed PMID: 19945651. Pubmed Central PMCID: 2799246. Epub 2009/12/01. eng.

[58] Badawi N, Kurinczuk JJ, Keogh JM, Alessandri LM, O'Sullivan F, Burton PR, et al., Intrapartum risk factors for newborn encephalopathy: the Western Australian case-control study. *Bmj.* 1998 Dec 5;317 (7172):1554-8. PubMed PMID: 9836653.

[59] Low JA, Boston RW, Pancham SR. Fetal asphyxia during the intrapartum period in intrauterine growth-retarded infants. *American journal of obstetrics and gynecology.* 1972 Jul 1;113 (3):351-7. PubMed PMID: 4637026.

[60] Berg AT. Indices of fetal growth-retardation, perinatal hypoxia-related factors and childhood neurological morbidity. *Early human development.* 1989 Jul;19 (4):271-83. PubMed PMID: 2806156.

[61] Low JA, Handley-Derry MH, Burke SO, Peters RD, Pater EA, Killen HL, et al., Association of intrauterine fetal growth retardation and learning deficits at age 9 to 11 years. *American journal of obstetrics and gynecology.* 1992 Dec;167 (6):1499-505. PubMed PMID: 1471654.

[62] Larroque B, Bertrais S, Czernichow P, Leger J. School difficulties in 20-year-olds who were born small for gestational age at term in a regional cohort study. *Pediatrics.* 2001 Aug;108 (1):111-5. PubMed PMID: 11433062.

[63] Blair E, Stanley F. Intrauterine growth and spastic cerebral palsy. I. Association with birth weight for gestational age. *American journal of obstetrics and gynecology.* 1990 Jan;162 (1):229-37. PubMed PMID: 2301497.

[64] Blair E, Stanley F. Intrauterine growth and spastic cerebral palsy II. The association with morphology at birth. *Early human development.* 1992 Feb;28 (2):91-103. PubMed PMID: 1587228.

[64a] Walker CK, Krakowiak P, Baker A, Hansen RL, Ozonoff S, Hertz-Picciotto I. Preeclampsia, placental insufficiency, and autism spectrum disorder or developmental delay. JAMA pediatrics. 2015 Feb;169(2):154-62. PubMed PMID: 25485869. Pubmed Central PMCID: 4416484.

[65] Morgane PJ, Mokler DJ, Galler JR. Effects of prenatal protein malnutrition on the hippocampal formation. *Neuroscience and biobehavioral reviews.* 2002 Jun;26 (4):471-83. PubMed PMID: 12204193.

[66] Smith GN, Flynn SW, McCarthy N, Meistrich B, Ehmann TS, MacEwan GW, et al., Low birthweight in schizophrenia: prematurity or poor fetal growth? *Schizophr. Res.* 2001 Mar 1;47 (2-3):177-84. PubMed PMID: 11278135.

[67] Gomez R, Romero R, Ghezzi F, Yoon BH, Mazor M, Berry SM. The fetal inflammatory response syndrome. *American journal of obstetrics and gynecology.* 1998 Aug;179 (1):194-202. PubMed PMID: 9704787.

[68] Yoon BH, Romero R, Moon JB, Oh SY, Han SY, Kim JC, et al., The frequency and clinical significance of intra-amniotic inflammation in patients with a positive cervical fetal fibronectin. *American journal of obstetrics and gynecology.* 2001 Nov;185 (5):1137-42. PubMed PMID: 11717647.

[69] Yoon BH, Romero R, Moon JB, Shim SS, Kim M, Kim G, et al., Clinical significance of intra-amniotic inflammation in patients with preterm labor and intact membranes. *American journal of obstetrics and gynecology.* 2001 Nov;185 (5):1130-6. PubMed PMID: 11717646.

[70] Yoon BH, Romero R, Park JS, Kim CJ, Kim SH, Choi JH, et al., Fetal exposure to an intra-amniotic inflammation and the development of cerebral palsy at the age of three years. *American journal of obstetrics and gynecology.* 2000 Mar;182 (3):675-81. PubMed PMID: 10739529.

[71] Yoon BH, Romero R, Park JS, Kim M, Oh SY, Kim CJ, et al., The relationship among inflammatory lesions of the umbilical cord (funisitis), umbilical cord plasma interleukin

6 concentration, amniotic fluid infection, and neonatal sepsis. *American journal of obstetrics and gynecology.* 2000 Nov;183 (5):1124-9. PubMed PMID: 11084553.

[72] Chau V, McFadden DE, Poskitt KJ, Miller SP. Chorioamnionitis in the pathogenesis of brain injury in preterm infants. *Clinics in perinatology.* 2014 Mar;41 (1):83-103. PubMed PMID: 24524448.

[73] Back SA, Han BH, Luo NL, Chricton CA, Xanthoudakis S, Tam J, et al., Selective vulnerability of late oligodendrocyte progenitors to hypoxia-ischemia. *The Journal of neuroscience: the official journal of the Society for Neuroscience.* 2002 Jan 15;22 (2):455-63. PubMed PMID: 11784790.

[74] Volpe JJ, Kinney HC, Jensen FE, Rosenberg PA. The developing oligodendrocyte: key cellular target in brain injury in the premature infant. *International journal of developmental neuroscience: the official journal of the International Society for Developmental Neuroscience.* 2011 Jun;29 (4):423-40. PubMed PMID: 21382469. Pubmed Central PMCID: 3099053. Epub 2011/03/09. eng.

[75] Golan HM, Lev V, Hallak M, Sorokin Y, Huleihel M. Specific neurodevelopmental damage in mice offspring following maternal inflammation during pregnancy. *Neuropharmacology.* 2005 May;48 (6):903-17. PubMed PMID: 15829260.

[76] Back SA, Miller SP. Brain injury in premature neonates: A primary cerebral dysmaturation disorder? *Annals of neurology.* 2014 Apr;75 (4):469-86. PubMed PMID: 24615937.

[77] Peebles DM, Wyatt JS. Synergy between antenatal exposure to infection and intrapartum events in causation of perinatal brain injury at term. *BJOG: an international journal of obstetrics and gynaecology.* 2002 Jul;109 (7):737-9. PubMed PMID: 12135207.

[78] Wang X, Stridh L, Li W, Dean J, Elmgren A, Gan L, et al., Lipopolysaccharide sensitizes neonatal hypoxic-ischemic brain injury in a MyD88-dependent manner. *Journal of immunology.* 2009 Dec 1;183 (11):7471-7. PubMed PMID: 19917690. Epub 2009/11/18. eng.

[79] Shankaran S, Laptook AR, Ehrenkranz RA, Tyson JE, McDonald SA, Donovan EF, et al., Whole-body hypothermia for neonates with hypoxic-ischemic encephalopathy. *The New England journal of medicine.* 2005 Oct 13;353 (15):1574-84. PubMed PMID: 16221780.

[80] Azzopardi D, Brocklehurst P, Edwards D, Halliday H, Levene M, Thoresen M, et al., The TOBY Study. Whole body hypothermia for the treatment of perinatal asphyxial encephalopathy: a randomised controlled trial. *BMC pediatrics.* 2008;8:17. PubMed PMID: 18447921. Pubmed Central PMCID: 2409316.

[81] Azzopardi D, Strohm B, Edwards AD, Halliday H, Juszczak E, Levene M, et al., Treatment of asphyxiated newborns with moderate hypothermia in routine clinical practice: how cooling is managed in the UK outside a clinical trial. *Archives of disease in childhood Fetal and neonatal edition.* 2009 Jul;94 (4):F260-4. PubMed PMID: 19060009. Epub 2008/12/09. eng.

[82] Jacobs SE, Berg M, Hunt R, Tarnow-Mordi WO, Inder TE, Davis PG. Cooling for newborns with hypoxic ischaemic encephalopathy. *Cochrane Database Syst. Rev.* 2013;1:CD003311. PubMed PMID: 23440789.

[83] Jacobs SE, Morley CJ, Inder TE, Stewart MJ, Smith KR, McNamara PJ, et al., Whole-body hypothermia for term and near-term newborns with hypoxic-ischemic

[83] encephalopathy: a randomized controlled trial. *Archives of pediatrics & adolescent medicine.* 2011 Aug;165 (8):692-700. PubMed PMID: 21464374.

[84] Rice JE, 3rd, Vannucci RC, Brierley JB. The influence of immaturity on hypoxic-ischemic brain damage in the rat. *Annals of neurology.* 1981 Feb;9 (2):131-41. PubMed PMID: 7235629.

[85] Lachmann PJ. The penumbra of thalidomide, the litigation culture and the licensing of pharmaceuticals. *QJM.* 2012 Dec;105 (12):1179-89. PubMed PMID: 22908318. Pubmed Central PMCID: 3516063.

[86] Ikonomidou C, Bittigau P, Koch C, Genz K, Hoerster F, Felderhoff-Mueser U, et al., Neurotransmitters and apoptosis in the developing brain. *Biochemical pharmacology.* 2001 Aug 15;62 (4):401-5. PubMed PMID: 11448448.

[87] Ikonomidou C, Bosch F, Miksa M, Bittigau P, Vockler J, Dikranian K, et al., Blockade of NMDA receptors and apoptotic neurodegeneration in the developing brain. *Science.* 1999 Jan 1;283 (5398):70-4. PubMed PMID: 9872743.

[88] Fahey JW, Talalay P. Antioxidant functions of sulforaphane: a potent inducer of Phase II detoxication enzymes. *Food Chem. Toxicol.* 1999 Sep-Oct;37 (9-10):973-9. PubMed PMID: 10541453.

[89] Fahey JW, Zalcmann AT, Talalay P. The chemical diversity and distribution of glucosinolates and isothiocyanates among plants. *Phytochemistry.* 2001 Jan;56 (1):5-51. PubMed PMID: 11198818. Epub 2001/02/24. eng.

[90] Fahey JW, Zhang Y, Talalay P. Broccoli sprouts: an exceptionally rich source of inducers of enzymes that protect against chemical carcinogens. *Proceedings of the National Academy of Sciences of the United States of America.* 1997 Sep 16;94 (19):10367-72. PubMed PMID: 9294217.

[91] Heiss WD, Thiel A, Grond M, Graf R. Which targets are relevant for therapy of acute ischemic stroke? *Stroke; a journal of cerebral circulation.* 1999 Jul;30 (7):1486-9. PubMed PMID: 10390327.

[92] Wu L, Ashraf MH, Facci M, Wang R, Paterson PG, Ferrie A, et al., Dietary approach to attenuate oxidative stress, hypertension, and inflammation in the cardiovascular system. *Proceedings of the National Academy of Sciences of the United States of America.* 2004 May 4;101 (18):7094-9. PubMed PMID: 15103025.

[93] Wu L, Noyan Ashraf MH, Facci M, Wang R, Paterson PG, Ferrie A, et al., Dietary approach to attenuate oxidative stress, hypertension, and inflammation in the cardiovascular system. *Proceedings of the National Academy of Sciences of the United States of America.* 2004 May 4;101 (18):7094-9. PubMed PMID: 15103025.

[94] Noyan-Ashraf MH, Wu L, Wang R, Juurlink BH. Dietary approaches to positively influence fetal determinants of adult health. *FASEB journal: official publication of the Federation of American Societies for Experimental Biology.* 2006 Feb;20 (2):371-3. PubMed PMID: 16354723.

[95] Wu L, Juurlink BH. The impaired glutathione system and its up-regulation by sulforaphane in vascular smooth muscle cells from spontaneously hypertensive rats. *J. Hypertens.* 2001 Oct;19 (10):1819-25. PubMed PMID: 11593102.

[96] Juurlink BH. Therapeutic potential of dietary phase 2 enzyme inducers in ameliorating diseases that have an underlying inflammatory component. *Canadian journal of physiology and pharmacology.* 2001 Mar;79 (3):266-82. PubMed PMID: 11294604.

[97] Juurlink BH. Can dietary intake of phase 2 protein inducers affect the rising epidemic of diseases such as Type 2 diabetes? *MedGenMed*. 2003 Dec 5;5 (4):25. PubMed PMID: 14745372.

[98] Shapiro TA, Fahey JW, Wade KL, Stephenson KK, Talalay P. Chemoprotective glucosinolates and isothiocyanates of broccoli sprouts: metabolism and excretion in humans. *Cancer epidemiology, biomarkers & prevention: a publication of the American Association for Cancer Research, cosponsored by the American Society of Preventive Oncology*. 2001 May;10 (5):501-8. PubMed PMID: 11352861.

[99] Noyan-Ashraf MH, Sadeghinejad Z, Juurlink BH. Dietary approach to decrease aging-related CNS inflammation. *Nutr Neurosci*. 2005 Apr;8 (2):101-10. PubMed PMID: 16053242.

[100] Wu L, Juurlink BH. Increased methylglyoxal and oxidative stress in hypertensive rat vascular smooth muscle cells. *Hypertension*. 2002 Mar 1;39 (3):809-14. PubMed PMID: 11897769.

[101] Zhao J, Kobori N, Aronowski J, Dash PK. Sulforaphane reduces infarct volume following focal cerebral ischemia in rodents. *Neuroscience letters*. 2006 Jan 30;393 (2-3):108-12. PubMed PMID: 16233958. Epub 2005/10/20. eng.

[102] Black AM, Armstrong EA, Scott O, Juurlink BJ, Yager JY. Broccoli sprout supplementation during pregnancy prevents brain injury in the newborn rat following placental insufficiency. *Behavioural brain research*. 2015 Sep 15;291:289-98. PubMed PMID: 26014855.

[103] Lane RH, Ramirez RJ, Tsirka AE, Kloesz JL, McLaughlin MK, Gruetzmacher EM, et al., Uteroplacental insufficiency lowers the threshold towards hypoxia-induced cerebral apoptosis in growth-retarded fetal rats. *Brain research*. 2001 Apr 23;895 (1-2):186-93. PubMed PMID: 11259777.

[104] Schober ME, McKnight RA, Yu X, Callaway CW, Ke X, Lane RH. Intrauterine growth restriction due to uteroplacental insufficiency decreased white matter and altered NMDAR subunit composition in juvenile rat hippocampi. *American journal of physiology Regulatory, integrative and comparative physiology*. 2009 Mar;296 (3):R681-92. PubMed PMID: 19144756.

[105] Rousset CI, Chalon S, Cantagrel S, Bodard S, Andres C, Gressens P, et al., Maternal exposure to LPS induces hypomyelination in the internal capsule and programmed cell death in the deep gray matter in newborn rats. *Pediatric research*. 2006 Mar;59 (3):428-33. PubMed PMID: 16492984.

[106] Bona E, Johansson BB, Hagberg H. Sensorimotor function and neuropathology five to six weeks after hypoxia-ischemia in seven-day-old rats. *Pediatric research*. 1997 Nov;42 (5):678-83. PubMed PMID: 9357943.

[107] Scott O, Galicia-Connolly E, Adams D, Surette S, Vohra S, Yager JY. The safety of cruciferous plants in humans: a systematic review. *Journal of biomedicine & biotechnology*. 2012;2012:503241. PubMed PMID: 22500092. Pubmed Central PMCID: 3303573. Epub 2012/04/14. eng.

[108] Zwaigenbaum L, Szatmari P, Jones MB, Bryson SE, MacLean JE, Mahoney WJ, et al., Pregnancy and birth complications in autism and liability to the broader autism phenotype. *Journal of the American Academy of Child and Adolescent Psychiatry*. 2002 May;41 (5):572-9. PubMed PMID: 12014790.

[109] Zwaigenbaum L. The intriguing relationship between cerebral palsy and autism. *Developmental medicine and child neurology.* 2014 Jan;56 (1):7-8. PubMed PMID: 24116659.

[110] Wolff JJ, Gu H, Gerig G, Elison JT, Styner M, Gouttard S, et al., Differences in white matter fiber tract development present from 6 to 24 months in infants with autism. *The American journal of psychiatry.* 2012 Jun;169 (6):589-600. PubMed PMID: 22362397. Pubmed Central PMCID: 3377782.

[111] Pinelli J, Zwaigenbaum L. Chorioamnionitis, gestational age, male sex, birth weight, and illness severity predicted positive autism screening scores in very-low-birth-weight preterm infants. *Evidence-based nursing.* 2008 Oct;11 (4):122. PubMed PMID: 18815334.

[112] Bjorgaas HM, Elgen I, Boe T, Hysing M. Mental health in children with cerebral palsy: does screening capture the complexity? *TheScientificWorldJournal.* 2013;2013:468402. PubMed PMID: 23690745. Pubmed Central PMCID: 3654290.

[113] Bjorgaas HM, Hysing M, Elgen I. Psychiatric disorders among children with cerebral palsy at school starting age. *Research in developmental disabilities.* 2012 Jul-Aug;33 (4):1287-93. PubMed PMID: 22502856.

In: Broccoli
Editor: Bernhard H. J. Juurlink

ISBN: 978-1-63484-313-3
© 2016 Nova Science Publishers, Inc.

Chapter 10

THE MULTIFACETED ROLE OF SULFORAPHANE IN PROTECTION AGAINST UV RADIATION-MEDIATED SKIN DAMAGE

Andrea L. Benedict[1], Elena V. Knatko[2], Rumen V. Kostov[2], Ying Zhang[2], Maureen Higgins[2], Sukirti Kalra[2], Jed W. Fahey[1,3], Sally H. Ibbotson[4], Charlotte M. Proby[2], Paul Talalay[1] and Albena T. Dinkova-Kostova[1,2,5,]*

[1]Lewis B. and Dorothy Cullman Chemoprotection Center, Department of Pharmacology and Molecular Sciences, Johns Hopkins University School of Medicine, Baltimore, MD, US
[2]Division of Cancer Research, Medical Research Institute, University of Dundee, Dundee, Scotland, UK
[3]Center for Human Nutrition, Department of International Health, Johns Hopkins University Bloomberg School of Public Health, Baltimore, MD, US
[4]Photobiology Unit, Ninewells Hospital and Medical School, University of Dundee, Dundee, Scotland, UK
[5]Department of Medicine, Johns Hopkins University School of Medicine, Baltimore, MD, US

ABSTRACT

Ultraviolet radiation (UVR), the most abundant carcinogen in our environment, is the major factor in the etiology of skin damage and photocarcinogenesis. Common preventive measures, such as sunscreens and general sun avoidance, are not sufficiently effective, and skin cancer is the most common human cancer. Furthermore, cutaneous squamous cell carcinomas are among the most highly mutated human malignancies, carrying 1 mutation per ~30,000 bp of coding sequence. Such extraordinary mutation

---

[*] Corresponding author: Email: A.DinkovaKostova@dundee.ac.uk.

burden makes the possibility for success of a single-target therapy questionable and highlights the need for agents capable of affecting multiple hallmarks of cancer. UVR causes direct DNA damage, generation of reactive oxygen species (ROS), inflammation, and immunosuppression. These deleterious biological insults are counteracted by an elaborate network of cellular defense mechanisms. The isothiocyanate sulforaphane is a potent inducer of these defenses, which include cytoprotective antioxidant and anti-inflammatory enzymes and glutathione. Sulforaphane-containing broccoli sprout extracts, administered either topically or in the diet, protect SKH-1 hairless mice against UVR-mediated skin damage and tumor formation. In humans, application of these extracts to the skin of healthy subjects reduces susceptibility to erythema arising from acute exposure to UVR. Many of the protective effects of sulforaphane are due to the potent ability of the isothiocyanate to activate transcription factor Nrf2, and are lost in cells and animals that are Nrf2-deficient. In addition, sulforaphane provides Nrf2-independent protection, such as suppression of NFκB signaling and direct inhibition of the activity of macrophage migration inhibitory factor (MIF), a pro-inflammatory cytokine implicated in UVR-mediated skin damage and carcinogenesis. Thus, sulforaphane provides a paradigm for a dietary small molecule indirect antioxidant which plays a multifaceted role in protection against the damaging effects of oxidative stress and inflammation.

Keywords: chemoprotection, Keap1, MIF, Nrf2, photodamage, skin cancer

INTRODUCTION

Ultraviolet Radiation (UVR)-Induced Skin Damage and Carcinogenesis

Non-melanoma skin cancer is the most common human malignancy, with more than two million new cases diagnosed globally each year [1]. Exome sequencing of human primary cutaneous squamous cell carcinomas and matched normal tissue has revealed an extraordinary large mutation burden of about 1,300 somatic single-nucleotide variants per exome (1 per ~30,000 bp of coding sequence) [2]. Ultraviolet radiation (UVR) is the major causative factor for skin cancer. It acts as a complete carcinogen that can cause the initiation, promotion and progression of squamous cell and basal cell carcinomas. Following UVR exposure, cells display diverse damage, including direct modification of DNA bases, inflammation, morphological changes, and generation of ROS, which in turn leads to oxidative stress [3, 4]. New strategies of molecular protection are being explored as a method to protect the cells of the skin from the damaging effects of UVR, as the standard practices of sun avoidance and sunscreens have not proven adequately effective in decreasing the global incidence of skin cancer. Molecular protectors that are capable of boosting multiple intracellular defense mechanisms, thereby defending against the many types of deleterious biological insults of UVR, would be particularly advantageous [5].

The UVR-spectrum has two physiologically relevant wavelength components: UVB (280-315 nm) and UVA (315-400 nm) (Figure 1) [6]. While UVB wavelengths only represent about 5% of the solar radiation energy that reaches the surface of the Earth, they are largely responsible for causing erythema, photoaging, and cancer [1]. UVB penetrates the epidermis, which consists mainly of differentiated and proliferating keratinocytes [7]. These wavelengths damage DNA directly, promoting cross-linking between DNA bases with the formation of cyclobutane-pyrimidine dimers and pyrimidine [6-4] pyrimidone photoproducts [8, 9]. The resulting mutations (characterized by C to T or CC to TT transitions) are known as "signatures" of sun exposure [10]. UVB wavelengths are also known to produce an acute inflammatory response culminating in edema and erythema. This response is accompanied by release of pro-inflammatory cytokines and upregulation of cyclooxygenase-2 (COX-2) and inducible nitric oxide synthase (iNOS), promoting prostaglandin-E2 (PG-E2) and nitric oxide (NO) synthesis [3]. This process signals the recruitment of leukocytes, leading to secondary tissue injury through the generation of reactive oxygen species (ROS) [6]. Evidence also suggests that UVB-induced DNA damage may play a role in initiating the inflammatory response and erythema by triggering IL-1 release [3].

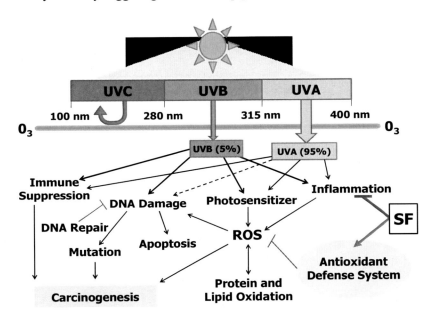

Figure 1. Sulforaphane has the potential to protect skin cells from UVR. The UVR-spectrum comprises UVC (100-280 nm), UVB (280-315 nm), and UVA (315-400 nm). UVC wavelengths are filtered by the ozone layer, thus UVB and UVA wavelengths are responsible for the physiological changes in skin and skin cells after exposure to solar radiation. These wavelengths are capable of producing direct damage to cellular macromolecules, generating ROS, increasing inflammation, as well as suppressing the immune system. These damaging effects are all important factors in the multistep carcinogenesis process. Sulforaphane (SF) has the potential to attenuate UV-induced damage by upregulating the antioxidant phase 2 defense system and suppressing pro-inflammatory processes. Modified from Svobodova et al. (2006).

UVA comprises ~95% of the terrestrial solar radiation energy, but it penetrates deeper into the dermis than does UVB, reaching the dermal fibroblast population, generating ROS and therefore indirectly oxidizing cellular proteins, lipids, polysaccharides, and DNA [4, 7]. In addition to damaging DNA indirectly resulting primarily in the formation of 8-oxo-7,8-dihydro-2'-deoxyguanosine, exposure of human skin to UVA also generates cyclobutane pyrimidine dimers, typical UVB-induced DNA lesions [11]. At high doses, UVA also initiates inflammatory responses within the skin [3]. Both UVA and UVB wavelengths thus induce inflammation, although wavelengths in the UVB region are more effective than those in the UVA region in inducing an erythemic response [6]. This may be a result of the ability of UVB to cause direct damage to the DNA in the cells of the epidermis, subsequently triggering a release of the pro-inflammatory cytokines IL-1β and TNF-α from keratinocytes [7, 12]. In turn, these soluble factors regulate the release of IL-6 and IL-8 from dermal fibroblasts, inducing a dermal inflammatory response resulting in edema and erythema [13]. UVA and UVB wavelengths also cause DNA damage, through both direct modification and oxidative damage to DNA bases, leading to increased risk of mutations in the genome. When mutations occur in the tumor suppressor gene sequences, such as the *p53* gene, the ability of the cells to undergo apoptosis is impaired, leading to survival of cells with mutations that can potentially progress to skin cancer [4].

Exposure to UVA radiation can also sensitize the skin of those individuals who are undergoing certain therapies, notably treatments with the anti-inflammatory and immunosuppressive thiopurines. Indeed, long-term use of thiopurines (azathioprine, 6-mercaptopurine, and 6-thioguanine) is associated with increased risk (by more than 100-fold) for the development of very aggressive multiple squamous cell carcinomas of the skin [14-16]. During replication, the active metabolite of the thiopurines, 6-thioguanine nucleotide, is incorporated into DNA. Interestingly, oral treatment with azathioprine in mice leads to a much greater incorporation of 6-thioguanine in DNA of skin than liver [17]. Peter Karran and his colleagues have elegantly demonstrated that unlike guanine, 6-thioguanine absorbs in the UVA region of the solar spectrum, generating reactive oxygen species (ROS) and 6-thioguanine photo-oxidation products that damage DNA and proteins, including DNA repair proteins [18-20]. The combination of 6-thioguanine and UVA radiation is synergistically mutagenic in cells [21]. Treatment with azathioprine increases the skin photosensitivity to UVA radiation in humans [21], whereas replacement of azathioprine with mycophenolate in organ transplant recipients leads to reversal of this sensitization [22]. Therefore, oxidative stress and the inflammation produced by UVR are potential targets for intervention to alleviate the cellular damage that may lead to skin cancer.

Antioxidant Defenses

Many of the damaging processes initiated by UVR are counteracted by the intrinsic cellular antioxidant defenses. Superoxide dismutase (SOD), a widely distributed enzyme that converts superoxide to hydrogen peroxide at diffusion-controlled rates, together with catalase and peroxidases that then dispose of hydrogen peroxide, exemplify three critical endogenous enzymatic protective antioxidants. Cells are also equipped with small molecules with direct antioxidant functions, including reduced glutathione (GSH), ascorbic acid (vitamin C), tocopherols, lipoic acid, ubiquinol, and carotenes, which participate in redox reactions directly and scavenge oxidants. In addition to these housekeeping antioxidant systems, cells have evolved other elaborate and complex protective mechanisms, such as the inducible phase 2 cytoprotective enzymes and GSH, which act to detoxify harmful electrophiles and ROS [23]. In the case of excess UVR, the cells are overwhelmed by oxidative stress and the innate defenses are insufficient for protection [4]. Increasing the antioxidant capacity of the cell helps to protect it from oxidative damage. Direct antioxidants, such as (−)-epicatechin-3-gallate and carotenoids (i.e., β-carotene and lycopene), are themselves oxygen radical scavengers and protect skin cells from ROS-induced damage [24-26]. Nevertheless, their protective effects are short-lived and they can also have pro-oxidant effects [27]. A more efficient and long-lasting protective strategy is the upregulation of the intrinsic antioxidant defense system through the Keap1/Nrf2 pathway.

The Keap1/Nrf2 Pathway

Keap1 (Kelch-like ECH-associated protein 1) mediates the ubiquitination of Nrf2 (NF-E2-related factor 2) by Cullin3 (Cul3)-based E3 ligase, and the subsequent degradation of the transcription factor by the 26S proteasome [28-32]. It does so by using a cyclic sequential attachment and regeneration mechanism whereby the Keap1-Nrf2 protein complex sequentially adopts two distinct conformations, "open," in which Nrf2 interacts with one molecule of Keap1, followed by "closed," in which Nrf2 binds to both members of the Keap1 dimer, allowing Nrf2 ubiquitination; the ubiquitinated Nrf2 is degraded by the proteasome, and Keap1 is regenerated (Figure 2) [33]. Oxidants and electrophiles modify reactive cysteine residues on Keap1 and disrupt the ability of Keap1 to target Nrf2 for degradation. Nrf2 then accumulates, translocates to the nucleus, where it dimerizes with small Maf proteins, and binds to cis-acting antioxidant response elements (AREs) in the 5'-flanking regions of Nrf2-dependent genes. These genes encode proteins and enzymes that have antioxidant and detoxification activities which promote removal of damaging ROS and reactive nitrogen species, electrophiles, toxins, and damaged proteins, lipids, and nucleic acids. Nrf2-dependent genes that provide these protective effects include: 1) conjugating enzymes, such as glutathione transferases (GSTs) and UDP-glucuronosyltransferases (UGTs); 2) enzymes involved in the GSH synthesis and utilization, including γ-glutamylcysteine synthetase (γ-GCS), glutathione peroxidase, and glutathione reductase; 3) antioxidant enzymes and proteins, such as NAD(P)H:quinone oxidoreductase 1 (NQO1), heme oxygenase 1 (HMOX1), superoxidase dismutase (SOD), catalase, thioredoxin (TRX), and thioredoxin reductase (TRXR). The coordinate upregulation of these systems, termed the phase 2 response, provides protection against a wide array of challenges and onset of disease [34].

SULFORAPHANE: DISCOVERY AS AN INDUCER OF THE PHASE 2 RESPONSE

A natural, electrophilic compound isolated from broccoli extracts, sulforaphane (SF) [1-isothiocyanato-(4R)-(methylsulfinyl) butane] (Figure 3), is a potent inducer of the phase 2 cytoprotective response. The discovery and isolation of SF as an inducer was made by Yuesheng Zhang and colleagues [35] during the quest to find the factor(s) within vegetables that upregulate the phase 2 response and confer protection against carcinogenesis. The correlation between high consumption of certain vegetables and a lower risk for developing cancer had long been observed in humans and in animal studies [36-39]. These studies led to the conclusion that many green and yellow vegetables protect against colorectal cancer, lung cancer, and possibly prostate cancer. It was found that broccoli and other members of the Cruciferae family were especially rich sources of phase 2-inducer activity and that 3-day-old broccoli sprouts contain 20 to 50 times higher levels of SF than does the mature plant [40].

SF is naturally found in the form of an inert glucosinolate (β-thioglucoside *N*-hydroxysulfate) precursor called glucoraphanin. Glucosinolates, like glucoraphanin, are enzymatically converted to their biologically-active forms by thioglucoside glucohydrolases, also known as myrosinases (EC 3.2.1.147) (Figure 3) [41]. Enzyme and substrate are compartmentalized within plants and, when the plant tissue is damaged, they come in contact giving rise to a range of hydrolytic products, including SF [42-44]. Myrosinases are also present in fungi and bacteria. Of specific importance, microflora of the animal and human gastrointestinal tract can efficiently convert glucosinolates to isothiocyanates [45-48].

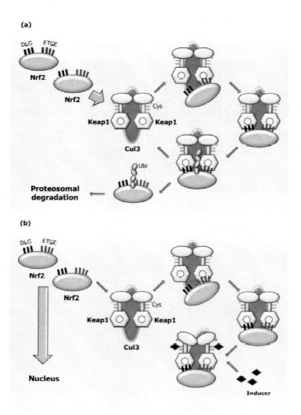

Figure 2. The cyclic sequential binding and regeneration model for Keap1-mediated degradation of Nrf2. (A) Nrf2 (purple) binds sequentially to a free Keap1 dimer (blue): first through its high-affinity ETGE motif (red) to one member of the Keap1 dimer to form the open conformation of the Keap1-Nrf2 complex, and then through its low-affinity DLG motif (black) to the second member of the Keap1 dimer to form the closed conformation of the complex. In the closed conformation, Nrf2 undergoes ubiquitination (yellow) by Cullin3 (green)/Rbx1 ubiquitin ligase. Ubiquitinated Nrf2 is released from Keap1 and degraded by the proteosome, free Keap1 is regenerated and able to bind to newly translated Nrf2, and the cycle begins again. (B) Inducers react with sensor cysteines of Keap1 (orange) leading to a conformational change resulting in inability for degradation. Consequently, the complex accumulates in the closed conformation, free Keap1 is not regenerated, and the newly-synthesized Nrf2 accumulates and translocates to the nucleus where, as a heterodimer with a small Maf transcription factor (not shown), Nrf2 binds to promoter sequences and activates expression of its target cytoprotective genes.

The central carbon of the isothiocyanate (-N=C=S) group is highly reactive with sulfhydryl groups, forming dithiocarbamate products. In animal tissues, SF is metabolized by the enzymes of the mercapturic acid pathway, ultimately forming reversible N-acetylcysteine-SF conjugates. Conjugation with glutathione, by action of cellular GSTs, sequesters SF within cells and this accumulation increases the inducer potency of SF [49-52]. Since its discovery as a phase 2 inducer, SF has been shown to be protective against many forms of cancers, traumatic injury, age-related diseases, and in many other disease and injury models. Together with the ability to initiate Nrf2-dependent phase 2 response, SF also suppresses pro-inflammatory processes and induces the heat shock response through Nrf2-dependent and -independent mechanisms [53-57]. At high concentrations, SF can also inhibit phase 1 enzymes, which activate procarcinogens to ultimate carcinogens, stimulate cell cycle arrest and apoptosis, and inhibit angiogenesis [58]. The multifunctional protective mechanisms and the natural, dietary occurrence of SF have made it a very attractive candidate as a potential therapeutic and cytoprotective agent against many forms of cellular damage, including UVR.

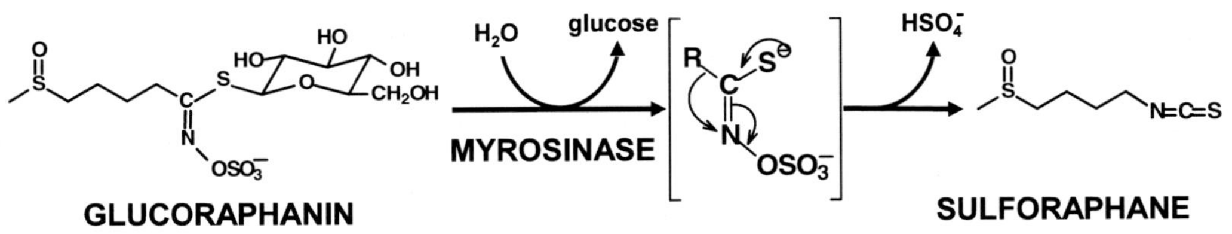

Figure 3. The general reaction in which glucoraphanin [(4-methylsulfinyl]butyl-glucosinolate; or thioglucoside N-hydroxysulfate, a glucosinolate], is converted to sulforaphane [1-isothiocyanato-(4R)-(methylsulfinyl)butane], is catalyzed by myrosinase (EC 3.2.1.147). This scheme in which a water soluble, relatively inactive, vacuole-bound precursor in a plant cell, is converted to a highly reactive, lachrymating, more lipophilic compound, is also known as the "mustard-oil bomb" - the enzyme is physically segregated from glucosinolates within the plant, but the two come into contact with each other upon tissue damage to the plant, such as by injury, cutting or chewing. The reaction involves enzymatic cleavage of the thioglucoside linkage, requires ascorbic acid as a co-factor, and is followed at neutral pH by rapid rearrangement of the unstable aglycone (a thiohydroximate-O-sulfonate) to form the cognate isothiocyanate. Under alternative conditions of pH, temperature, and metal cations, oxazolidine-2-thione may be formed, and with further specifier proteins a variety of other rearrangement products can also be formed (e.g., nitriles, epithionitriles, and thiocyanates).

CELL CULTURE AND NRF2-KNOCKOUT RESEARCH

Cell culture experiments and Nrf2-knockout mice have helped to define the protective role of Nrf2 and the SF-mediated induction of the Keap1/Nrf2 pathway on the damage caused by UVR insult. SF has been shown to induce NQO1 enzyme activity, the prototypic biomarker of the Nrf2-mediated phase 2 antioxidant response, and increase GSH levels in skin cell lines and primary culture, including human HaCaT keratinocytes, murine PE keratinocytes, and primary SKH-1 mouse keratinocytes and dermal fibroblasts [59, 60]. Prior treatment of the aforementioned cells with SF for 24 h before UVA irradiation protects the cells against UVA-induced oxidative stress by reducing levels of ROS. Protection by SF is also evident in cells that have 6-thioguanine in their genomic DNA and are hypersensitive to UVA radiation-mediated ROS formation [60]. At the same 6-thioguanine levels in their DNA, Keap1-knockout cells, in which Nrf2 is constitutively activated, are highly resistant to UVA radiation-induced oxidative stress, whereas cells that lack Nrf2 are more sensitive than their wild-type counterparts [61]. The protective effect of both SF and the Keap1-knockout genotype is completely lost in the absence of Nrf2 (i.e., in Nrf2-knockout or Keap1/Nrf2-double knockout cells), implying that protection is due to induction of Nrf2-dependent target genes [60, 61].

Curiously, in SKH-1 hairless mice the time of day of exposure to UVR is a contributing factor to its carcinogenicity, correlating with the circadian rhythmicity of the rate of excision repair in the murine skin [62]. SF does not appear to affect the extent of direct DNA damage in skin cells in culture. Primary SKH-1 keratinocytes and dermal fibroblasts treated for 24 h with 1 µM SF before broadband UVB radiation did not show reduction in the formation of cyclobutane pyrimidine dimers (CPDs) or 6,4-photoproducts (6,4-PPs) [60]. Oxidative DNA damage in skin cells caused by both UVA and UVB radiation has the potential to be affected by the SF-mediated upregulation in antioxidant capacity of the cells and has yet to be explored. Studies in Nrf2-knockout mice have shown that oxidative DNA damage and inflammation in ear tissue were increased with chronic UVB exposure as compared to wild-type mice, but this did not result in differences in tumor incidence or multiplicity between Nrf2-knockout and wild-type mice on the dorsal skin [63]. This study highlights the importance of this pathway in protection against oxidative stress and inflammation, but also indicates that there are other factors involved in addition to the Nrf2 pathway in preventing UVR-induced carcinogenesis. Another study on the impact of the Nrf2 pathway and SF treatment on UVR-induced damage also found photoprotective effects [64]. When Nrf2 wild-type and knockout mice were irradiated with 300 mJ/cm^2 UVB broad-band radiation, Nrf2-knockout animals were more susceptible than were wild-type mice to sunburn and apoptotic cell formation, increased skin thickness, and had higher levels of the pro-inflammatory cytokines, IL-1β and IL-6. When the mice were treated topically for 4 to 5 days with a low dose of SF (100 nmol), the wild-type mice showed a 43% protection against UVB-induced increase in skin thickness, whereas Nrf2-knockout mice had a variable 18% reduction in skin thickness 8 h after irradiation. These findings suggest that the Nrf2 pathway plays an important role in protection against UV-insult and that SF-mediated upregulation of this pathway could lead to reduction of oxidative DNA damage and inflammatory response induced by UVB and UVA wavelengths. Therefore, SF is a potential protective agent against UVR-induced skin damage by its ability to modulate oxidative stress, inflammation, and other skin cancer initiation and promotion effects at the molecular level.

PROTECTION OF MITOCHONDRIAL INTEGRITY

UVR causes mitochondrial dysfunction manifesting as a decrease in mitochondrial membrane potential and an increase in superoxide production [65]. Cells isolated from Nrf2-knockout animals have higher basal levels of superoxide than do their wild-type counterparts [66]. Furthermore, under conditions of Nrf2 deficiency, mitochondria are depolarized, respiration is impaired, and cellular ATP levels are decreased. Conversely, in cells with constitutive activation of Nrf2 (by Keap1-knockdown or knockout), the mitochondrial membrane potential, ATP levels, rate of respiration and efficiency of oxidative phosphorylation are all increased [66, 67]. Together, these findings suggest that enhanced mitochondrial activity under conditions of Nrf2 activation may be contributing to the Nrf2-mediated cytoprotection.

Mitochondria isolated from brain and liver of rats treated with a single dose of SF were resistant to opening of the mitochondrial permeability transition pore (PTP) caused by the oxidant *tert*-butyl hydroperoxide [68, 69]. Interestingly, PTP, a complex that allows the mitochondrial inner membrane to become permeable to solutes with molecular masses up to ~1500 Da, was recently found to be formed from dimers of the FoF1-ATP synthase [70]. The SF-mediated resistance to PTP opening correlated with increased antioxidant defenses, and the levels of mitochondrial GSH, glutathione peroxidase 1 (GPX1), malic enzyme 3 (ME3), and thioredoxin 2 (TRX2) were all upregulated in mitochondrial fractions isolated from the SF-treated animals [69]. Mitochondrial protein damage and impairment in respiration caused by the electrophilic lipid peroxidation product 4-hydroxy-2-nonenal were attenuated in mitochondria isolated from the cerebral cortex of SF-treated mice [71]. In rat renal epithelial cells and in kidney, SF protected against cisplatin- and gentamicin-induced toxicity and loss in mitochondrial membrane potential [72-74]. Protection against a panel of oxidants (superoxide, hydrogen peroxide, peroxynitrite) and electrophiles (4-hydroxy-2-nonenal, and acrolein), and an increase in mitochondrial antioxidant defenses were also observed when rat aortic smooth muscle cells were treated with SF [75].

In addition to protecting mitochondria by increasing the endogenous antioxidant defenses, SF also stimulates mitochondrial biogenesis, a process which is largely controlled by two classes of nuclear transcriptional regulators: transcription factors, such as nuclear respiratory factor-1 and 2, and transcriptional coactivators, such as peroxisome proliferator-activated receptor γ coactivator-1α and β (PGC1α and PGC1β) [76-80]. The Nrf2-dependent transcriptional upregulation and nuclear accumulation of nuclear respiratory factor-1 promotes mitochondrial biogenesis and protects against the cytotoxicity of the cardiotoxic anthracycline chemotherapeutic agent doxorubicin [81]. SF treatment of human fibroblasts causes an increase in mitochondrial mass and induction of PGC1α and PGC1β [82]; however, the dependence on Nrf2 has not been examined. Although further work is required to establish the precise relation between the Nrf2 status and the expression of the PGC1 coactivators, current findings suggest that preservation of mitochondrial integrity, through both increased endogenous antioxidant capacity and enhanced mitochondrial function, contributes to the cytoprotective effects of SF.

SKH-1 MOUSE STUDIES

Several studies have shown that SF-containing broccoli sprout extracts (BSE) are capable of protecting the skin of SKH-1 hairless mice against the damaging effects of UVR and UVR-induced carcinogenesis. Among rodents, the hairless but immunologically competent SKH-1 mouse, lacking a transcriptional co-repressor essential for hair follicle regeneration, is a highly relevant model for human skin cancer [83]. After 16-20 weeks of bi-weekly exposure to relatively low-dose UVB (30 mJ/cm^2), this mouse develops multiple skin tumors during the subsequent 12-16 weeks [84]. Topical application of a single dose of SF-containing BSE (100 nmol SF/cm^2) to the dorsal skin of these mice caused a 1.6-fold induction of NQO1 activity and increased the protein levels of NQO1, HMOX1 and GSTA1, indicating induction of the Nrf2 pathway in skin cells [85]. Treatment of SKH-1 mouse skin with the same dose of SF-containing BSE for 3 days resulted in an even greater (2.7-fold) induction of NQO1 activity [85].

To confirm that the induction of the Nrf2 pathway was solely due to the SF and not some other constituent of the BSE, as well as whether UVB wavelengths would affect induction of the Nrf2 pathway, synthetic SF and BSE containing equivalent amounts of SF were applied topically to SKH-1 hairless mouse dorsal skin at a dose of 100 nmol/cm^2, once daily for 3 days, followed by irradiation with a single dose of 700 mJ/cm^2 UVB narrow-band (311 nm) 24 h after the last topical treatment [53]. Twenty-four hours after irradiation, the NQO1 activity was found to be slightly depressed in control-treated dorsal skin compared to non-irradiated control levels, and treatment with either synthetic SF or equivalent concentrations of SF in BSE for 3 days before irradiation resulted in nearly identical ~40% induction in NQO1 activity compared to control levels. This study provides evidence that the phase 2 inducer activities of SF-containing BSE are entirely attributable to their SF content.

To determine the effect of SF on tumor formation after UV exposure, SKH-1 mice were chronically irradiated with UVB broad-band wavelengths (30 mJ/cm^2; bi-weekly), and were subsequently topically treated once daily, 5 days a week, for 11 weeks with BSE delivering 1.0 µmol SF [59]. It was found that topical treatment with SF-containing BSE resulted in a significant decrease in tumor incidence, multiplicity, and burden by ~50% when compared to control-treated animals. Another study showed that feeding daily doses of broccoli sprout powder containing 10 µmol of the SF-precursor glucoraphanin to SKH-1 mice, that had received chronic bi-weekly UVB exposure, also led to a decrease in tumor incidence, multiplicity and volume [86], indicating that dietary intake of the precursor of SF is capable of being converted to SF by the gut microflora of mice and is subsequently bioavailable to skin cells.

To address the ability of SF to provide protection against the damaging effects of UVR before UVR exposure, SKH-1 mice were pretreated with synthetic SF (1 or 2.5 µmol SF) for 1 week prior to UVB exposure and then 1 h before each irradiation, which resulted in a reduction in tumor multiplicity and burden at both doses of SF over the 25 week study [87]. In another pretreatment experiment, synthetic SF (5.6 and 14.1 µmol) was given orally once a day for 14 days and SKH-1 mice were irradiated with UVB wavelengths on days 9, 11, and 13 [88]. Oral SF pretreatment reduced gross skin thickness, number of cell layers in the epidermis and protein levels of COX-2 in the skin 24 h after the last UVB exposure. These studies in the SKH-1 hairless mouse have provided significant evidence that SF, administered both topically and orally and in the form of BSE rich in SF or pure SF, can protect the skin against the damaging effects of UVR and prevent or reduce tumor formation when treatments are given before or after UVR insult.

We have recently generated SKH-1 hairless mice in which Nrf2 is either deleted or constitutively activated by back-crossing Nrf2-knockout [89, 90] and Keap1-knockdown [91] C57BL/6 mice onto the SKH-1 hairless genetic background over six generations. Compared to wild-type, skin and liver samples isolated from Nrf2-knockout SKH-1 hairless animals have lower enzyme activity levels of the Nrf2-dependent enzyme NQO1, whereas those isolated from their Keap1-knockdown SKH-1 hairless counterparts, have higher enzyme activity levels (Figure 4A, B). Interestingly, the contribution of Nrf2 to the basal levels of NQO1 in the skin and liver is vastly different. Thus, in wild-type animals, the NQO1 activity is 2.8-fold greater in the skin than in the liver. Furthermore, whereas the NQO1 activity in the liver of Nrf2-knockout mice is only ~20% of their wild-type counterparts (Figure 4B), the NQO1 activity in the knockout mouse skin is ~80% of that in wild-type skin (Figure 4A). In agreement with the differential effect of Nrf2 in the two organs, the levels of NQO1 in the skin and liver of Keap1-knockdown mice are ~2-fold and ~10-fold greater than that in the wild-type animals. The finding that the skin of the Nrf2-knockout mice contains higher basal levels of NQO1 than the liver could indicate the existence of compensatory mechanism(s) for the absence of Nrf2, such as those mediated by Nrf1, Nrf3, or p45NEF2 [92] in the skin that may not be present and/or activated in the liver. Indeed, the levels mRNA of Nrf3 are elevated in the skin of Nrf2-knockout mice [93, 94]. This organ-specific difference in basal levels of NQO1 suggests that skin cells may have adapted alternate antioxidant response mechanisms that help them to maintain homeostasis in the face of environmental stresses.

Primary dermal fibroblasts from SKH-1 hairless mice displayed potent and robust NQO1 induction 48 h after SF treatment (~8-fold at 5 µM SF), whereas their counterparts isolated from hairless Nrf2-knockout mice showed no inducible NQO1 activity (Figure 4C). When SKH-1 and hairless Nrf2-knockout mouse dorsal skin was treated in vivo topically with 100 nmol/cm^2 SF, once daily for 3 days, the NQO1 activity in the SKH-1 skin increased ~2-fold with the SF treatment, whereas an identical treatment of hairless Nrf2-knockout mice did not induce NQO1 (Figure 4D).

Skin isolated from Keap1-knockdown SKH-1 hairless mice has ~3-fold higher levels of Nrf2 compared to SKH-1 hairless mouse skin [94]. In addition to NQO1, the levels of GST, HMOX, and GCLC are also upregulated. Keap1-knockdown mice showed a profound reduction in induction of erythema and the inflammatory marker IL-6 expression provoked by solar-simulated UVR. Furthermore, Keap1-knockdown SKH-1 hairless mice were substantially protected against the carcinogenic effects of solar-simulated UVR. Thus, compared to SKH-1 hairless mice, the tumor incidence was reduced by 40%, and the tumor multiplicity by ~5-fold in the Keap1-knockdown SKH-1 hairless mice. The total tumor volume per mouse was also profoundly reduced (by 80%) by the genetic upregulation of Nrf2. The Nrf2-knockout and Keap1-knockdown SKH-1 hairless mice provide important tools for mechanistic studies of the role of Nrf2 in protection against photodamage and photocarcinogenesis.

HUMAN STUDIES

In healthy human subjects, topical SF treatment has been shown to upregulate the phase 2 response and guard against the erythema caused by acute exposure to UVR. When a single dose of BSE containing 170 or 340 nmol of SF was applied to small circular areas (1 cm in diameter) on the skin of three healthy human subjects, NQO1 enzyme activity increased by ~1.5-fold 24 h after treatment in a 3-mm punch biopsy taken from the center of the area, compared to control-treated skin (80% acetone, v/v) [85]. The effects of three repeated topical applications, given at 24-h intervals, was also examined with cumulative doses of 150, 300, and 450 nmol SF in BSE, resulting in an average increase of NQO1 specific activity by ~4.5-

fold for the 450 nmol SF dose over control skin 24 h after the last treatment. In an independent study, SF, and the related phenethylisothiocyanate (PEITC), were reported to upregulate the mRNA levels for Nrf2 and increase the expression of its downstream target genes NQO1, HMOX1, γGCS, and catalase, and to protect against UVR-mediated structural damage in organ cultures of explants from full-thickness human skin [95].

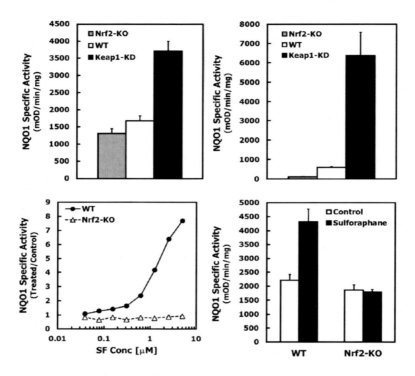

Figure 4. Compared to SKH-1 hairless mice, Nrf2-knockout SKH-1 hairless mice have lower and uninducible levels of NQO1, whereas the levels of this Nrf2-target enzyme are higher in their Keap1-knockdown counterparts. (A,B) The NQO1 enzyme activity was determined in homogenate supernatants prepared from dorsal skin (A) and liver (B) of male SKH-1 (WT), Nrf2-knockout (Nrf2-KO), and Keap1-knockdown (Keap1-KD) mice (n=3 for each genotype). Average values ± SD are shown. In the WT animals, the basal activity of NQO1 are higher in skin than in liver. The effect of the Nrf2 genotype are much more pronounced in liver than in skin. (C) Primary dermal fibroblasts were isolated from 2-day-old SKH-1 (WT) or hairless Nrf2-knockout (Nrf2-KO) mice. Cells were plated at 20,000 cells per well in 96-well plates and 24 h later were exposed to serial dilutions of SF for a further 48 h. NQO1 activity is expressed as mean ratios of treated over control specific activities using eight replicate wells for each SF concentration. The standard deviation for all points was less than 10%. SF induced dose-dependently the NQO1 enzyme activity in SKH-1 (WT) dermal fibroblasts, but not in the hairless Nrf2-knockout (Nrf2-KO) cells. (D) The dorsal skin of female SKH-1 (WT) mice or hairless Nrf2-knockout (Nrf2-KO) mice (n=3 for each genotype) was treated topically, on the right- or left-hand side of the back, with 3 daily doses of: (i) 50 μL of 80% acetone/20% water (control), and (ii) 0.5 μmol of SF (in 50 μL of 80% acetone, v/v). The animals were euthanized 24 h later. NQO1 specific activity was measured in total skin homogenate supernatants. Average values ± SD are shown. SF treatment increased NQO1 activity ~2-fold over control treatment in the SKH-1 mice, but no NQO1 induction was detected in the Nrf2-KO mice.

The potential ability of SF to protect against skin photodamage in healthy human subjects was evaluated by measuring the susceptibility to erythema arising from narrow-band (311 nm) UVB radiation [53]. Six healthy human volunteers (three males and three females) received on 3 consecutive days at 24-h intervals BSE containing 200 or 400 nmol SF or vehicle (80% acetone, v/v) applied topically to small circular areas (2 cm in diameter) on their back skin that had not been previously exposed to UVR. Twenty-four hours after the last dose, these small areas of the skin were exposed to narrow-band (311 nm) UVB radiation. Erythema development was objectively determined 24 h after irradiation by using reflectance spectroscopy and was found to be reduced by ~40% at sites that received BSE containing SF compared with vehicle-treated sites.

A randomized, double-blind, placebo-controlled study compared the response of the skin of 24 healthy human volunteers to different wavebands of monochromator UVR, solar-simulated UV waveband radiation, and visible light after topical application of extracts containing either sulforaphane (200 nmol/cm^2, active) or glucoraphanin (200 nmol/cm^2, placebo), with each subject acting as their own control [94]. The extracts were applied in a randomized fashion to the right or the left half of the mid-upper back skin of each volunteer, 3 times, 24 h apart. Small areas of the skin (approximately 1 cm^2) within the extract-treated areas were exposed to a range of doses of monochromatic UVR or visible light, or solar-simulated UVR 24 h after the last extract applications, and skin erythema responses were assessed afer a further 24 h. Erythema was determined by using both a semi-quantitative visual scale as well as erythema meter for objective quantification. Although there were no significant differences in threshold responses, i.e., minimal erythemal dose (MED), at any of the wavelengths, the mean of the sum of erythema across all doses after exposure to solar-simulated UVR for the SF-treated sites was reduced by 35% compared to the placebo-treated areas. Therefore, SF has been shown to offer a degree of photoprotection against UVB and solar-simulated UVR-induced erythema, supporting a role in the protection against the deleterious effects of solar radiation.

NRF2-INDEPENDENT MECHANISMS OF SULFORAPHANE PROTECTION

Sulforaphane also mediates Nrf2-independent events that can contribute to the protection to skin cells. SF has been shown to reduce the inflammatory response in vitro and in vivo, and this activity could play a significant role in the protective effects of SF against UV-induced inflammation. In HaCaT keratinocytes, pretreatment with SF 24 h before UVB radiation reduced the gene expression of IL-1β, IL-6, and COX-2, decreased protein expression of COX-2 and PGE2, and inhibited phosphorylation and activation of the MAPK pathway [88]. Studies have also shown that UVB radiation can induce an NF-κB-mediated inflammatory response in murine 308 keratinocytes [96]. SF treatment reduces LPS- and IFN-γ-induced NF-κB-mediated inflammation [57, 59]. Although it has not been directly demonstrated, one possibility is that SF reacts with cysteine residues in the DNA binding domain of NF-κB and/or in the IKK kinase complex (e.g., IKKβ) (Figure 5A), as has been shown for the cysteine-reactive triterpenoids [97-100]. Some aspects of the anti-inflammatory actions of SF may involve Nrf2-dependent mechanisms, as studies utilizing MEF cells and primary peritoneal macrophages isolated from Nrf2-knockout mice show SF and other Nrf2 activators (e.g., the triterpenoid TP-225) are much less effective at inhibiting IFN-γ- and TNF-α-stimulated NO production in the Nrf2-knockout cells, compared to WT cells [55], which could indicate that this inflammatory response is through a pathway other than NF-κB (e.g., the JAK/STAT pathway).

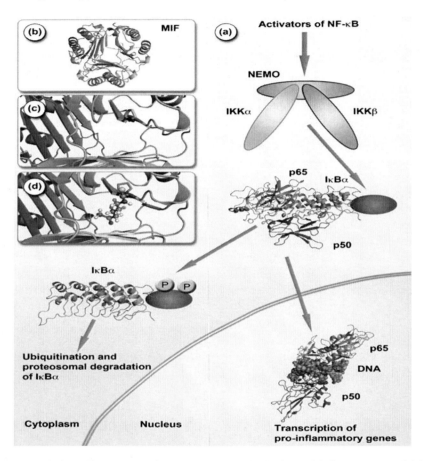

Figure 5. Examples of protein targets and processes that underlie the anti-inflammatory activities of sulforaphane. (A) The NF-κB pathway. In the absence of a stimulus, IκBα (green) negatively regulates transcription factor NF-κB by binding both subunits (p65, red, and p50, blue) of NF-κB and precludes its transfer to the nucleus (pdb data from 1IKN file). Activators of the NF-κB pathway include bacterial and viral products, inflammatory cytokines, reactive oxygen species, and ultraviolet radiation. These stimuli activate a kinase complex (IKKα, IKKβ, NEMO) resulting in IκBα phosphorylation, followed by ubiquitination and proteasomal degradation (pdb data from 1IKN file). Consequently, NF-κB translocates to the nucleus where its p50-p65 heterodimers bind specific DNA sequences of the promoter regions of its target genes (pdb data from ILE5 file). Following transcription, NF-κB is removed from its gene promoters through association with nuclear IκBα (not shown), restoring the pre-activation state. SF may inhibit this pathway by binding to cysteine residues of the kinase complex (e.g., IKKβ) or NF-κB itself. (B) Crystal structure of the macrophage migration inhibitory factor (MIF) trimer (generated with the program Pymol based on pdb file 1MIF). (C) Closeup of the MIF protein subunit showing the N-terminal active site proline. (D) In silico model of the binding of SF to the active site N-terminal proline of MIF. To generate the model, the data from the pdb file 3CE4 and the program Pymol were used.

Another Nrf2-independent inflammatory mechanism that has been correlated with UVR-induced skin damage and carcinogenesis is the increase of the levels of macrophage migration inhibitory factor (MIF). MIF is a pleiotropic cytokine also possessing catalytic tautomerase activity, and both UVA and UVB wavelengths have been shown to increase MIF production in dermal fibroblasts and keratinocytes, respectively [101-103]. Studies in MIF-knockout and MIF-overexpressing transgenic mice have suggested that MIF plays a role in skin cancer by increasing inflammation and inhibiting the p53-dependent apoptotic process of eliminating damaged cells [104, 105]. MIF has also been shown to be increased in skin biopsies of actinic keratosis and cutaneous squamous cell carcinoma patients [103]. Inactivation of MIF catalytic activity has been implicated to have anti-inflammatory effects in vitro and in vivo [106, 107]. SF modifies MIF by binding to its N-terminal proline residue in the enzymatic active site, leading to loss of catalytic tautomerase activity and causing conformational changes in protein structure (Figure 5B-D) [108]. Studies have shown that MIF tautomerase activity was detectable in human urine, and that oral administration of broccoli sprout preparations as a source of the SF precursor, glucoraphanin, to human volunteers almost completely abolished urinary tautomerase activity [109]. This inhibitory action of SF on the catalytic activity of MIF in human subjects makes it an attractive candidate for further studies on the anti-inflammatory properties mediated by this inactivation.

Sulforaphane has also been shown to prevent UVB-induced DNA binding and activation of activator protein-1 (AP-1) both in vitro and in vivo, potentially by directly modifying cysteine residues in the DNA binding sites of cFos and cJun [87]. Activation of AP-1 by UVR leads to changes in proliferation, apoptosis and differentiation, and inhibition of AP-1 activation has been shown to reduce UVB-induced carcinogenesis [110]. Using an AP-1 reporter mouse, a topical formulation of SF in polyethylene glycol (PEG) ointment base has been recently developed and shown to be stable and effective in reducing AP-1 activation after UVR stimulation [111]. SF also modulates the heat shock response. The heat shock response is primarily regulated by the transcription factor heat shock factor-1 (HSF1), which upon stimulation dissociates from heat shock protein (Hsp) 90 complex, trimerizes, and binds to heat shock elements (HSEs) and drives expression of target genes that upregulate molecular chaperone proteins, Hsp90, Hsp72, and Hsp27, which direct refolding of denatured proteins [112]. This response could be critical in eliminating proteins that have been damaged by UVR. SF has been shown to activate HSF1, upregulating the expression of Hsp27 and increasing proteasome activity [56]. There is also evidence that SF can increase the expression of 26S proteasomal subunits through an Nrf2-dependent mechanism, which protected murine neuroblastoma cells from hydrogen peroxide-mediated toxicicity [113]. These findings indicate a possible overlap in function between the HSF1-mediated heat shock response and the Nrf2 pathway.

CONCLUSION

Sulforaphane was identified as a potent inducer of the phase 2 response, via activation of the Nrf2 pathway. SF also harnesses many other protective mechanisms, which make it an ideal candidate as a cytoprotector against the many forms of cellular damage and injury that occur in skin exposed to UVR. Many of the protective responses activated by SF are overlapping, and crosstalk among the cellular signaling pathways is not well understood. The process of evolution has provided cells with interconnected mechanisms of protection that are wired to respond to the environment that we are now only starting to unravel. The advantages of using SF as inducer are that it is a dietary component and exerts most of its effects via the transcriptional enhancement of the synthesis of proteins, most of which are enzymes that have long-lasting, catalytic effects. There is strong indication that SF, and other inducers of the Nrf2 pathway, are protective against UVR-induced skin damage by means of reducing oxidative stress and inflammation, which ultimately can lead to carcinogenesis. The Nrf2-dependent and -independent aspects of this protection are not completely understood and the stage is set for further investigation into the mechanisms of SF-mediated protective effects against UVR and the role of the Nrf2 pathway in this protection.

ACKNOWLEDGMENTS

We are extremely grateful to all of the healthy volunteers for their participation in our human studies, to Cancer Research UK (C20953/A10270 and C20953/A18644) and the Lewis B. and Dorothy Cullman Chemoprotection Foundation for financial support, and to Pamela Talalay for editorial comments.

REFERENCES

[1] Narayanan, DL; Saladi, RN; Fox, JL. Ultraviolet radiation and skin cancer. *International journal of dermatology.*, 2010, 49, 978-86.

[2] Durinck, S; Ho, C; Wang, NJ; Liao, W; Jakkula, LR; Collisson, EA; et al. Temporal dissection of tumorigenesis in primary cancers. *Cancer discovery.*, 2011, 1, 137-43.

[3] Clydesdale, GJ; Dandie, GW; Muller, HK. Ultraviolet light induced injury: immunological and inflammatory effects. *Immunology and cell biology.*, 2001, 79, 547-68.

[4] Svobodova, A; Walterova, D; Vostalova, J. Ultraviolet light induced alteration to the skin. *Biomed Pap Med Fac Univ Palacky Olomouc Czech Repub.*, 2006, 150, 25-38.

[5] Ichihashi, M; Ueda, M; Budiyanto, A; Bito, T; Oka, M; Fukunaga, M; et al. UV-induced skin damage. *Toxicology.*, 2003, 189, 21-39.

[6] Terui, T; Okuyama, R; Tagami, H. Molecular events occurring behind ultraviolet-induced skin inflammation. *Curr Opin Allergy Clin Immunol.*, 2001, 1, 461-7.

[7] Young, AR. Acute effects of UVR on human eyes and skin. *Progress in biophysics and molecular biology.*, 2006, 92, 80-5.

[8] Setlow, RB; Carrier, WL. Pyrimidine dimers in ultraviolet-irradiated DNA's. *J Mol Biol.*, 1966, 17, 237-54.

[9] Cadet, J; Sage, E; Douki, T. Ultraviolet radiation-mediated damage to cellular DNA. *Mutat Res.*, 2005, 571, 3-17.

[10] Sarasin, A. The molecular pathways of ultraviolet-induced carcinogenesis. *Mutat Res.*, 1999, 428, 5-10.

[11] Mouret, S; Baudouin, C; Charveron, M; Favier, A; Cadet, J; Douki, T. Cyclobutane pyrimidine dimers are predominant DNA lesions in whole human skin exposed to UVA radiation. *Proc Natl Acad Sci U S A.*, 2006, 103, 13765-70.

[12] Spiekstra, SW; Breetveld, M; Rustemeyer, T; Scheper, RJ; Gibbs, S. Wound-healing factors secreted by epidermal keratinocytes and dermal fibroblasts in skin substitutes. Wound repair and regeneration: *official publication of the Wound Healing Society [and] the European Tissue Repair Society.*, 2007, 15, 708-17.

[13] Boxman, IL; Ruwhof, C; Boerman, OC; Lowik, CW; Ponec, M. Role of fibroblasts in the regulation of proinflammatory interleukin IL-1, IL-6 and IL-8 levels induced by keratinocyte-derived IL-1. *Archives of dermatological research.*, 1996, 288, 391-8.

[14] Karran, P; Attard, N. Thiopurines in current medical practice: molecular mechanisms and contributions to therapy-related cancer. *Nat Rev Cancer.*, 2008, 8, 24-36.

[15] Setshedi, M; Epstein, D; Winter, TA; Myer, L; Watermeyer, G; Hift, R. Use of thiopurines in the treatment of inflammatory bowel disease is associated with an increased risk of non-melanoma skin cancer in an at-risk population: a cohort study. *J Gastroenterol Hepatol.*, 2012, 27, 385-9.

[16] Harwood, CA; Mesher, D; McGregor, JM; Mitchell, L; Leedham-Green, M; Raftery, M; et al. A surveillance model for skin cancer in organ transplant recipients: a 22-year prospective study in an ethnically diverse population. *Am J Transplant.*, 2013, 13, 119-29.

[17] Kalra, S; Zhang, Y; Knatko, EV; Finlayson, S; Yamamoto, M; Dinkova-Kostova, AT. Oral Azathioprine Leads to Higher Incorporation of 6-Thioguanine in DNA of Skin than Liver: The Protective Role of the Keap1/Nrf2/ARE Pathway. *Cancer Prev Res (Phila).*, 2011.

[18] Ren, X; Li, F; Jeffs, G; Zhang, X; Xu, YZ; Karran, P. Guanine sulphinate is a major stable product of photochemical oxidation of DNA 6-thioguanine by UVA irradiation. *Nucleic Acids Res.*, 2010, 38, 1832-40.

[19] Gueranger, Q; Kia, A; Frith, D; Karran, P. Crosslinking of DNA repair and replication proteins to DNA in cells treated with 6-thioguanine and UVA. *Nucleic Acids Res.*, 2011, 39, 5057-66.

[20] Brem, R; Karran, P. Multiple forms of DNA damage caused by UVA photoactivation of DNA 6-thioguanine. *Photochem Photobiol.*, 2012, 88, 5-13.

[21] O'Donovan, P; Perrett, CM; Zhang, X; Montaner, B; Xu, YZ; Harwood, CA; et al. Azathioprine and UVA light generate mutagenic oxidative DNA damage. *Science.*, 2005, 309, 1871-4.

[22] Hofbauer, GF; Attard, NR; Harwood, CA; McGregor, JM; Dziunycz, P; Iotzova-Weiss, G; et al. Reversal of UVA skin photosensitivity and DNA damage in kidney transplant recipients by replacing azathioprine. *Am J Transplant.*, 2012, 12, 218-25.

[23] Marrot, L; Jones, C; Perez, P; Meunier, JR. The significance of Nrf2 pathway in (photo)-oxidative stress response in melanocytes and keratinocytes of the human epidermis. *Pigment Cell Melanoma Res.*, 2008, 21, 79-88.

[24] Huang, CC; Fang, JY; Wu, WB; Chiang, HS; Wei, YJ; Hung, CF. Protective effects of (-)-epicatechin-3-gallate on UVA-induced damage in HaCaT keratinocytes. *Archives of dermatological research.*, 2005, 296, 473-81.

[25] Stahl, W; Sies, H. Carotenoids and protection against solar UV radiation. *Skin Pharmacol Appl Skin Physiol.*, 2002, 15, 291-6.

[26] Sies, H; Stahl, W. Carotenoids and UV protection. *Photochem Photobiol Sci.*, 2004, 3, 749-52.
[27] Dinkova-Kostova, AT; Talalay, P. Direct and indirect antioxidant properties of inducers of cytoprotective proteins. *Mol Nutr Food Res.*, 2008, 52 Suppl 1, S128-38.
[28] Kobayashi, M; Yamamoto, M. Molecular mechanisms activating the Nrf2-Keap1 pathway of antioxidant gene regulation. *Antioxid Redox Signal.*, 2005, 7, 385-94.
[29] Kensler, TW; Wakabayashi, N; Biswal, S. Cell survival responses to environmental stresses via the Keap1-Nrf2-ARE pathway. *Annu Rev Pharmacol Toxicol.*, 2007, 47, 89-116.
[30] Hayes, JD; Dinkova-Kostova, AT. The Nrf2 regulatory network provides an interface between redox and intermediary metabolism. *Trends Biochem Sci.*, 2014, 39, 199-218.
[31] Villeneuve, NF; Lau, A; Zhang, DD. Regulation of the Nrf2-Keap1 antioxidant response by the ubiquitin proteasome system: an insight into cullin-ring ubiquitin ligases. *Antioxid Redox Signal.*, 2010, 13, 1699-712.
[32] Suzuki, T; Motohashi, H; Yamamoto, M. Toward clinical application of the Keap1-Nrf2 pathway. *Trends in pharmacological sciences.*, 2013, 34, 340-6.
[33] Baird, L; Lleres, D; Swift, S; Dinkova-Kostova, AT. Regulatory flexibility in the Nrf2-mediated stress response is conferred by conformational cycling of the Keap1-Nrf2 protein complex. *Proc Natl Acad Sci U S A.*, 2013, 110, 15259-64.
[34] Talalay, P. Chemoprotection against cancer by induction of phase 2 enzymes. *Biofactors.*, 2000, 12, 5-11.
[35] Zhang, Y; Talalay, P; Cho, CG; Posner, GH. A major inducer of anticarcinogenic protective enzymes from broccoli: isolation and elucidation of structure. *Proc Natl Acad Sci U S A.*, 1992, 89, 2399-403.
[36] Wattenberg, LW; Hanley, AB; Barany, G; Sparnins, VL; Lam, LK; Fenwick, GR. Inhibition of carcinogenesis by some minor dietary constituents. *Princess Takamatsu Symp.*, 1985, 16, 193-203.
[37] Boyd, JN; Babish, JG; Stoewsand, GS. Modification of beet and cabbage diets of aflatoxin B1-induced rat plasma alpha-foetoprotein elevation, hepatic tumorigenesis, and mutagenicity of urine. *Food Chem Toxicol.*, 1982, 20, 47-52.
[38] Colditz, GA; Branch, LG; Lipnick, RJ; Willett, WC; Rosner, B; Posner, BM; et al. Increased green and yellow vegetable intake and lowered cancer deaths in an elderly population. *Am J Clin Nutr.*, 1985, 41, 32-6.
[39] Block, G; Patterson, B; Subar, A. Fruit, vegetables, and cancer prevention: a review of the epidemiological evidence. *Nutr Cancer.*, 1992, 18, 1-29.
[40] Fahey, JW; Zhang, Y; Talalay, P. Broccoli sprouts: an exceptionally rich source of inducers of enzymes that protect against chemical carcinogens. *Proc Natl Acad Sci U S A.*, 1997, 94, 10367-72.
[41] Fahey, JW; Zalcmann, AT; Talalay, P. The chemical diversity and distribution of glucosinolates and isothiocyanates among plants. *Phytochemistry.*, 2001, 56, 5-51.
[42] Dinkova-Kostova, AT; Kostov, RV. Glucosinolates and isothiocyanates in health and disease. *Trends Mol Med.*, 2012, 18, 337-47.
[43] Halkier, BA; Gershenzon, J. Biology and biochemistry of glucosinolates. *Annu Rev Plant Biol.*, 2006, 57, 303-33.
[44] Matusheski, NV; Swarup, R; Juvik, JA; Mithen, R; Bennett, M; Jeffery, EH. Epithiospecifier protein from broccoli (Brassica oleracea L. ssp. italica) inhibits

formation of the anticancer agent sulforaphane. *J Agric Food Chem.*, 2006, 54, 2069-76.

[45] Shapiro, TA; Fahey, JW; Wade, KL; Stephenson, KK; Talalay, P. Human metabolism and excretion of cancer chemoprotective glucosinolates and isothiocyanates of cruciferous vegetables. *Cancer Epidemiol Biomarkers Prev.*, 1998, 7, 1091-100.

[46] Shapiro, TA; Fahey, JW; Wade, KL; Stephenson, KK; Talalay, P. Chemoprotective glucosinolates and isothiocyanates of broccoli sprouts: metabolism and excretion in humans. *Cancer Epidemiol Biomarkers Prev.*, 2001, 10, 501-8.

[47] Egner, PA; Chen, JG; Wang, JB; Wu, Y; Sun, Y; Lu, JH; et al. Bioavailability of Sulforaphane from two broccoli sprout beverages: results of a short-term, cross-over clinical trial in Qidong, China. *Cancer Prev Res (Phila).*, 2011, 4, 384-95.

[48] Li, F; Hullar, MA; Beresford, SA; Lampe, JW. Variation of glucoraphanin metabolism in vivo and ex vivo by human gut bacteria. *Br J Nutr.*, 2011, 106, 408-16.

[49] Zhang, Y; Talalay, P. Mechanism of differential potencies of isothiocyanates as inducers of anticarcinogenic Phase 2 enzymes. *Cancer Res.*, 1998, 58, 4632-9.

[50] Zhang, Y. Role of glutathione in the accumulation of anticarcinogenic isothiocyanates and their glutathione conjugates by murine hepatoma cells. *Carcinogenesis.*, 2000, 21, 1175-82.

[51] Zhang, Y. Molecular mechanism of rapid cellular accumulation of anticarcinogenic isothiocyanates. *Carcinogenesis.*, 2001, 22, 425-31.

[52] Ye, L; Zhang, Y. Total intracellular accumulation levels of dietary isothiocyanates determine their activity in elevation of cellular glutathione and induction of Phase 2 detoxification enzymes. *Carcinogenesis.*, 2001, 22, 1987-92.

[53] Talalay, P; Fahey, JW; Healy, ZR; Wehage, SL; Benedict, AL; Min, C; et al. Sulforaphane mobilizes cellular defenses that protect skin against damage by UV radiation. *Proc Natl Acad Sci U S A.*, 2007, 104, 17500-5.

[54] Kerns, ML; DePianto, D; Dinkova-Kostova, AT; Talalay, P; Coulombe, PA. Reprogramming of keratin biosynthesis by sulforaphane restores skin integrity in epidermolysis bullosa simplex. *Proc Natl Acad Sci U S A.*, 2007, 104, 14460-5.

[55] Liu, H; Dinkova-Kostova, AT; Talalay, P. Coordinate regulation of enzyme markers for inflammation and for protection against oxidants and electrophiles. *Proc Natl Acad Sci U S A.*, 2008, 105, 15926-31.

[56] Gan, N; Wu, YC; Brunet, M; Garrido, C; Chung, FL; Dai, C; et al. Sulforaphane activates heat shock response and enhances proteasome activity through up-regulation of Hsp27. *J Biol Chem.*, 2010, 285, 35528-36.

[57] Heiss, E; Herhaus, C; Klimo, K; Bartsch, H; Gerhauser, C. Nuclear factor kappa B is a molecular target for sulforaphane-mediated anti-inflammatory mechanisms. *J Biol Chem.*, 2001, 276, 32008-15.

[58] Juge, N; Mithen, RF; Traka, M. Molecular basis for chemoprevention by sulforaphane: a comprehensive review. *Cell Mol Life Sci.*, 2007, 64, 1105-27.

[59] Dinkova-Kostova, AT; Jenkins, SN; Fahey, JW; Ye, L; Wehage, SL; Liby, KT; et al. Protection against UV-light-induced skin carcinogenesis in SKH-1 high-risk mice by sulforaphane-containing broccoli sprout extracts. *Cancer Lett.*, 2006, 240, 243-52.

[60] Benedict, AL; Knatko, EV; Dinkova-Kostova, AT. The indirect antioxidant sulforaphane protects against thiopurine-mediated photooxidative stress. *Carcinogenesis.*, 2012.

[61] Kalra, S; Knatko, EV; Zhang, Y; Honda, T; Yamamoto, M; Dinkova-Kostova, AT. Highly potent activation of Nrf2 by topical tricyclic bis(cyano enone): implications for protection against UV radiation during thiopurine therapy. *Cancer Prev Res (Phila).*, 2012, 5, 973-81.

[62] Gaddameedhi, S; Selby, CP; Kaufmann, WK; Smart, RC; Sancar, A. Control of skin cancer by the circadian rhythm. *Proc Natl Acad Sci U S A.*, 2011, 108, 18790-5.

[63] Kawachi, Y; Xu, X; Taguchi, S; Sakurai, H; Nakamura, Y; Ishii, Y; et al. Attenuation of UVB-induced sunburn reaction and oxidative DNA damage with no alterations in UVB-induced skin carcinogenesis in Nrf2 gene-deficient mice. *J Invest Dermatol.*, 2008, 128, 1773-9.

[64] Saw, CL; Huang, MT; Liu, Y; Khor, TO; Conney, AH; Kong, AN. Impact of Nrf2 on UVB-induced skin inflammation/photoprotection and photoprotective effect of sulforaphane. *Mol Carcinog.*, 2011, 50, 479-86.

[65] Paz, ML; Gonzalez Maglio, DH; Weill, FS; Bustamante, J; Leoni, J. Mitochondrial dysfunction and cellular stress progression after ultraviolet B irradiation in human keratinocytes. *Photodermatol Photoimmunol Photomed.*, 2008, 24, 115-22.

[66] Holmstrom, KM; Baird, L; Zhang, Y; Hargreaves, I; Chalasani, A; Land, JM; et al. Nrf2 impacts cellular bioenergetics by controlling substrate availability for mitochondrial respiration. *Biology open.*, 2013, 2, 761-70.

[67] Kovac, S; Angelova, PR; Holmstrom, KM; Zhang, Y; Dinkova-Kostova, AT; Abramov, AY. Nrf2 regulates ROS production by mitochondria and NADPH oxidase. *Biochim Biophys Acta.*, 2014, 1850, 794-801.

[68] Greco, T; Fiskum, G. Brain mitochondria from rats treated with sulforaphane are resistant to redox-regulated permeability transition. *J Bioenerg Biomembr.*, 2010, 42, 491-7.

[69] Greco, T; Shafer, J; Fiskum, G. Sulforaphane inhibits mitochondrial permeability transition and oxidative stress. *Free Radic Biol Med.*, 2011.

[70] Giorgio, V; von Stockum, S; Antoniel, M; Fabbro, A; Fogolari, F; Forte, M; et al. Dimers of mitochondrial ATP synthase form the permeability transition pore. *Proc Natl Acad Sci U S A.*, 2013, 110, 5887-92.

[71] Miller, DM; Singh, IN; Wang, JA; Hall, ED. Administration of the Nrf2-ARE activators sulforaphane and carnosic acid attenuates 4-hydroxy-2-nonenal-induced mitochondrial dysfunction ex vivo. *Free Radic Biol Med.*, 2013, 57, 1-9.

[72] Guerrero-Beltran, CE; Calderon-Oliver, M; Pedraza-Chaverri, J; Chirino, YI. Protective effect of sulforaphane against oxidative stress: Recent advances. *Exp Toxicol Pathol.*, 2010.

[73] Negrette-Guzman, M; Huerta-Yepez, S; Tapia, E; Pedraza-Chaverri, J. Modulation of mitochondrial functions by the indirect antioxidant sulforaphane: a seemingly contradictory dual role and an integrative hypothesis. *Free Radic Biol Med.*, 2013, 65, 1078-89.

[74] Negrette-Guzman, M; Huerta-Yepez, S; Medina-Campos, ON; Zatarain-Barron, ZL; Hernandez-Pando, R; Torres, I; et al. Sulforaphane attenuates gentamicin-induced nephrotoxicity: role of mitochondrial protection. *Evid Based Complement Alternat Med.*, 2013, 2013, 135314.

[75] Zhu, H; Jia, Z; Strobl, JS; Ehrich, M; Misra, HP; Li, Y. Potent induction of total cellular and mitochondrial antioxidants and phase 2 enzymes by cruciferous sulforaphane in rat

aortic smooth muscle cells: cytoprotection against oxidative and electrophilic stress. *Cardiovasc Toxicol.*, 2008, 8, 115-25.

[76] Scarpulla, RC. Nuclear control of respiratory chain expression by nuclear respiratory factors and PGC-1-related coactivator. *Ann N Y Acad Sci.*, 2008, 1147, 321-34.

[77] Scarpulla, RC. Transcriptional paradigms in mammalian mitochondrial biogenesis and function. *Physiol Rev.*, 2008, 88, 611-38.

[78] Vercauteren, K; Gleyzer, N; Scarpulla, RC. PGC-1-related coactivator complexes with HCF-1 and NRF-2beta in mediating NRF-2(GABP)-dependent respiratory gene expression. *J Biol Chem.*, 2008, 283, 12102-11.

[79] Scarpulla, RC. Metabolic control of mitochondrial biogenesis through the PGC-1 family regulatory network. *Biochim Biophys Acta.*, 2011, 1813, 1269-78.

[80] Finck, BN; Kelly, DP. PGC-1 coactivators: inducible regulators of energy metabolism in health and disease. *J Clin Invest.*, 2006, 116, 615-22.

[81] Piantadosi, CA; Carraway, MS; Babiker, A; Suliman, HB. Heme oxygenase-1 regulates cardiac mitochondrial biogenesis via Nrf2-mediated transcriptional control of nuclear respiratory factor-1. *Circ Res.*, 2008, 103, 1232-40.

[82] Brose, RD; Shin, G; McGuinness, MC; Schneidereith, T; Purvis, S; Dong, GX; et al. Activation of the stress proteome as a mechanism for small molecule therapeutics. *Hum Mol Genet.*, 2012, 21, 4237-52.

[83] Benavides, F; Oberyszyn, TM; VanBuskirk, AM; Reeve, VE; Kusewitt, DF. The hairless mouse in skin research. *J Dermatol Sci.*, 2009, 53, 10-8.

[84] Lu, YP; Lou, YR; Xie, JG; Peng, QY; Liao, J; Yang, CS; et al. Topical applications of caffeine or (-)-epigallocatechin gallate (EGCG) inhibit carcinogenesis and selectively increase apoptosis in UVB-induced skin tumors in mice. *Proc Natl Acad Sci U S A.*, 2002, 99, 12455-60.

[85] Dinkova-Kostova, AT; Fahey, JW; Wade, KL; Jenkins, SN; Shapiro, TA; Fuchs, EJ; et al. Induction of the phase 2 response in mouse and human skin by sulforaphane-containing broccoli sprout extracts. *Cancer Epidemiol Biomarkers Prev.*, 2007, 16, 847-51.

[86] Dinkova-Kostova, AT; Fahey, JW; Benedict, AL; Jenkins, SN; Ye, L; Wehage, SL; et al. Dietary glucoraphanin-rich broccoli sprout extracts protect against UV radiation-induced skin carcinogenesis in SKH-1 hairless mice. *Photochem Photobiol Sci.*, 2010, 9, 597-600.

[87] Dickinson, SE; Melton, TF; Olson, ER; Zhang, J; Saboda, K; Bowden, GT. Inhibition of activator protein-1 by sulforaphane involves interaction with cysteine in the cFos DNA-binding domain: implications for chemoprevention of UVB-induced skin cancer. *Cancer Res.*, 2009, 69, 7103-10.

[88] Shibata, A; Nakagawa, K; Yamanoi, H; Tsuduki, T; Sookwong, P; Higuchi, O; et al. Sulforaphane suppresses ultraviolet B-induced inflammation in HaCaT keratinocytes and HR-1 hairless mice. *J Nutr Biochem.*, 2010, 21, 702-9.

[89] Itoh, K; Chiba, T; Takahashi, S; Ishii, T; Igarashi, K; Katoh, Y; et al. An Nrf2/small Maf heterodimer mediates the induction of phase II detoxifying enzyme genes through antioxidant response elements. *Biochem Biophys Res Commun.*, 1997, 236, 313-22.

[90] Higgins, LG; Hayes, JD. The cap'n'collar transcription factor Nrf2 mediates both intrinsic resistance to environmental stressors and an adaptive response elicited by

chemopreventive agents that determines susceptibility to electrophilic xenobiotics. *Chem Biol Interact.*, 2011, 192, 37-45.

[91] Taguchi, K; Maher, JM; Suzuki, T; Kawatani, Y; Motohashi, H; Yamamoto, M. Genetic analysis of cytoprotective functions supported by graded expression of Keap1. *Mol Cell Biol.*, 2010, 30, 3016-26.

[92] Biswas, M; Chan, JY. Role of Nrf1 in antioxidant response element-mediated gene expression and beyond. *Toxicol Appl Pharmacol.*, 2010, 244, 16-20.

[93] Braun, S; Hanselmann, C; Gassmann, MG; auf dem Keller, U; Born-Berclaz, C; Chan, K; et al. Nrf2 transcription factor, a novel target of keratinocyte growth factor action which regulates gene expression and inflammation in the healing skin wound. *Mol Cell Biol.*, 2002, 22, 5492-505.

[94] Knatko, EV; Ibbotson, SH; Zhang, Y; Higgins, M; Fahey, JW; Talalay, P; et al. Nrf2 Activation Protects against Solar-Simulated Ultraviolet Radiation in Mice and Humans. *Cancer Prev Res (Phila).*, 2015, 8, 475-86.

[95] Kleszczynski, K; Ernst, IM; Wagner, AE; Kruse, N; Zillikens, D; Rimbach, G; et al. Sulforaphane and phenylethyl isothiocyanate protect human skin against UVR-induced oxidative stress and apoptosis: role of Nrf2-dependent gene expression and antioxidant enzymes. *Pharmacol Res.*, 2013, 78, 28-40.

[96] Cooper, S; Ranger-Moore, J; Bowden, TG. Differential inhibition of UVB-induced AP-1 and NF-kappaB transactivation by components of the jun bZIP domain. *Mol Carcinog.*, 2005, 43, 108-16.

[97] Ahmad, R; Raina, D; Meyer, C; Kharbanda, S; Kufe, D. Triterpenoid CDDO-Me blocks the NF-kappaB pathway by direct inhibition of IKKbeta on Cys-179. *J Biol Chem.*, 2006, 281, 35764-9.

[98] Yore, MM; Liby, KT; Honda, T; Gribble, GW; Sporn, MB. The synthetic triterpenoid 1-[2-cyano-3,12-dioxooleana-1,9(11)-dien-28-oyl]imidazole blocks nuclear factor-kappaB activation through direct inhibition of IkappaB kinase beta. *Mol Cancer Ther.*, 2006, 5, 3232-9.

[99] Lee, JH; Koo, TH; Yoon, H; Jung, HS; Jin, HZ; Lee, K; et al. Inhibition of NF-kappa B activation through targeting I kappa B kinase by celastrol, a quinone methide triterpenoid. *Biochem Pharmacol.*, 2006, 72, 1311-21.

[100] Gupta, SC; Prasad, S; Reuter, S; Kannappan, R; Yadav, VR; Ravindran, J; et al. Modification of cysteine 179 of IkappaBalpha kinase by nimbolide leads to down-regulation of NF-kappaB-regulated cell survival and proliferative proteins and sensitization of tumor cells to chemotherapeutic agents. *J Biol Chem.*, 2010, 285, 35406-17.

[101] Shimizu, T; Abe, R; Ohkawara, A; Nishihira, J. Ultraviolet B radiation upregulates the production of macrophage migration inhibitory factor (MIF) in human epidermal keratinocytes. *J Invest Dermatol.*, 1999, 112, 210-5.

[102] Watanabe, H; Shimizu, T; Nishihira, J; Abe, R; Nakayama, T; Taniguchi, M; et al. Ultraviolet A-induced production of matrix metalloproteinase-1 is mediated by macrophage migration inhibitory factor (MIF) in human dermal fibroblasts. *J Biol Chem.*, 2004, 279, 1676-83.

[103] Heise, R; Vetter-Kauczok, CS; Skazik, C; Czaja, K; Marquardt, Y; Lue, H; et al. Expression and function of macrophage migration inhibitory factor in the pathogenesis

of UV-induced cutaneous nonmelanoma skin cancer. *Photochem Photobiol.*, 2012, 88, 1157-64.

[104] Honda, A; Abe, R; Yoshihisa, Y; Makino, T; Matsunaga, K; Nishihira, J; et al. Deficient deletion of apoptotic cells by macrophage migration inhibitory factor (MIF) overexpression accelerates photocarcinogenesis. *Carcinogenesis.*, 2009, 30, 1597-605.

[105] Martin, J; Duncan, FJ; Keiser, T; Shin, S; Kusewitt, DF; Oberyszyn, T; et al. Macrophage migration inhibitory factor (MIF) plays a critical role in pathogenesis of ultraviolet-B (UVB) -induced nonmelanoma skin cancer (NMSC). *Faseb J.*, 2009, 23, 720-30.

[106] Al-Abed, Y; Dabideen, D; Aljabari, B; Valster, A; Messmer, D; Ochani, M; et al. ISO-1 binding to the tautomerase active site of MIF inhibits its pro-inflammatory activity and increases survival in severe sepsis. *J Biol Chem.*, 2005, 280, 36541-4.

[107] Garai, J; Lorand, T. Macrophage migration inhibitory factor (MIF) tautomerase inhibitors as potential novel anti-inflammatory agents: current developments. *Curr Med Chem.*, 2009, 16, 1091-114.

[108] Brown, KK; Blaikie, F; Smith, RA; Tyndall, JD; Lue, H; Bernhagen, J; et al. Direct modification of the proinflammatory cytokine macrophage migration inhibitory factor by dietary isothiocyanates. *J Biol Chem.*, 2009, 284, 32425-33.

[109] Healy, ZR; Liu, H; Holtzclaw, WD, Talalay P. Inactivation of tautomerase activity of macrophage migration inhibitory factor by sulforaphane: a potential biomarker for anti-inflammatory intervention. *Cancer Epidemiol Biomarkers Prev.*, 2011, 20, 1516-23.

[110] Cooper, SJ; Bowden, GT. Ultraviolet B regulation of transcription factor families: roles of nuclear factor-kappa B (NF-kappaB) and activator protein-1 (AP-1) in UVB-induced skin carcinogenesis. *Curr Cancer Drug Targets.*, 2007, 7, 325-34.

[111] Franklin, SJ; Dickinson, SE; Karlage, KL; Bowden, GT; Myrdal, PB. Stability of sulforaphane for topical formulation. *Drug development and industrial pharmacy.*, 2013.

[112] Westerheide, SD; Morimoto, RI. Heat shock response modulators as therapeutic tools for diseases of protein conformation. *J Biol Chem.*, 2005, 280, 33097-100.

[113] Kwak, MK; Cho, JM; Huang, B; Shin, S; Kensler, TW. Role of increased expression of the proteasome in the protective effects of sulforaphane against hydrogen peroxide-mediated cytotoxicity in murine neuroblastoma cells. *Free Radic Biol Med.*, 2007, 43, 809-17.

In: Broccoli
Editor: Bernhard H. J. Juurlink

ISBN: 978-1-63484-313-3
© 2016 Nova Science Publishers, Inc.

Chapter 11

PRECLINICAL STUDIES ON THE EFFECT OF SULFORAPHANE ON CARDIOVASCULAR DISEASE AND FETAL DETERMINANTS OF ADULT HEALTH

*Ali Banigesh[1] and Bernhard H. J. Juurlink[2,]**

[1]Department of Pharmacology, College of Medicine, University of Saskatchewan, Saskatoon, SK, Canada
[2]Department of Anatomy & Cell Biology, College of Medicine, University of Saskatchewan, Saskatoon, SK, Canada

ABSTRACT

This chapter outlines some of the basic mechanisms, in particular oxidative stress and inflammation that drive atherogenesis and hypertension. We review the experiments where consumption of either glucoraphanin-rich broccoli sprouts or sulforaphane show a decrease in oxidative stress and inflammation that is associated with: better blood pressure, a decrease monocyte infiltration of blood vessels and better ability of hearts to cope with ischemia and reperfusion. We also review the experiments that demonstrate that a reduction in oxidative stress and inflammation accompanied by better blood pressure have positive effects on fetal determinants of adult health and normalize the kidney epigenome as determined by examining for global cytosine methylation.

Keywords: animal models, atherosclerosis, blood pressure, broccoli sprouts, epigenetics, fetal determinants of adult health, hypertension, oxidative stress

INTRODUCTION

Atherosclerosis and hypertension are major diseases of the cardiovascular system in the developed and developing world [1]. Both are diseases associated with increasing age and

---

* Corresponding author: Email: bernhard.juurlink@usask.ca.

poor life style [1]: major drivers include lack of exercise [2-4] and inadequate intake of fruits and vegetables [5-8]. Disturbances in redox homeostasis is a driver for both atherosclerosis [9, 10] and hypertension [11, 12]. This chapter deals with the potential of Nrf2 activators such as sulforaphane in ameliorating cardiovascular problems.

MECHANISMS DRIVING ATHEROSCLEROSIS AND HYPERTENSION

Atherosclerosis

A critical factor in the development of an atherosclerotic lesion is the oxidation of unsaturated lipids found mainly in low-density lipoprotein (LDL) particles [13, 14]. Associated with LDL oxidation is the arterial subendothelial accumulation of oxidized-LDL (OxLDL), inflammatory changes in the endothelium resulting in expression of cell adhesion molecules and chemokines/cytokines as well as activation and infiltration of blood monocytes that phagocytose OxLDL giving rise to foam cells. Arterial atherosclerotic lesions tend to occur at arterial branch points that are associated with turbulence. The activation of the endothelium and monocytes is due, at least in part, by interaction of the OxLDL with a number of scavenger receptors, including the low density lipoprotein receptor-1 (LOX1) [14, 15] present on endothelial cells, monocytes as well as smooth muscle cells. Interaction of OxLDL with some of the scavenger receptors such as LOX1 activates the NAD(P)H oxidase complex resulting in the generation of more reactive oxygen species (ROS) [16, 17]. As outlined in Chapter 5, oxidative stress results in activation of several signalling pathways (e.g., nuclear factor kappa B) resulting in expression of pro-inflammatory genes such as cell adhesion molecules and pro-inflammatory cytokines and chemokines.

As the lesion develops there is increasing accumulation of OxLDL-laden foam cells within the tunica intima of the artery, infiltration of smooth muscle cells from the tunica media; these smooth muscle cells proliferate within the atherosclerotic lesion. There is production of a variety of hydrolytic enzymes such as matrix metalloproteinases that digest collagen resulting in the weakening of the structural integrity of the tunica intima [14, 15]. The increasing size of the atherosclerotic lesion limits blood flow and the atherosclerotic lesion may rupture resulting in the formation of thrombi that can completely block blood flow to the tissues served by that vessel. The coronary arteries of the heart are common sites of atherosclerotic lesions that often lead to "heart attacks."

The above description of atherosclerotic lesion formation as represented in Figure 1 is a bit simplistic but it does illustrate the important role of LDL and ROS in atherosclerotic lesion formation. Increasing plasma levels of LDL increase the probability of LDL unsaturated lipids being oxidized and increasing production of ROS increases the probability of LDL unsaturated lipids being oxidized. Hence the rationale for decreasing plasma LDL levels and the clinical trials aimed at decreasing oxidative stress. Clinical trials examining the effects of anti-oxidants such as vitamin E have had disappointing results [18]. The reason for this likely has to do with the fact that anti-oxidants such as vitamin E and vitamin C have very limited, although very important, roles in the anti-oxidant defense system (see Chapter 5). Nrf2 activators that increase multiple facets of the anti-oxidant defense of cells (see

Chapter 6) ought to have a much greater impact in ameliorating conditions that have an underlying oxidative stress component to them.

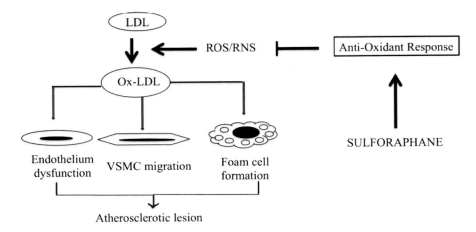

Figure 1. Diagram illustrating the potential roles of reactive oxygen species (ROS) and reactive nitrogen species (RNS) in driving the formation of atherosclerotic lesions. Oxidation of low density lipoprotein (LDL) unsaturated fatty acids results in oxidized LDL (Ox-LDL) that in turn results in inflammatory changes in the vascular endothelium and activation and infiltration of monocytes/macrophages that phagocytose the Ox-LDL forming foam cells. These inflammatory changes are also associated with migration of vascular smooth muscle cells to the tunica intima. Sulforaphane by activating the anti-oxidant response decreases formation of the ROS/RNS, thereby decreasing the probability of atherogenesis.

Hypertension

An increase in systemic blood pressure (hypertension) is commonly seen with age [19]. Hypertension leads to a number of serious problems such as cognitive decline and dementia [20, 21] as well as cardiac and renal disease [22].

Blood pressure is regulated by the extent of contraction/relaxation of the smooth muscle cells of the arterial tunica media and by the volume of blood enclosed in the arterial system: these factors are governed by both autonomic nerves and endocrine hormones. Regulation of blood pressure is complex and there is no intention here to thoroughly review the mechanisms that control blood pressure, rather the focus will be on a few mechanisms that may be influenced by the redox state of the cells. The reader may then have some appreciation on how diet may have the potential to positively influence blood pressure.

Hypertension is usually due to an increased contractile state of the smooth muscle cells of the tunica media, i.e., by an imbalance of relaxation and contraction forces. A major vasorelaxation molecule is the nitric oxide free radical (NO·) [23]. The signalling pathway that results in NO· production is diagrammed in Figure 2. Acetylcholine released from parasympathetic nerve endings acts upon muscarinic cholinergic G protein-coupled receptors present in the plasmalemma of endothelial cells. Activation of these receptors results in activation of phospholipase C that causes release of inositol 1,4,5-triphosphate (IP$_3$). IP$_3$ then acts upon receptors on the endoplasmic reticulum resulting in Ca^{2+} stored in the endoplasmic reticulum flowing into the cytosol. The rising levels of cytosolic Ca^{2+} results in Ca^{2+} binding to calmodulin with the Ca^{2+}-calmodulin complex binding to and activating endothelial nitric oxide synthase (eNOS), an enzyme that converts arginine to citrulline and NO˙. The NO˙ diffuses from the endothelium and some of the NO˙ molecules will bind to the heme moiety of cyclic guanosine monophosphate (cGMP) synthase, thereby activating it to produce cGMP from guanosine triphosphate. The cGMP will activate protein kinase G (PKG) that in turn will phosphorylate myosin light chain kinase (MLCK), thereby inhibiting the ability of MLCK to phosphorylate myosin; phosphorylation of myosin light chains is the critical step in smooth muscle contraction.

An increased production of the superoxide anion ($O_2^{-˙}$) will result in $O_2^{-˙}$ reacting with NO˙ to form peroxynitrite ($ONOO^-$), a very powerful oxidant. There are thus two dire consequences of the reaction of $O_2^{-˙}$ with NO˙: a decrease in NO˙ for vasorelaxation (Figure 3) and an increase in powerful oxidants that can cause cellular damage and promote inflammation (see Chapter 5). A decreased production of $O_2^{-˙}$ or an increased ability to scavenge oxidants will promote better blood pressure. Decreased availability of NO˙ for smooth muscle relaxation is referred to as endothelial dysfunction [24] and such endothelial dysfunction is implicated not only in hypertension but also in atherosclerosis [25]. Such a decreased availability of NO˙ may be due to decreased levels of eNOS or increased production of $O_2^{-˙}$.

The major driver for vasoconstriction is the peptide angiotensin II (ANGII). ANGII acts on angiotensin receptor-1 (AT1R) to activate the G-protein coupled phospholipase C (PLC) signalling pathway that increases intracellular Ca^{2+}. Three cell types that express AT1R will be considered: vascular smooth muscle cells, vascular endothelial cells and adrenal cortical zona glomerulosa cells [26, 27] as shown in Figure 3. Figure 3 looks complex; however, we have already considered the NO˙ vasorelaxation pathway and the effect of $O_2^{-˙}$.

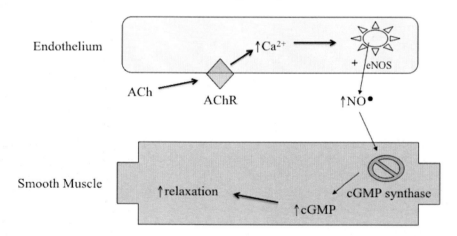

Figure 2. Diagram illustrating the activation of the muscarinic receptor (AChR) by acetylcholine (ACh) that results in increased cytosolic Ca^{2+}. The Ca^{2+} binds to calmodulin thereby activating endothelial nitric oxide synthase (eNOS) resulting in the formation of the nitric oxide radical (NO˙). NO˙ diffuses and binds to the heme of cyclic guanosine monophosphate (cGMP) synthase increasing production of cGMP that, in turn, activates protein kinase G that then phosphorylates myosin light chain kinase, thus inhibiting its kinase activity, thereby leading to smooth muscle relaxation. Smooth muscle relaxation results in lowered blood pressure.

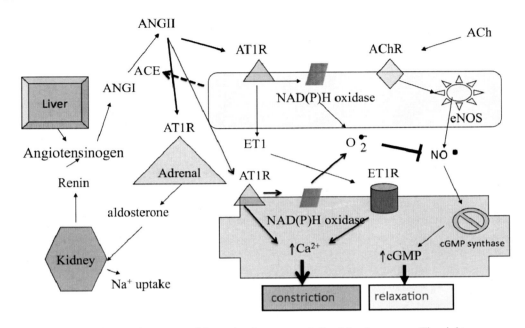

Figure 3. Diagram illustrating some of the major factors regulating blood pressure. The right component of the diagram dealing with NO· has been outlined previously in Figure 2. The left component of the diagram deals with the angiotensin control of blood pressure. The liver produces angiotensinogen that is cleaved by the renal secreted enzyme renin into angiotensin I (ANGI). Angiotensin converting enzyme (ACE) released by endothelial cells converts ANGI to ANGII. ANGII acts upon angiotensin receptor-1 (AT1R). Activation of AT1R on endothelial cells activates NAD(P)H that results in increased $O_2^{·-}$ production and promotes secretion of endothelin-1 (ET1), both promote vasoconstriction: $O_2^{·-}$ will react with NO· producing the powerful oxidant peroxynitrite which amongst other things decreases NO· available for vasorelaxation activity while ET1 will act on ET1 receptors (ET1R) on vascular smooth muscle cells to initiate signalling that increases cytosolic Ca^{2+}, thus promoting vasoconstriction. ANGII will also act on AT1R on vascular smooth muscle to also cause signalling that increases cytosolic Ca^{2+}, thus promoting vasoconstriction. ANGII will also act on AT1R on adrenal cortical cells resulting in the release of aldosterone with aldosterone promoting Na^+ reuptake by the kidneys, thereby increasing blood volume and thus increasing blood pressure.

ANGII acting on AT1R on vascular smooth muscle cells causes a PLC driven increase in IP_3 that in turns causes release of Ca^{2+} from endoplasmic reticular stores. This results in Ca^{2+} binding to calmodulin with the Ca^{2+}-calmodulin binding to MLCK that in turn now phosphorylates myosin light chain, the critical step in smooth muscle contraction. Activation of AT1R also results in a signalling to NAD(P)H oxidase resulting in the formation of $O_2^{·-}$; this free radical has a number of effects including reacting with NO·, thereby decreasing the vasorelaxation activity of NO·. This linking of receptor activity with activation of NAD(P)H oxidase is seen in a number of signalling pathways (see Chapter 5).

ANGII acting on AT1R on endothelial cells results in a number of effects. The AT1R is also linked to a G-protein coupled activation of PLC resulting in a rise in intracellular Ca^{2+}, similar to what is seen in the activation of the cholinergic muscarinic receptors. This may seem confusing but keep in mind that signalling is very spatially localized (see Chapter 5) with muscarinic signalling occurring at sites distinct from angiotensin signalling. Endothelial

AT1R-coupled signalling is also linked to NAD(P)H oxidase resulting in increased O_2^- production with the O_2^- decreasing the availability of $NO^.$ for vasorelaxation activity. Another consequence of AT1R-coupled signalling is secretion of the protein endothelin-1 (ET1). There are ET1 receptors (ET1R) vascular smooth muscle cells that are linked to the G protein-coupled PLC pathway that cause an increase in intracellular Ca^{2+} and thus vasocontraction. Thus ET1 acts as a vasoconstrictor when it acts on ET1R on smooth muscle cells.

ANGII acting on AT1R on zona glomerulosa cells of the adrenal cortex results in the synthesis and secretion of aldosterone. Aldosterone promotes Na^+ reuptake by the kidneys, thereby increasing blood volume and thus blood pressure.

Besides regulating blood volume through controlling the amount of Na^+ taken up, the kidneys also play another critical role in regulating blood pressure: in response to a reduction in Na^+ concentration in the kidney filtrate (generally due to low blood pressure) the kidneys secrete renin. Renin plays a critical role in in the formation of ANGII. The precursor protein for ANGII is angiotensinogen, a protein produced and secreted by the liver. Renin cleaves angiotensinogen into angiotensin I (ANGI). Angiotensin converting enzyme (ACE), secreted by endothelial cells, then converts ANGI to angiotensin II, i.e., ANGII, the vasoactive peptide (see Figure 3). There is a continual formation and secretion of angiotensinogen by the liver and there is a continual synthesis of ACE; hence, secretion of renin by the kidney is the rate-limiting step in ANGII formation. A major cause of hypertension is over-secretion of renin by the kidneys [28] with therapies aimed at blocking the AT1R, blocking the action of ACE or more recently blocking renin secretion by the kidneys. The kidney is the main determinate in regulation of blood pressure; indeed, the blood pressure of renal transplant patients is determined by the blood pressure of the donor, not the recipient [29]. Furthermore, the probability of kidneys being pro-hypertensive can be developmentally programmed [30].

There is an abundance of evidence that oxidative stress is associated with hypertension, not only at the level of the endothelium but also at the level of the kidneys [31]. How oxidative stress at the level of the kidneys affects blood pressure is complex [32], but in part it involves changes in renal hemodynamics that affects the tubule-glomerular feedback mechanisms that regulate renin secretion. Renin secretion is regulated by signalling pathways that are susceptible oxidant over-activation (see Chapter 5 for effects of oxidants on kinase cascades) and this, likely is one way that oxidative stress affects the renin-angiotensin-aldosterone axis.

Comments

The above descriptions of atherogenesis and mechanisms that lead to hypertension are a bit simplistic but do outline ways in how oxidative stress promote both atherosclerosis and hypertension. One can understand how Nrf2 activators such as sulforaphane, by promoting the expression of genes that increase oxidant scavenging pathways or decrease the probability of strong oxidant formation, ought to decrease the probability of developing atherosclerosis (e.g., Figure 1) or of developing hypertension.

PRECLINICAL STUDIES OF THE EFFECTS OF SULFORAPHANE ON THE CARDIOVASCULAR SYSTEM

Findings from Our Laboratory on Therapeutic Effects of Sulforaphane

In our experiments we used spontaneously hypertensive stroke-prone rats (SHRsp) and Sprague Dawley rats, the latter as the normal physiology strain. The SHRsp develop severe hypertension and usually die of stroke if left to live out their natural days [33]. The first set of experiments were performed on male rats [34] and the second set of experiments were preformed on female rats [35]. In these experiments the rat chow used was the defined AIN-93 without tertiary-butylhydroquinone. In the third set of experiments rats were administered by gavage either sulforaphane in corn oil or just corn oil.

In our first two sets of experiments rats were fed daily from the age of 5 weeks one of the following dietary supplements: i) 200 mg dried Calabrese broccoli sprouts with intact glucosinolates containing 5.5 µmoles sulforaphane equivalents; ii) 200 mg dried Calabrese broccoli sprouts that had been frozen and thawed before drying thus destroying most of the glucosinolates with only 0.46 µmoles sulforaphane equivalents remaining; or iii) no supplement [34]. The Calabrese sprouts were chosen because they had a favourable glucosinolate (GS) profile with: glucoiberin, 3-(methylsulfinyl) propyl-GS, 13.4%; glucoraphanin, 4-(methylsulfinyl) butyl-GS, 35.1%; glucobrassicanapin, 4-pentenyl-GS, 8.0%; and gluconasturtiin, 2-phenethyl-GS, 14.1%, sinigrin (2-propenyl-GS,1.0%). The anti-nutritive GS progoitrin (2-hydroxy-3-butenyl-GS) was only a minor component (2.8%) as were the two unknowns (6.53% and 3.3%).

The animals were caged separately, thus ensuring each animal ate the 200 mg of supplement daily (Figure 4).

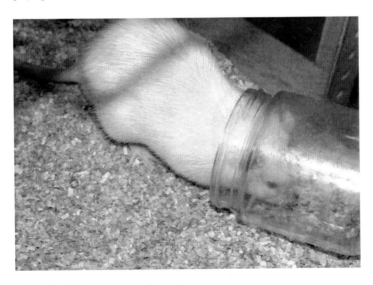

Figure 4. SHRsp eating its daily sprout supplement.

The following parameters were measured after 14 weeks (i.e., at 19 weeks of age): glutathione (GSH) and oxidized-glutathione (GSSG) as well as glutathione peroxidase and glutathione reductase activities in aorta, carotid artery, heart and kidneys [34, 35]. In addition, endothelial function was measured in the thoracic aorta and macrophage infiltration of the kidneys was examined.

Consumption of Glucoraphanin-Rich Broccoli Sprouts Moderates the Rise in Blood Pressure in SHRsp

Dietary intervention had no measureable effect in the normal-physiology Sprague Dawley rats as measured at 19 weeks. This suggests to us that there are sufficient feedback mechanisms in place that large increases in consumption of dietary Nrf2 activators will not result alterations of the normal redox balance of cells and tissues. The various tissues examined in male Sprague Dawley rats had GSH:GSSG ratios of 17 to 21 regardless of diet whilst male SHRsp on low glucosinolate broccoli sprouts had ratios ranging from 4 to 7 [34]. In contrast, SHRsp consuming broccoli sprouts with intact glucosinolates had increased the GSH:GSSG ratios from 11 to14, thus approaching, but not reaching the ratios seen in the normal physiology Sprague Dawley. The change in ratio of GSH:GSSG seen with the SHRsp was due both to an increase in tissue GSH as well as a decrease in tissue GSSG. There were also no statistically significant differences in parameters measured between SHRsp on sprouts with depleted glucosinolates compared to animals with no supplementation; therefore, the remaining measurements were done on SHRsp and Sprague Dawley on the control diet with no supplementation in comparison with rats supplemented with broccoli sprouts containing intact glucosinolates.

Both glutathione peroxidase and glutathione reductase were significantly lower in SHRsp on control diet than in the Sprague Dawley rats [34, 35]. Consumption of broccoli sprouts with intact glucosinolates significantly increased these enzyme activities but they did not reach the levels of the normal physiology Sprague Dawley rats except for kidney glutathione peroxidase activity in male SHRsp.

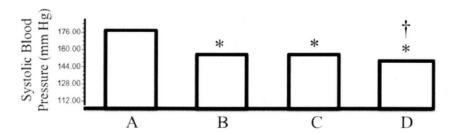

Figure 5. Systolic blood pressures of female SHRsp at 14 weeks of age. Female Sprague Dawley systolic blood pressure (not shown) is around 112 mm Hg. Column 'A' represents the blood pressure of SHRsp on control diet. Column 'B' represents the blood pressure of SHRsp on a glucoraphanin-enriched broccoli sprout supplement. Columns 'C' and 'D' are from female offspring whose mothers were on a glucoraphanin-enriched broccoli sprout supplemented diet with column 'C' representing SHRsp offspring on the control diet from weaning onwards while column 'D' represents offspring on a diet supplemented with glucoraphanin-enriched broccoli sprouts. Figure is drawn from data represented in Figure 1 as well as Supplementary Figure 1 from Noyan-Ashraf et al. [35]. * P< 0.001 compared to column 'A'; † significantly different (P<0.01) from Column 'C.'

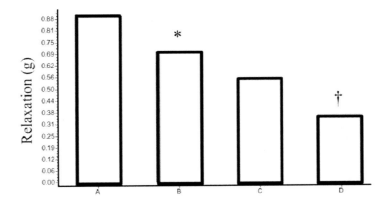

Figure 6. After 14 weeks of the experimental period male SHRsp and Sprague Dawley rats were euthanized and thoracic aortae obtained to examine vasorelaxation responses to acetylcholine. Graphs depict data of relaxation in response to 10 μM acetylcholine. Column 'A' represents Sprague Dawley on control diet. Columns 'B' to 'D' represent SHRsp on various diets. Column 'C' represents SHRsp on diet supplemented with broccoli sprout with depleted glucosinolates. Column 'D' represents SHRsp on control diet. Figure created from data represented in Figure 5 of Wu et al. [34]. * Significantly different (P <0.001) from Column 'D'; † Significantly different (P<0.001) from Column 'A.'

Immunochemistry and Western blot analyses demonstrated SHRsp on control diet had nuclear localization of p65 (indicative of nuclear factor kappa B [NFκB] activation) in tissues examined (arteries, heart and kidneys). This was associated with increased intercellular adhesion molecule-1 (ICAM1), inducible nitric oxide synthase (iNOS) expression as well as macrophage infiltration of the inner intimal layers of the heart, aorta, carotid artery as well as kidney tubules. Both activation of NFκB and inflammatory parameters such as ICAM1, iNOS and macrophage infiltration were significantly reduced in SHRsp consuming broccoli sprouts with intact glucosinolates [34, 35].

SHRsp on control diet also had inflammation in other tissues such as the central nervous system and consumption of broccoli sprouts with intact glucosinolates also decreased such inflammation [36]. As expected, broccoli consumption led to an increased localization of Nrf2 in nuclei, particularly the nuclei of vascular endothelial cells [36]. Nuclear localization of Nrf2 is an indicator of Nrf2 activation.

This decrease in oxidative stress in the cardiovascular and renal systems was associated with a significant moderation in the rise of blood pressure that is normally seen in SHRsp (Figure 5, compare columns 'A' with "B'). In female SHRsp, the increase in blood pressure plateaued after two weeks on the broccoli diet (Figure 5) and in males it plateaued after 4 weeks on the broccoli diet.

This moderation in the rise of blood pressure is due, at least in part, by better endothelial function as determined by relaxation of the thoracic aorta in response to acetylcholine (Figure 6). As mentioned above, the major vasorelaxant factor in arteries is NO˙ produced in response to acetylcholine signalling. This NO˙ is greatly influenced by local concentrations of O_2^{-}, i.e., local oxidative stress. It is clear from Figure 6 that SHRsp supplemented with glucosinolate-depleted diet had a vasorelaxant response to acetylcholine intermediate between that of the rats on control diet and rats on diet supplemented with glucoraphanin-enriched broccoli sprouts. This effect may be due to the 0.46 μmoles of sulforaphane equivalent inducers still present in the supplement or it may be due to other factors such as the flavonoids present in the broccoli sprouts. Regardless, the better endothelium function seen in this group of rats did not affect blood pressure, as these animals had the same blood pressure as SHRsp on control diet with no supplementation.

Concluding Comments

Our experiments have thus shown that consumption of broccoli sprouts with intact glucosinolates had no measurable effect on the normal-physiology Sprague Dawley male or female rats but decreased oxidative stress in the male and female SHRsp. This decrease in oxidative stress was associated with decreased inflammation in all tissues examined as well as a moderation in the rise of blood pressure. This moderation in the rise of blood pressure was associated with better endothelial function as determined by vascular smooth muscle vasorelaxant responses to acetylcholine. How relevant are these experiments to combatting human essential hypertension? Both hypertension in SHRsp and in humans have an oxidative stress component to them; hence, one can argue that the results obtained in SHRsp forms a rationale for human clinical trials. A major criticism is that our experiments dealt with the prevention in the rise of blood pressure and we did not examine the effects of glucoraphanin-rich broccoli sprouts on SHRsp with already established hypertension.

Effect of Consumption of Broccoli Sprouts on Epigenetics

Effect on Fetal Determinants of Adult Health

In one set of experiments female SHRsp that consumed a daily supplement of glucoraphanin-enriched broccoli sprouts from the age of 5 weeks were mated at 8 weeks. The pregnant rats were maintained on the broccoli supplement during pregnancy and while nursing. At weaning the offspring were placed either on a normal rat chow without supplements or on rat chow with the glucoraphanin-enriched broccoli sprout supplement until they reached 15 weeks of age [35]. The offspring of mothers consuming broccoli sprouts, regardless whether the offspring were placed on rat chow with no broccoli supplementation or rat chow with glucoraphanin-enriched broccoli had the same blood pressure as their mothers that were on a glucoraphanin-enriched broccoli sprout supplemented diet. The offspring, like their mothers had a systolic blood pressure 20 mm Hg lower than their cousins whose mothers were fed only rat chow (Figure 5, Columns 'C' and 'D'). The offspring that were on glucoraphanin-enriched broccoli sprout supplementation (Figure 5, Column 'D' had slightly, but significantly, better blood pressures than their siblings placed on regular rat chow (Figure 5, Column 'C'). We conclude that lower oxidative stress, inflammation and blood pressure in pregnant SHRsp results in positive effects of fetal determinants of adult health.

The lower blood pressure in the offspring was also associated with even less oxidative stress and inflammation than in the maternal generation consuming high glucoraphanin-containing broccoli sprouts in organs examined. Figure 7 illustrates quantification of inducible nitric oxide synthase (iNOS) protein content of female SHRsp kidneys. Expression of iNOS is an indicator of inflammation. It can be seen that consumption of broccoli sprouts enriched in glucoraphanin decreases iNOS protein content (compare Column 'A' with 'B'). Offspring of rats placed on control diet with no supplementation but whose mothers consumed broccoli sprouts enriched in glucoraphanin had an even lower iNOS protein content (Column 'C' while offspring supplemented with glucoraphanin-enriched broccoli sprouts (Column 'D') had yet a lower iNOS protein content.

Reducing oxidative stress, inflammation and blood pressure results in positive effects on fetal determinants of adult health. Up to now we have been interpreting the effects of glucoraphanin-enriched broccoli sprout supplementation as due to the activation of the Nrf2 signalling system but have no direct evidence that the positive health effects are due to the actions of molecules such as sulforaphane on the Nrf2 signalling system.

The Health Promoting Effects of Broccoli Sprouts Can Be Attributed to Sulforaphane and Such Effects Do Have a Positive Effect on the Epigenome

Our last set of experiments examined the effect of daily administration by gavage sulforaphane (10 μmoles) in corn oil or just corn oil to young female SHRsp and Sprague Dawley rats [37]. The experiment was started at 5 weeks of age and continuing for 4 months. In this study an external catheter was used to measure blood pressure in the anesthetized rat just before the animals were euthanized while previous experiments used a tail cuff to measure blood pressure.

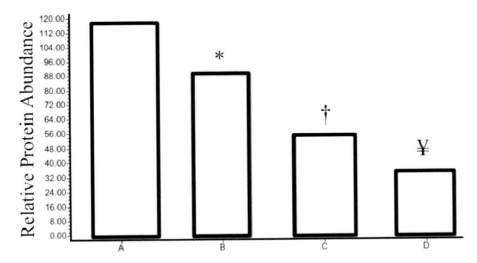

Figure 7. Graph depicting Western blot data of inducible nitric oxide synthase (iNOS) in kidneys of female SHRsp on control diet consisting only of rat chow (Column 'A'), first generation females on rat chow supplemented with glucoraphanin-enriched broccoli sprouts (Column 'B'), female offspring of female rats on glucoraphanin-enriched broccoli sprout supplementation but offspring placed on chow with no supplementation (Column 'C') and female offspring of female rats on glucoraphanin-enriched broccoli sprout supplementation and with offspring placed on broccoli sprout supplementation (Column 'D'). * significantly different ($P<0.01$) from Column 'A'; † significantly different ($P<0.01$) from Column 'B'; ¡ ¥ significantly different ($P<0.05$) from Column 'C.' Graph drawn from data represented in Supplementary Figure 6C from Noyan-Ashraf et al. [35].

Sulforaphane administration significantly decreased the rise in blood pressure normally seen in the SHRsp but had no effect on the blood pressure of Sprague Dawley rats. Thus, one can conclude that a major effect of the broccoli sprout supplementation in the previous experiments can be attributed to sulforaphane. The SHRsp on sulforaphane supplementation also had a significantly decreased oxidative stress and associated inflammation in the tissues examined (kidneys and blood vessels). This can be attributed, at least in part, to the induction of phase 2 protein genes as evidenced by the increase in γ-glutamyl-cysteine ligase (rate-limiting enzyme in glutathione synthesis) protein content [37].

Epigenetic changes have been implicated in renal disease [38]. Methylation of cytosines in cytosine-guanosine repeats is a major component of the epigenetic modification of the genome. Total methylated cytosine content was lower in the SHRsp kidneys compared to Sprague Dawley rats [37]. Interestingly, there were no differences in global cytosine methylation in livers between SHRsp and Sprague Dawley rats. Sulforaphane supplementation resulted in total methylated cytosine content in SHRsp kidneys to be indistinguishable from that of Sprague Dawley rats. Sulforaphane supplementation had no effect on total cytosine methylation in Sprague Dawley rat kidneys, nor in livers of SHRsp and Sprague Dawley rats. We conclude that sulforaphane administration had positive effects on the renal epigenome in SHRsp. This is in line with the positive fetal determinants of adult health seen previously in our experiments feeding broccoli sprouts pregnant and nursing SHRsp.

Findings from Other Laboratories on Therapeutic Effects of Sulforaphane

Elbarbry and colleagues demonstrated that incorporation of sulforaphane into the drinking water of young male spontaneously hypertensive rats (SHR) moderated the rise in blood pressure typically seen in this strain of rat [39], essentially confirming the findings of our laboratory on the effect of sulforaphane on SHRsp blood pressure. They also showed that arachidonic acid metabolism in the kidney was affected in a manner that promoted the formation of vasorelaxant eicosanoids, specifically sulforaphane was associated with decreased cytochrome P450 4A (CYP4A) which is associated with the formation of vasoconstrictor eicosanoids and decreased epoxide hydrolase activity; epoxide hydrolase breaks down vasorelaxant eicosanoids.

Akhlaghi and Bandy [40] placed male Wistar rats on a defined AIN-93G diet with either no supplements or supplemented with dried 6-day-old Calabrese broccoli sprouts (2 g per 100 g AIN-93G) for 10 days. Hearts were then removed and placed in a Langendorff apparatus and subjected to ischemia for 20 minutes followed by reperfusion for 2 hr.

Following ischemia and reperfusion, hearts from rats on broccoli sprouts had significantly less damage as determined by lower cellular lactate dehydrogenase release, lower caspase 3 activation (marker of apoptosis), less malondialdehyde formation (marker of lipid peroxidation) and increased aconitase activity (marker of mitochondrial health. Interestingly, the liver, but not the heart of these broccoli sprout fed-animals had higher γ-glutamyl-cysteine ligase activity and higher GSH levels. This is in keeping with our previous observations that cells with a high oxidative metabolism do not respond to oxidative stress by activation of the anti-oxidant response [41].

There are no publications, to date, examining the effects of sulforaphane on animal models of atherosclerosis, although there are a number of *in vitro* studies examining atherosclerosis-relevant aspects, e.g., [42, 43]. Nallasamy and colleagues [43] also examined the ability of sulforaphane, taken through the diet, to influence tumour necrosis factor-α (TNFα)-induced monocyte adhesion to the endothelium. Monocyte adhesion to the endothelium and subsequent infiltration of the tunica intima is a critical step in atherosclerotic lesion development. In these experiments mice were fed AIN-93G diet containing either 300 ppm sulforaphane or no added sulforaphane. After one week the mice were intraperitoneally administered TNFα daily for 1 week.

TNFα administration to mice on control diet resulted in increases in the blood levels of several chemokines (monocyte chemotactic protein-1 and keratinocyte chemokine) and several soluble forms of cell adhesion molecules (soluble intercellular adhesion molecule-1 [sICAM1] and soluble E-Selectin) and increased the expression of cell-associated vascular cell adhesion molecule-1 (VCAM1). In addition, there was a great increase in monocyte adhesion to the endothelium and infiltration of the intima. Mice on sulforaphane had significantly lower blood chemokine levels, lower soluble cell adhesion molecules as well as lower VCAM1 levels, lower monocyte adhesion and infiltration of the intima. Lower infiltration of monocytes also resulted in better structural integrity of the arteries [43].

Although the animal model used by Nallasamy and colleagues is not a model of atherosclerosis, it does feature significant aspects of atherosclerosis: increased chemokine and cytokine levels, expression of cell adhesion molecules and adhesion and infiltration of monocytes/macrophages. Is 300 ppm sulforaphane achievable in the diet? The authors report that intake of AIN-93G containing 300 ppm sulforaphane results in sulforaphane plasma levels reaching 0.57 µM. Such blood levels can certainly be achieved in humans consuming high-glucoraphanin-containing broccoli sprouts [44]. Perhaps a better rodent model of atherosclerosis is the LDL receptor -/-, apolipoprotein B transgenic mouse that has been used in examining the effect of green and yellow vegetable intake on atherosclerotic lesions [45].

CONCLUSION

More studies are required, both with animal models of cardiovascular diseases, in particular models of atherosclerosis, as well as human clinical trials. The human clinical trials to date have shown no adverse effects of consuming broccoli sprouts rich in glucoraphanin, other than minor ones such as increase in flatulence in some individuals. There have been a few clinical trials examining the effect of glucoraphanin-rich broccoli sprout consumption, particularly on the cardiovascular system in the context of Type 2 diabetes (see Chapter 12) and one study aimed at reducing blood pressure (see Chapter 13).

I trust that this chapter has outlined the rationale for why sulforaphane (and other Nrf2 activators) and broccoli sprouts enriched in glucoraphanin may have cardiovascular therapeutic properties. We were struck, in particular, by the positive effects of pregnant and nursing rats consuming glucoraphanin-rich broccoli sprouts on fetal determinants of adult health [35]. There is a large literature negative maternal conditions can have a negative effect on fetal determinants of adult health, both in animal models as well as in humans [46-49]. We believe this is the first study showing positive effects on fetal determinants of adult health.

REFERENCES

[1] Wong, MC; Zhang de, X; Wang, HH. Rapid emergence of atherosclerosis in Asia: a systematic review of coronary atherosclerotic heart disease epidemiology and implications for prevention and control strategies. *Curr Opin Lipidol*, 2015, 26, 257-69.

[2] Palmefors, H; DuttaRoy, S; Rundqvist, B; Borjesson, M. The effect of physical activity or exercise on key biomarkers in atherosclerosis--a systematic review. *Atherosclerosis*, 2014, 235, 150-61.

[3] Cleroux, J; Feldman, RD; Petrella, RJ. Lifestyle modifications to prevent and control hypertension. 4. Recommendations on physical exercise training. Canadian Hypertension Society, Canadian Coalition for High Blood Pressure Prevention and Control, Laboratory Centre for Disease Control at Health Canada, Heart and Stroke Foundation of Canada. *CMAJ*, 1999, 160, S21-8.

[4] Figueira, FR; Umpierre, D; Cureau, FV; et al. Association between physical activity advice only or structured exercise training with blood pressure levels in patients with Type 2 diabetes: a systematic review and meta-analysis. *Sports Med*, 2014, 44, 1557-72.

[5] Mahe, G; Ronziere, T; Laviolle, B; et al. An unfavorable dietary pattern is associated with symptomatic ischemic stroke and carotid atherosclerosis. *J Vasc Surg*, 2010, 52, 62-8.

[6] Zhang, X; Shu, XO; Xiang, YB; et al. Cruciferous vegetable consumption is associated with a reduced risk of total and cardiovascular disease mortality. *Am J Clin Nutr*, 2011, 94, 240-6.

[7] Saneei, P; Salehi-Abargouei, A; Esmaillzadeh, A; Azadbakht, L. Influence of Dietary Approaches to Stop Hypertension (DASH) diet on blood pressure: a systematic review and meta-analysis on randomized controlled trials. *Nutr Metab Cardiovasc Dis*, 2014, 24, 1253-61.

[8] Siervo, M; Lara, J; Chowdhury, S; Ashor, A; Oggioni, C; Mathers, JC. Effects of the Dietary Approach to Stop Hypertension (DASH) diet on cardiovascular risk factors: a systematic review and meta-analysis. *Br J Nutr*, 2014, 1-15.

[9] Alexander, RW. The Jeremiah Metzger Lecture. Pathogenesis of atherosclerosis: redox as a unifying mechanism. *Trans Am Clin Climatol Assoc*, 2003, 114, 273-304.

[10] Juurlink, BH. Dietary Nrf2 activators inhibit atherogenic processes. *Atherosclerosis*, 2012, 225, 29-33.

[11] Lee, MY, Griendling KK. Redox signaling, vascular function, and hypertension. *Antioxid Redox Signal*, 2008, 10, 1045-59.

[12] Majzunova, M; Dovinova, I; Barancik, M; Chan, JY. Redox signaling in pathophysiology of hypertension. *J Biomed Sci*, 2013, 20, 69.

[13] Hulsmans, M; Holvoet, P. The vicious circle between oxidative stress and inflammation in atherosclerosis. *J Cell Mol Med*, 2010, 14, 70-8.

[14] Maiolino, G; Rossitto, G; Caielli, P; Bisogni, V; Rossi, GP; Calo, LA. The role of oxidized low-density lipoproteins in atherosclerosis: the myths and the facts. *Mediators Inflamm*, 2013, 2013, 714653.

[15] Pirillo, A; Norata, GD; Catapano, AL. LOX-1, OxLDL, and atherosclerosis. *Mediators Inflamm*, 2013, 2013, 152786.

[16] Ashraf, MZ; Sahu, A. Scavenger receptors: a key player in cardiovascular diseases. *Biomol Concepts*, 2012, 3, 371-80.

[17] Yang, HY; Bian, YF; Zhang, HP; et al. LOX1 is implicated in oxidized lowdensity lipoproteininduced oxidative stress of macrophages in atherosclerosis. *Mol Med Rep*, 2015.

[18] Badimon, L; Vilahur, G; Padro, T. Nutraceuticals and atherosclerosis: human trials. *Cardiovasc Ther*, 2010, 28, 202-15.

[19] Robles, NR; Macias, JF. Hypertension in the elderly. *Cardiovasc Hematol Agents Med Chem*, 2015, 12, 136-45.

[20] Gasecki, D; Kwarciany, M; Nyka, W; Narkiewicz, K. Hypertension, brain damage and cognitive decline. *Curr Hypertens Rep*, 2013, 15, 547-58.

[21] Nelson, L; Gard, P; Tabet, N. Hypertension and inflammation in Alzheimer's disease: close partners in disease development and progression! *J Alzheimers Dis*, 2014, 41, 331-43.

[22] Jia, G; Aroor, AR; Sowers, JR. Arterial Stiffness: A Nexus between Cardiac and Renal Disease. *Cardiorenal Med*, 2014, 4, 60-71.

[23] Palmer, RM; Ferrige, AG; Moncada, S. Nitric oxide release accounts for the biological activity of endothelium-derived relaxing factor. *Nature*, 1987, 327, 524-6.

[24] Higashi, Y; Kihara, Y; Noma, K. Endothelial dysfunction and hypertension in aging. *Hypertens Res*, 2012, 35, 1039-47.

[25] Karnik, SS; Unal, H; Kemp, JR; et al. Angiotensin receptors: Interpreters of pathophysiological angiotensinergic stimuli. *Pharmacol Rev*, 2015, 67, 754-819.

[26] MacKenzie, A. Endothelium-derived vasoactive agents, AT1 receptors and inflammation. *Pharmacol Ther*, 2011, 131, 187-203.

[27] Tran, LT; Yuen, VG; McNeill, JH. The fructose-fed rat: a review on the mechanisms of fructose-induced insulin resistance and hypertension. *Mol Cell Biochem*, 2009, 332, 145-59.

[28] Ferrari, R; Boersma, E. The impact of ACE inhibition on all-cause and cardiovascular mortality in contemporary hypertension trials: a review. *Expert Rev Cardiovasc Ther*, 2013, 11, 705-17.

[29] Rettig, R; Grisk, O. The kidney as a determinant of genetic hypertension: evidence from renal transplantation studies. *Hypertension*, 2005, 46, 463-8.

[30] Tomat, AL; Salazar, FJ. Mechanisms involved in developmental programming of hypertension and renal diseases. Gender differences. *Horm Mol Biol Clin Investig,*, 2014, 18, 63-77.

[31] Luo, H; Wang, X; Chen, C; et al. Oxidative stress causes imbalance of renal renin angiotensin system (RAS) components and hypertension in obese Zucker rats. *J Am Heart Assoc*, 2015, 4.

[32] Araujo, M; Wilcox, CS. Oxidative stress in hypertension: role of the kidney. *Antioxid Redox Signal*, 2014, 20, 74-101.

[33] Nabika, T; Ohara, H; Kato, N; Isomura, M. The stroke-prone spontaneously hypertensive rat: still a useful model for post-GWAS genetic studies? *Hypertens Res*, 2012, 35, 477-84.

[34] Wu, L; Noyan Ashraf, MH; Facci, M; et al. Dietary approach to attenuate oxidative stress, hypertension, and inflammation in the cardiovascular system. *Proc Natl Acad Sci U S A*, 2004, 101, 7094-9.

[35] Noyan-Ashraf, MH; Wu, L; Wang, R; Juurlink, BH. Dietary approaches to positively influence fetal determinants of adult health. *FASEB J*, 2006, 20, 371-3.

[36] Noyan-Ashraf, MH; Sadeghinejad, Z; Juurlink, BH. Dietary approach to decrease aging-related CNS inflammation. *Nutr Neurosci*, 2005, 8, 101-10.

[37] Senanayake, GV; Banigesh, A; Wu, L; Lee, P; Juurlink, BH. The dietary phase 2 protein inducer sulforaphane can normalize the kidney epigenome and improve blood pressure in hypertensive rats. *Am J Hypertens*, 2012, 25, 229-35.

[38] Reddy, MA; Natarajan, R. Recent developments in epigenetics of acute and chronic kidney diseases. *Kidney Int*, 2015, 88, 250-61.

[39] Elbarbry, F; Vermehren-Schmaedick, A; Balkowiec, A. Modulation of arachidonic Acid metabolism in the rat kidney by sulforaphane: implications for regulation of blood pressure. *ISRN Pharmacol*, 2014, 2014, 683508.

[40] Akhlaghi, M; Bandy, B. Dietary broccoli sprouts protect against myocardial oxidative damage and cell death during ischemia-reperfusion. *Plant Foods Hum Nutr*, 2010, 65, 193-9.

[41] Eftekharpour, E; Holmgren, A; Juurlink, BH. Thioredoxin reductase and glutathione synthesis is upregulated by t-butylhydroquinone in cortical astrocytes but not in cortical neurons. *Glia*, 2000, 31, 241-8.

[42] Kwon, JS; Joung, H; Kim, YS; et al. Sulforaphane inhibits restenosis by suppressing inflammation and the proliferation of vascular smooth muscle cells. *Atherosclerosis*, 2012, 225, 41-9.

[43] Nallasamy, P; Si, H; Babu, PV; et al. Sulforaphane reduces vascular inflammation in mice and prevents TNF-alpha-induced monocyte adhesion to primary endothelial cells through interfering with the NF-kappaB pathway. *J Nutr Biochem*, 2014, 25, 824-33.

[44] Ye, L; Dinkova-Kostova, AT; Wade, KL; Zhang, Y; Shapiro, TA; Talalay, P. Quantitative determination of dithiocarbamates in human plasma, serum, erythrocytes and urine: pharmacokinetics of broccoli sprout isothiocyanates in humans. *Clin Chim Acta*, 2002, 316, 43-53.

[45] Adams, MR; Golden, DL; Chen, H; Register, TC; Gugger, ET. A diet rich in green and yellow vegetables inhibits atherosclerosis in mice. *J Nutr*, 2006, 136, 1886-9.

[46] Skogen, JC; Overland, S. The fetal origins of adult disease: a narrative review of the epidemiological literature. *JRSM Short Rep*, 2012, 3, 59.

[47] Reusens, B; Ozanne, SE; Remacle, C. Fetal determinants of Type 2 diabetes. *Curr Drug Targets*, 2007, 8, 935-41.

[48] Alexander, BT; Dasinger, JH; Intapad, S. Fetal programming and cardiovascular pathology. *Compr Physiol*, 2015, 5, 997-1025.

[49] Klimek, P; Leitner, M; Kautzky-Willer, A; Thurner, S. Effect of fetal and infant malnutrition on metabolism in older age. *Gerontology*, 2014, 60, 502-7.

In: Broccoli
Editor: Bernhard H. J. Juurlink

ISBN: 978-1-63484-313-3
© 2016 Nova Science Publishers, Inc.

Chapter 12

BENEFICIAL EFFECTS OF BROCCOLI SPROUTS AND ITS BIOACTIVE COMPOUND SULFORAPHANE IN MANAGEMENT OF TYPE 2 DIABETES

Zahra Bahadoran[1] *and Parvin Mirmiran*[2,*]

[1]Nutrition and Endocrine Research Center, Research Institute for Endocrine Sciences, Shahid Beheshti University of Medical Sciences, Tehran, Iran
[2]Department of Clinical Nutrition and Dietetics, Faculty of Nutrition Sciences and Food Technology, National Nutrition and Food Technology Research Institute, Shahid Beheshti University of Medical Sciences, Tehran, Iran

ABSTRACT

Young broccoli sprouts are rich sources of many bioactive compounds, especially sulforaphane (SFN). Studies have shown that SFN has the potential to activate the antioxidant response signaling pathway, thereby inducing phase 2 enzymes. This will attenuate oxidative stress as well as inflammation. SFN, by activating the antioxidant response, also regulates lipid metabolism and glucose homeostasis. Anti-hypertensive, anti-cancer, cardio-protective, hypo-cholesterolemic capacity and antibactericidal properties against *Helicobacter Pylori* have also been reported for SFN. Clinical studies with high-SFN broccoli sprouts have shown increased total antioxidant capacity of plasma and a decrease in the following: the oxidative stress index, lipid peroxidation, serum triglycerides, oxidized-LDL/LDL-C ratio, serum insulin, insulin resistance, and serum high sensitive C reactive protein. Thus SFN has the potential to prevent diabetic vascular complications. Potential therapeutic efficacy of SFN and probably other bioactive components present in young broccoli sprouts make it as an excellent choice for supplementary treatment in Type 2 diabetes.

Keywords: broccoli sprouts, sulforaphane, insulin resistance, oxidative stress, diabetes complications

---

[*] Corresponding author: E-mail: mirmiran@endocrine.ac.ir.

INTRODUCTION

Young broccoli sprouts (3 to 4-day old broccoli sprouted seeds) are enriched in a wide variety of bioactive compounds including flavonoids, other polyphenolics, carotenoids, antioxidant vitamins such as vitamin C and E, selenium and especially some important antioxidant and chemoprotective metabolites including glucosinolates and isothiocyanates [1, 2]. Bioactive phytochemicals in broccoli sprouts appear to play an important role in the prevention and treatment of some chronic diseases. Sulforaphane (SFN; 1-isothiocyanato-4-methylsulfinylbutane), a hydrolysis product of glucoraphanin via myrosinase, is a determinant nutraceutical present in young broccoli sprouts [3]. There is a growing interest regarding the potential properties of SFN and its underlying mechanisms. One of the best known biological property of SFN is upregulatation of phase II detoxifying enzymes including superoxide dismutase, catalase, nicotinamide adenine dinucleotide phosphate (NADPH):quinone oxidoreductase 1, γ-glutamyl-cysteine ligase (rate-limiting enzyme for glutathione synthesis), glutathione peroxidase, glutathione reductase and glutathione S-transferases. These are the main endogenous defense systems responsible for inactivation and clearance of reactive oxygen species and carcinogens [4, 5]. Sulforaphane can also down-regulate cytochrome P450 3A4 (CYP3A4) expression in hepatocytes: CYP3A4 is responsible for the hepatic and intestinal metabolism of numerous protoxicants, pharmaceutical compounds, and endogenous sterols [6]. SFN induces anti-inflammatory pathways via activation of NF-E2-related factor-2 (Nrf2) dependent antioxidant response signaling pathway that suppresses a key modulator of inflammatory pathways, nuclear factor κB (NF-κB) [7, 8]. Other interesting effects of SFN include induction of thioredoxin (part of the antioxidant response and is a cardioprotective protein) [9], antibactericidal properties against *Helicobacter pylori* [10], protection of dopaminergic cells [11], enhancement of natural killer cell activity and other markers of immune function [12]. Furthermore, SFN acts as a inducer of peroxisome proliferator activated receptors (PPARs), PPAR-binding proteins and PPAR co-activators that contribute to lipid metabolism and glucose homeostasis [13]. SFN may also exhibit antiobesity effects through inhibitition of adipogenesis by down-regulation of PPARγ and CCAAT/enhancer-binding protein α and by suppression of lipogenesis via activation of the AMP-activated protein kinase α (AMPKα) pathway [13]. In non-alcholic fatty liver disease, SFN prevents elevation of liver enzymes and liver injury through activation of Nrf2-antioxidant response element (ARE) pathway and enhancement of antioxidant defense system [14]. The protective effect of high-SFN broccoli sprouts against fructose-induced metabolic and liver disoders may be considered as another important benefit of this bioactive compounds [15].

Considering to the potential efficacies of SFN and probably other bioactive components, it seems that young broccoli sprouts may be an excellent complementary treatment in Type 2 diabetes and its related metabolic disorders [16].

POTENTIAL THERAPEUTIC ACTIONS OF SULFORAPHANE IN THE CONTEXT OF TYPE 2 DIABETES

Sulforaphane has the potential to ameliorate Type 2 diabetes in a number of ways that are reviewed in this chapter. These include increasing the capacity to inactivate oxidants, promoting better insulin function, improved lipid metabolism, improved renal function, improved vascular function and better outcomes with *Helicobacter pylori* infections.

Antioxidative Properties of Broccoli Sprouts and SFN

Increased oxidative stress has a determinant role in the development and progression of micro and macro vascular complications in diabetes. Increased generation of free radicals and an impaired antioxidant defense system in diabetic conditions induces an imbalance of the oxidant/antioxidant status [17-19]. It has been proposed that inhibition of such oxidative stress could prevent the onset and the development of long-term diabetic complications [19, 20]. SFN induces phase II anti-oxidative enzymes that counteract oxidative species, including free radicals, mainly through glutathione-mediated mechanisms [21].

It is noteworthy that anti-oxidative effects of SFN are mainly observed in relation to activation of Nrf2 and antioxidant response element (ARE)-linked gene expression [4]. Nrf2 is a transcription factor that induces the expression of various genes encoding antioxidant enzymes, and plays a physiological role in the regulation of oxidative stress [22] – also see Chapter 6. Compounds that target Nrf2 are now considered for potential therapeutic interventions for oxidative-stress related conditions [23]. Activation of Nrf2 is facilitated by Kelch-like ECH associated protein 1 (KEAP1), a cysteine-rich protein. SFN interacts with specific cysteine residues of KEAP1, and consequently induces translocation of Nrf2 to the nucleus and activates ARE-dependent genes (see Chapter 6). This KEAP1/Nrf2/ARE pathway increases the capacity of the cells to counter oxidative species [21].

In the hyperglycemic state seen with Type 2 diabetes, SFN is predicted to prevent mitochondrial dysfunction and formation of reactive oxygen species and attenuate hyperglycemia-induced activation of hexosamine and protein kinase C (PKC) pathways and protein glycation. Considering the determinant role of increased PKC activity, overproduction of advanced glycation end products (AGEs), the aldose reductase pathway, and oxidative/nitrosative/ carbonyl stress in the development of vascular complocations in diabetes, this property of SFN may be considered as a novel strategy to suppress endothelial cell dysfunction and development of vascular disease [4].

Indeed, in an *in vitro* study where rat aortic smooth muscle cells were incubated with 0.25 - 5 µM, SFN induced important cellular antioxidants and phase II enzymes, including superoxide dismutase (SOD), catalase, glutathione peroxidase, glutathione reductase, glutathione S-transferase (GST), and NAD(P)H:quinine oxidoreductase 1 (NQO1) [5] as well as glutathione (GSH); these findings suggest that SFN could improve resistance of vascular cells against oxidative and electrophilic stress *in vivo*. Furthermore, oral administration of 100 or 200 mg/kg broccoli extract to diabetic rats resulted in a significant reduction in serum thiobarbituric acid-reactive substances; thiobarbituric acid-reactive substances are markers of lipid peroxidation [24]. Administration of 200 mg/d dried broccoli sprouts to rats decreased oxidative stress as shown by increased GSH, a critical endogenous antioxidant for scavenging peroxides and other lipid derived oxidants [25]. The above findings in animal models suggest that human studies are warranted in Type 2 diabetic humans.

Riedl et al., in a clinical study on healthy subjects who received 25, 100, 125, 150, 175 or 200 g of homogenized broccoli sprouts *vs*. 200 g alfalfa sprouts for 3 days, showed a dose-dependent increase in expression of phase II antioxidant enzymes including glutathione-S-transferase, glutathione-S-transferase, NADPH quinone oxidoreductase, and heme oxyganase-1 in nasal lavage cells, with a maximal enzyme induction in dose of 200 g broccoli sprouts [26]. The 200 g dose contained 102 μmol SFN. This study has shown that broccoli sprout homogenates that contain sulforaphane can induce phase II enzymes in humans. The question arises whether broccoli sprout consumption can affect Type 2 diabetes in humans.

A 4-week supplementation trial with high SFN (~ 22.5 μmol/g) broccoli sprouts powder in dose of 10 g sprouts/d in Type 2 diabetic human patients resulted in significant decrease in serum concentrations of malondialdehyde (MDA) and oxidized-LDL cholesterol; both 5 and 10 g/d broccoli sprouts significantly increased total antioxidant capacity (TAC) and decreased the oxidative stress index, defined as total oxidant status to total antioxidant capacity ratio [27]. In another human study, consumption of 100 g/d fresh broccoli sprouts in healthy subjects reduced urinary 8-isoprostane and plasma phosphatidylcholine hydroperoxide and, as well, increased the CoQ10H2 (reduced form of coenzyme Q10)/coenzyme Q10 ratio [28]. This study showed that SFN also resulted in a better HDL/LDL ratio.

Effects of Broccoli Sprouts and SFN on Inflammatory Pathways

Subclinical low-grade inflammation contributes to the development of Type 2 diabetes and its complications. It is well known that adipocytokines and activated macrophage derivates including C-reactive protein (CRP), interleukin 6 (IL-6), and tumor necrosis factor α (TNF-α) have key roles in the cascade of inflammation, systemic insulin resistance, β cell dysfunction, atherosclerosis and cardiovascular events [29, 30]. Anti-inflammatory therapeutic approaches are now considered to be important in the management of Type 2 diabetes and prevention of micro and macro vascular diseases [31].

SFN has the potential to inhibit production of pro-inflammatory cytokines include interleukin-8, interleukin-1β, through the activation of the Nrf2 pathway and consequently induction of NADPH: quinone oxidoreductase 1 (NQO1), an antioxidant phase II protein [32]. In an *in vitro* model, Shan et al. investigated protective effects of SFN on inflammatory damage induced by lipopolysaccharide (LPS) in human vascular endothelial cells [33]. SFN could inhibit LPS-stimulated production of TNF-α and IL-1β, and also production of inflammatory mediators such as cytokines, prostaglandins and NO through inhibition of NF-κB transcriptional activity: NF-κB is a key modulator of pro-inflammatory processes [7, 34]. Further, it has been shown that SFN at a dose of 0.5 μM significantly inhibited TNF-α-induced adhesion of monocytes to endothelial cells, a determinent event in the pathogenesis of atherosclerosis; SFN also reduced vascular inflammation in mice and prevented TNF-α-induced monocyte adhesion to primary endothelial cells through interfering with the NF-κB pathway [35]. Moreover, SFN inhibits the expression of cyclooxygenase-2 (COX-2), inducible nitric oxide synthase (iNOS) and, as well, inhibits caspase-1 autoproteolytic activation, interleukin-1β maturation and secretion, and related inflammatory processes [36].

It is thought that these properties of SFN can be useful in chronic inflammatory conditions such as diabetes but there are limited data to confirm the hypothesis in human. In a recent human study, consumption of half (30 g) and full (60 g) servings of fresh broccoli sprouts resulted in decreased urinary concentrations of tetranor-PGEM (major urinary metabolite of prostaglandins E1 and E2), 11-dehydro-TXB2 (metabolite of thromboxane A2) and 11β-PGF2a (metabolite of prostaglandin D2) involved in a number of inflammatory processes [37]. Findings from a randomized clinical trial, conducted on Type 2 diabetic patients, showed that a 4-week supplementation with doses of 5 and 10 g/d high-SFN broccoli sprouts significantly decreased serum hs-CRP concentration (-20.5% and -16.4%), and led to non-significant decreases in serum IL-6 (-3.6% and -0.7%), and TNF-α concentration (-1.6% and -10.9%) with doses of 5 and 10 g/d, respectively [38].

Effects of Broccoli Sprouts and SFN on Insulin Homeostasis

Subclinical inflammation, increased oxidative stress and accumulation of lipid peroxidation metabolites in muscle, liver, adipocytes and pancreatic β cells contribute to development of insulin resistance, β cell dysfunction and development of Type 2 diabetes [39]. The use of antioxidant components along with common medications such as biguanides and thiazolidindiones is a new approach in management of insulin resistance. Studies suggest the beneficial effects of bioactive food components with antioxidant activity, including α-lipoic acid, antioxidant vitamins and flavonols, in increasing insulin sensitivity in Type 2 diabetes [40]. The effects of broccoli sprouts and bioactive compounds on insulin homeostasis have been less well documented. Fu et al. [41] in an *in vitro* model showed that incubation of INS-1(832/13) cells and isolated mouse islets with SFN dose-dependently stimulated insulin secretion; this study revealed that acute effect of SFN on insulin secretion was mediated by SFN-stimulated transient reative oxygen species accumulation. In contrast, prolonged SFN exposure attenuates glucose-stimulated ROS and glucose-stimulated insulin secretion due to activation of Nrf2 and induction of antioxidant signalling pathways. It has been suggested that as an Nrf2-activator, SFN may stimulate basal insulin release in fasted state, and inhibit postprandial glucose-stimulated insulin secretion [41]. Another important action of SFN is protection of β-cells against cytotoxicity induced by exogenous oxidative and electrophilic stress-induced cell damage [41]. In a clinical study, supplementation of Type 2 diabetic patients with high SFN content broccoli sprouts resulted in decreases in serum insulin level and decreases in insulin resistance as measured by the homeostasis model assessment of insulin resistance [42]. The anti-oxidative and anti-inflammatory properties of broccoli sprouts may be main reason for the observed effects. Moreover, SFN is involved in regulation of some important pathways related to glucose and insulin homeostasis. For example, SFN inhibits the NF-κB pathway, a key factor in the development of insulin resistance and pathogenesis of Type 2 diabetes and its complications. Studies have shown that inhibition of the NF-κB pathway in addition to *in vitro* protection of pancreatic β cells also increased insulin sensitivity [43]. SFN also activates peroxisome proliferator activated receptors (PPARs), the nuclear receptor super-family involved in lipid and carbohydrates metabolism. Recently the ability of PPAR-α receptor agonists to improve insulin sensitivity by multiple mechanisms including improvement of insulin signaling and decrease of circulating fatty acids and triglycerides has been investigated [44].

Effects of Broccoli Sprouts and SFN on Lipid Metabolism

Few studies have investigated the effect of broccoli sprouts on lipid profiles. Lee et al. examined the effect of an ethanolic broccoli sprout extract on rats fed a high fat diet [45].

In this study, a high-fat-induced diet increased levels of total cholesterol and triglycerides in the liver and adipose tissue and increased the activity of heparin-releasable lipoprotein lipase.

Administration of an ethanol extract of broccoli sprouts in two doses of 200 and 400 g/kg for 4 weeks in rats fed this high fat diet resulted in decreased levels of serum total cholesterol, LDL-C and triglycerides; this was associated with a decreased cardiac risk factor as shown by a decreased cholesterol/HDL-C ratio and increased HDL-C [45]. Furthermore, total extractable lipoprotein lipase in adipose tissue was significantly reduced.

Administration of broccoli sprouts to human Type 2 diabetics for 4-weeks resulted in an 18.7% decrease in serum triglyceride levels; a non-significant decrease in serum levels of total cholesterol and LDL-C was also observed. Another important outcome of broccoli sprout supplementation in diabetics was a significant, 52% reduction in the level of atherogenic index of plasma (defined as Logarithm of TG/HDL ratio); this index has recently been considered as a direct measure of lipoprotein particle size and as a measure of the risk for atherosclerosis [46].

One week consumption of fresh broccoli sprouts was also accompanied with increased levels of HDL-C and decrease in both total cholesterol and LDL-C [28]. In contrast in a double-blind clinical trial, ingestion of 10 g/d broccoli sprouts during 4 weeks intervention in patients with hypertension, had no effects on LDL-C, total cholesterol and HDL-C [47].

The mechanism for the effects of broccoli sprout extracts on lipid metabolism has not yet been clearly explained; one possible mechanism is that phytonutrient compounds in broccoli such as isothiocyanates, bind with bile acids and reduce fat absorption [48]. Broccoli sprout extracts also inhibits lipoprotein lipase activity in adipose tissue, decreases gene expression and the activity of key lipogenic enzymes, including diacylglycerol acyltransferases, fatty acid synthase, and acyl-CoA-cholesterol acyltransferase [49].

In addition, indole glucosinolates reduce apolipoprotein B secretion as a primary apolipoprotein of low-density lipoproteins [50]. Another mechanism in relation to the lipid-lowering effect of broccoli sprouts may be associated with SFN's capacity to induce the Nrf2 pathway. Nrf2 activation directly targets lipogenic gene expression such as PPARγ and subsequently modulates hepatic lipid homeostasis [51].

Interestingly recent studies suggest that activation of PPARγ may decrease atherosclerosis progression and increase insulin sensitivity, mechanism which are considered as potential therapeutic targets for the treatment of Type 2 diabetes and lipid disorders [52].

Effects of SFN on Prevention of Diabetic Nephropathy

Another important long-term complication of diabetes is nephropathy which mainly occurs due to hyperglycemia-induced oxidative stress and activation of glycogen synthase kinase 3beta (GSK3β) [53, 54]. It has been suggested that activation of Nrf2-dependent antioxidant response signaling pathway may be a preventive strategy for development of diabetic nephropathy [55]. Shang et al. reported that 12 weeks SFN administration in a dose of 5 mg/kg/d body weight prevented the increase in urine albumin excretion, matrix expansion, transforming growth factor-β1 expression, fibronectin and type IV collagen deposition in the experimental diabetic kidney; moreover, SFN-treated diabetic rats had a lower level of 8-oxo-deoxyguanosine, with a significant reduction GSK-3β/Fyn and Nrf2 signaling activity. Such findings suggeste that SFN could ameliorate experimental diabetic nephropathy [56]. Cui et al. recently showed that treatment of diabetic mouse model with 0.5 mg/kg body weight SFN for 3 months attenuated diabetes-increased albumin to creatinine ratio, prevented diabetes-induced renal fibrosis, inflammation, oxidative stress and protected diabetic nephropathy via up-regulation of renal Nrf2-dependent genes [57].

To date, there are no reported studies examining the effect of broccoli sprouts or sulforaphane in human diabetic nephropathy.

Effects of Broccoli Sprouts and SFN on Vascular Function

Increased oxidative stress and inflammatory processes in line with decreased endothelium-derived nitric oxide, over production of AGEs and increased plasma free fatty acids are main cause of endothelial damage and consequently micro and macro vascular complications in diabetic patients [58, 59]. Evans [60] in a recent review paper, discussed that a plasma concentration of SFN achieved by regular consumption of Brassica vegetables could affect the physiology of vascular and inflammatory cells; due to these capacities current data suggest that SFN may prevent cardiovascular disease. SFN inhibits inflammation-induced vascular endothelial damage via modulation of inflammatory signaling pathways including p38 mitogen-activated protein kinases and c-Jun N-terminal kinases [61]. Activation of Nrf2 and its target genes and suppression of vascular cell adhesion protein-1 (VCAM-1) are other protective effects of SFN on vascular endothelium [33, 62].

Moreover, SFN can attenuate hyperglycemia-induced endothelial damage via inhibition of mitochondrial ROS production and inactivation of the hexosamine and PKC pathways and protein glycation [63].

In an *in vitro* study, Li et al. showed that SFN protected the lysophosphatidylcholine-induced injury of vascular endothelial cell by enhanced endogenous antioxdant system mediated by Nrf2 activation [64]. In this study, incubation of EA.hy.926 cells with 0.5, 1.25, 2.5 µmol L(-1) SFN for 24 h in the presence of lysophosphatidylcholine, could restore superoxide dismutase (SOD) activity by 58%, 64%, and 123%, respectively; moreover, SFN restored and up-regulated the expressions of glutathione S-transferase, glutathione peroxidase and thioredoxin reductase both in a dose- and time-dependent mannaer [64].

In another *in vitro* model, Yoo et al. [65] investigated the inhibitory effects of SFN on vascular smooth muscle cell (VSMC) proliferation and neointimal formation in a rat carotid artery injury model. SFN at doses of 0.5, 1.0, and 2.0 µM significantly inhibited platelet-derived growth factor (PDGF)-BB-induced VSMC proliferation and also inhibited neointimal formation as measured by angiographic mean luminary diameters.

It is relevent to mention that VSMC proliferation and intimal thickening arterial walls have determinant roles in the development of vascular diseases such as atherosclerosis and restenosis artery angioplasty [66].

Kwon et al. [67], also reported that SFN inhibited the protein expression of vascular cell adhesion molecule 1 (VCAM-1) induced by tumor necrosis factor (TNF-α) in VSMCs; moreover, SFN exhibited a regulatory effect on migration and proliferation in VSMCs. Such observations confirm the hypothesis that SFN may be a potential therapeutic agent for preventing vascular abnormalities however there are insufficient data to confirm these effects in human.

In a clinical trial on human hypertensive subjects, 4-week administration of 10 g/d dried broccoli sprouts increased overall flow mediated dilation (FMD) (from 4% to 5.8% compared to 4% at baseline and 3.9% in control) as a measure of endothelial function; similarly, significant changes in blood pressure were not detected between or within groups [47].

Anti-Bactericidal Properties of Broccoli Sprouts and SFN against *H. Pylori* Infection

Recent studies report a bilateral relation between *H. pylori* infection and Type 2 diabetes; besides an increased susceptibility of diabetic patients to *H. pylori* infection, this infection is proposed to be a major contributing factor of developing insulin resistance and Type 2 diabetes [68].

H. pylori infection in diabetic patients can interfere with glycemic control, resulting in higher levels of glycosylated hemoglobin (HbA1c), increased inflammation and insulin resistance and development of long-term diabetes complications [69, 70]; hence, eradication of the infection in diabetic patients may improve glycemic control and prevent diabetes complications. *In vitro* and *in vivo* models showed that broccoli sprouts and SFN are able to reduce the *H. pylori* infection and improve *H. pylori*-induced oxidative stress and inflammation [71, 72].

In human epithelial cell lines, SFN exhibited a high inhibitory activity (minimal inhibitory concentration for 90% of the strains was ≤4 µg/ml) against *H. pylori* strains and more interestingly, SFN inhibited both clarithromycin- and metronidazol-resistant strains [10]. Administration of SFN-rich broccoli sprouts (~3 µmol/d SFN) to *H. pylori*-infected mice successfully reduced gastric bacterial colonization, attenuated mucosal gene expression of inflammatory markers including TNF-α and interleukin-1β, inhibited gastric atrophy and oxidative damage, and also mitigated corpus inflammation [72].

Fahey et al. [73] reported that SFN could inactivate urease, a major factor which allows the bacteria to survive in an acidic gastric environment, and contributes to pathologies induced by *H. pylori*. Haristoy et al. [74], in an *in vivo* study conducted using human gastric xenograft, showed that short-term administration of SFN (at a dose of 1.33 mg/d/xenograft, i.e., ~ 100 mg/d in the human diet) provided an eradication rate by 73%.

In a randomized clinical trial [75], conducted on Type 2 diabetic patients with positive *H. pylori* stool antigen test (HpSAg), the patients received one of the following treatment including standard triple therapy (omeprazole 20 mg, clarithromycin 500 mg, amoxicillin 1000 mg, twice a day for 14 days), broccoli sprouts powder (6 g/d for 28 days ~ 135 µmol/d SFN), or combination of standard therapy + broccoli sprouts.

The findings showed that the *H. pylori* eradication rates, assessed by urea breath test (UBT) and HpSAg, were 85.3% and 89.3% in standard triple therapy, 36.0% and 56.0% in broccoli treated, and 83.3% and 91.7% in combination treated groups, respectively.

There were no significant differences in serum pepsinogen I, pepsinogen II and pepsinogen I/pepsinogen II ratio, as an accurate surogate of gastric inflammation, and glucose homeostasis parameters between the three groups [75].

CONCLUSION

Type 2 diabetes, as a complicated metabolic disorder is also accompanied by other pathogenic conditions such as sub-clinical inflammation and oxidative stress that subsequently intensifies the insulin resistance and long-term diabetes complications. Considering current knowledge from *in vitro* and animal models as well as some human clinical trials, broccoli sprouts, a main source of bioactive components, especially SFN, may be an effective supplementary treatment for management of Type 2 diabetes and prevention of its long-term complications. Further studies with longer durations and various doses may shed more light on the importance of the therapeutic effects of broccoli sprout powder in Type 2 diabetic patients.

REFERENCES

[1] Moreno, D. A., Carvajal, M., Lopez-Berenguer, C., Garcia-Viguera, C. Chemical and biological characterisation of nutraceutical compounds of broccoli. *J. Pharm. Biomed. Anal.* 2006; 41: 1508-22.

[2] Pérez-Balibrea, S., Moreno, D. A., García-Viguera, C. Influence of light on health-promoting phytochemicals of broccoli sprouts. *Journal of the Science of Food and Agriculture* 2008; 88: 904-10.

[3] Keum, Y. S., Jeong, W. S., Kong, A. N. Chemoprevention by isothiocyanates and their underlying molecular signaling mechanisms. *Mutat. Res.* 2004; 555: 191-202.

[4] Xue, M., Qian, Q., Adaikalakoteswari, A., Rabbani, N., Babaei-Jadidi, R., Thornalley, P. J. Activation of NF-E2-related factor-2 reverses biochemical dysfunction of endothelial cells induced by hyperglycemia linked to vascular disease. *Diabetes* 2008; 57: 2809-17.

[5] Zhu, H., Jia, Z., Strobl, J. S., Ehrich, M., Misra, H. P., Li, Y. Potent induction of total cellular and mitochondrial antioxidants and phase 2 enzymes by cruciferous sulforaphane in rat aortic smooth muscle cells: cytoprotection against oxidative and electrophilic stress. *Cardiovasc. Toxicol.* 2008; 8: 115-25.

[6] Zhou, C., Poulton, E. J., Grun, F. et al. The dietary isothiocyanate sulforaphane is an antagonist of the human steroid and xenobiotic nuclear receptor. *Mol. Pharmacol.* 2007; 71: 220-9.

[7] Heiss, E., Herhaus, C., Klimo, K., Bartsch, H., Gerhäuser, C. Nuclear Factor κB Is a Molecular Target for Sulforaphane-mediated Anti-inflammatory Mechanisms. *Journal of Biological Chemistry* 2001; 276: 32008-15.

[8] Durham, A., Jazrawi, E., Rhodes, J. A. et al. The anti-inflammatory effects of sulforaphane are not mediated by the Nrf2 pathway. *European Respiratory Journal* 2014; 44.

[9] Mukherjee, S., Gangopadhyay, H., Das, D. K. Broccoli: a unique vegetable that protects mammalian hearts through the redox cycling of the thioredoxin superfamily. *J. Agric. Food Chem.* 2008; 56: 609-17.

[10] Fahey, J. W., Haristoy, X., Dolan, P. M. et al. Sulforaphane inhibits extracellular, intracellular, and antibiotic-resistant strains of Helicobacter pylori and prevents benzo[a]pyrene-induced stomach tumors. *Proc. Natl. Acad. Sci. US* 2002; 99: 7610-5.

[11] Han, J. M., Lee, Y. J., Lee, S. Y. et al. Protective effect of sulforaphane against dopaminergic cell death. *J. Pharmacol. Exp. Ther.* 2007; 321: 249-56.

[12] Thejass, P., Kuttan, G. Augmentation of natural killer cell and antibody-dependent cellular cytotoxicity in BALB/c mice by sulforaphane, a naturally occurring isothiocyanate from broccoli through enhanced production of cytokines IL-2 and IFN-gamma. *Immunopharmacol. Immunotoxicol.* 2006; 28: 443-57.

[13] Choi, K. M., Lee, Y. S., Kim, W. et al. Sulforaphane attenuates obesity by inhibiting adipogenesis and activating the AMPK pathway in obese mice. *J. Nutr. Biochem.* 2014; 25: 201-7.

[14] Zhao, H.-D., Zhang, F., Shen, G. et al. Sulforaphane protects liver injury induced by intestinal ischemia reperfusion through Nrf2-ARE pathway. *World journal of gastroenterology: WJG* 2010; 16: 3002.

[15] Zahra Bahadoran, P. M., Hanieh-Sadat Ejtahed, Mahshid Abd-Mishani, Fatemeh Bagheri pour, Maryam Tohidi, Fereidoun Azizi. Protective effects of broccoli sprout powder against fructose-induced metabolic and liver disorders in rats. *International Journal for Vitamin and Nutrition Research* 2015.

[16] Bahadoran, Z., Mirmiran, P., Azizi, F. Potential efficacy of broccoli sprouts as a unique supplement for management of Type 2 diabetes and its complications. *J. Med. Food* 2013; 16: 375-82.

[17] Opara, E. C. Oxidative stress, micronutrients, diabetes mellitus and its complications. *J. R. Soc. Promot. Health* 2002; 122: 28-34.

[18] Opara, E. C., Abdel-Rahman, E., Soliman, S. et al. Depletion of total antioxidant capacity in Type 2 diabetes. *Metabolism* 1999; 48: 1414-7.

[19] Perez-Matute, P., Zulet, M. A., Martinez, J. A. Reactive species and diabetes: counteracting oxidative stress to improve health. *Curr. Opin. Pharmacol.* 2009; 9: 771-9.

[20] Maritim, A. C., Sanders, R. A., Watkins, J. B., 3rd. Diabetes, oxidative stress, and antioxidants: a review. *J. Biochem. Mol. Toxicol.* 2003; 17: 24-38.

[21] Boddupalli, S., Mein, J. R., Lakkanna, S., James, D. R. Induction of phase 2 antioxidant enzymes by broccoli sulforaphane: perspectives in maintaining the antioxidant activity of vitamins a, C, and e. *Front. Genet.* 2012; 3: 7.

[22] Kaspar, J. W., Niture, S. K., Jaiswal, A. K. Nrf2:INrf2 (Keap1) signaling in oxidative stress. *Free Radic. Biol. Med.* 2009; 47: 1304-9.

[23] Hybertson, B. M., Gao, B., Bose, S. K., McCord, J. M. Oxidative stress in health and disease: the therapeutic potential of Nrf2 activation. *Mol. Aspects Med.* 2011; 32: 234-46.

[24] Cho, E. J., Lee, Y. A., Yoo, H. H., Yokozawa, T. Protective effects of broccoli (Brassica oleracea) against oxidative damage in vitro and in vivo. *J. Nutr. Sci. Vitaminol.* (Tokyo) 2006; 52: 437-44.

[25] Wu, L., Noyan Ashraf, M. H., Facci, M. et al. Dietary approach to attenuate oxidative stress, hypertension, and inflammation in the cardiovascular system. *Proc. Natl. Acad. Sci. US* 2004; 101: 7094-9.

[26] Riedl, M. A., Saxon, A., Diaz-Sanchez, D. Oral sulforaphane increases Phase II antioxidant enzymes in the human upper airway. *Clin. Immunol.* 2009; 130: 244-51.

[27] Bahadoran, Z., Mirmiran, P., Hosseinpanah, F., Hedayati, M., Hosseinpour-Niazi, S., Azizi, F. Broccoli sprouts reduce oxidative stress in Type 2 diabetes: a randomized double-blind clinical trial. *Eur. J. Clin. Nutr.* 2011; 65: 972-7.

[28] Murashima, M., Watanabe, S., Zhuo, X. G., Uehara, M., Kurashige, A. Phase 1 study of multiple biomarkers for metabolism and oxidative stress after one-week intake of broccoli sprouts. *Biofactors* 2004; 22: 271-5.

[29] Goldberg, R. B. Cytokine and cytokine-like inflammation markers, endothelial dysfunction, and imbalanced coagulation in development of diabetes and its complications. *J. Clin. Endocrinol. Metab.* 2009; 94: 3171-82.

[30] Sjoholm, A., Nystrom, T. Inflammation and the etiology of Type 2 diabetes. *Diabetes Metab. Res. Rev.* 2006; 22: 4-10.

[31] Ceriello, A., Testa, R. Antioxidant anti-inflammatory treatment in Type 2 diabetes. *Diabetes Care* 2009; 32 Suppl. 2: S232-6.

[32] Ritz, S. A., Wan, J., Diaz-Sanchez, D. Sulforaphane-stimulated phase II enzyme induction inhibits cytokine production by airway epithelial cells stimulated with diesel extract. *Am. J. Physiol. Lung Cell. Mol. Physiol.* 2007; 292: L33-9.

[33] Shan, Y., Zhao, R., Geng, W. et al. Protective effect of sulforaphane on human vascular endothelial cells against lipopolysaccharide-induced inflammatory damage. *Cardiovasc. Toxicol.* 2010; 10: 139-45.

[34] Lin, W., Wu, R. T., Wu, T., Khor, T. O., Wang, H., Kong, A. N. Sulforaphane suppressed LPS-induced inflammation in mouse peritoneal macrophages through Nrf2 dependent pathway. *Biochem. Pharmacol.* 2008; 76: 967-73.

[35] Nallasamy, P., Si, H., Babu, P. V. et al. Sulforaphane reduces vascular inflammation in mice and prevents TNF-alpha-induced monocyte adhesion to primary endothelial cells through interfering with the NF-kappaB pathway. *J. Nutr. Biochem.* 2014; 25: 824-33.

[36] Greaney, A. J., Maier, N. K., Leppla, S. H., Moayeri, M. Sulforaphane inhibits multiple inflammasomes through an Nrf2-independent mechanism. *J. Leukoc. Biol.* 2015.

[37] Medina, S., Dominguez-Perles, R., Moreno, D. A. et al. The intake of broccoli sprouts modulates the inflammatory and vascular prostanoids but not the oxidative stress-related isoprostanes in healthy humans. *Food Chem.* 2015; 173: 1187-94.

[38] Mirmiran, P., Bahadoran, Z., Hosseinpanah, F., Keyzad, A., Azizi, F. Effects of broccoli sprout with high sulforaphane concentration on inflammatory markers in Type 2 diabetic patients: A randomized double-blind placebo-controlled clinical trial. *Journal of Functional Foods* 2012; 4: 837-41.

[39] Henriksen, E. J., Diamond-Stanic, M. K., Marchionne, E. M. Oxidative stress and the etiology of insulin resistance and Type 2 diabetes. *Free Radic. Biol. Med.* 2011; 51: 993-9.

[40] Evans, J. L. Antioxidants: do they have a role in the treatment of insulin resistance? *Indian J. Med. Res.* 2007; 125: 355-72.

[41] Fu, J., Zhang, Q., Woods, C. G. et al. Divergent effects of sulforaphane on basal and glucose-stimulated insulin secretion in beta-cells: role of reactive oxygen species and induction of endogenous antioxidants. *Pharm. Res.* 2013; 30: 2248-59.

[42] Bahadoran, Z., Tohidi, M., Nazeri, P., Mehran, M., Azizi, F., Mirmiran, P. Effect of broccoli sprouts on insulin resistance in Type 2 diabetic patients: a randomized double-blind clinical trial. *Int. J. Food Sci. Nutr.* 2012; 63: 767-71.

[43] Patel, S., Santani, D. Role of NF-kappa B in the pathogenesis of diabetes and its associated complications. *Pharmacol. Rep.* 2009; 61: 595-603.

[44] Haluzik, M. M., Haluzik, M. PPAR-alpha and insulin sensitivity. *Physiol. Res.* 2006; 55: 115-22.

[45] Lee, J.-J., Shin, H.-D., Lee, Y.-M., Kim, A.-R., Lee, M.-Y. Effect of broccoli sprouts on cholesterol-lowering and anti-obesity effects in rats fed high fat diet. *Journal of the Korean Society of Food Science and Nutrition* 2009; 38: 309-18.

[46] Bahadoran, Z., Mirmiran, P., Hosseinpanah, F., Rajab, A., Asghari, G., Azizi, F. Broccoli sprouts powder could improve serum triglyceride and oxidized LDL/LDL-cholesterol ratio in Type 2 diabetic patients: a randomized double-blind placebo-controlled clinical trial. *Diabetes Res. Clin. Pract.* 2012; 96: 348-54.

[47] Christiansen, B., Bellostas Muguerza, N., Petersen, A. M. et al. Ingestion of broccoli sprouts does not improve endothelial function in humans with hypertension. *PLoS One* 2010; 5: e12461.

[48] Kahlon, T., Chapman, M., Smith, G. In vitro binding of bile acids by spinach, kale, brussels sprouts, broccoli, mustard greens, green bell pepper, cabbage and collards. *Food Chemistry* 2007; 100: 1531-6.

[49] Dunn, S. E., LeBlanc, G. A. Hypocholesterolemic properties of plant indoles: inhibition of acyl-coa: cholesterol acyltransferase activity and reduction of serum LDL/VLDL cholesterol levels by glucobrassicin derivatives. *Biochemical pharmacology* 1994; 47: 359-64.

[50] Maiyoh, G. K., Kuh, J. E., Casaschi, A., Theriault, A. G. Cruciferous indole-3-carbinol inhibits apolipoprotein B secretion in HepG2 cells. *J. Nutr.* 2007; 137: 2185-9.

[51] Huang, J., Tabbi-Anneni, I., Gunda, V., Wang, L. Transcription factor Nrf2 regulates SHP and lipogenic gene expression in hepatic lipid metabolism. *Am. J. Physiol. Gastrointest. Liver Physiol.* 2010; 299: G1211-21.

[52] Tavares, V., Hirata, M. H., Hirata, R. D. [Peroxisome proliferator-activated receptor gamma (PPARgamma): molecular study in glucose homeostasis, lipid metabolism and therapeutic approach]. *Arq. Bras. Endocrinol. Metabol.* 2007; 51: 526-33.

[53] Valk, E. J., Bruijn, J. A., Bajema, I. M. Diabetic nephropathy in humans: pathologic diversity. *Curr. Opin. Nephrol. Hypertens.* 2011; 20: 285-9.

[54] Kashihara, N., Haruna, Y., Kondeti, V. K., Kanwar, Y. S. Oxidative stress in diabetic nephropathy. *Curr. Med. Chem.* 2010; 17: 4256-69.

[55] Li, B. Y., Cheng, M., Gao, H. Q. et al. Back-regulation of six oxidative stress proteins with grape seed proanthocyanidin extracts in rat diabetic nephropathy. *J. Cell. Biochem.* 2008; 104: 668-79.

[56] Shang, G., Tang, X., Gao, P. et al. Sulforaphane attenuation of experimental diabetic nephropathy involves GSK-3 beta/Fyn/Nrf2 signaling pathway. *J. Nutr. Biochem.* 2015; 26: 596-606.

[57] Cui, W., Bai, Y., Miao, X. et al. Prevention of diabetic nephropathy by sulforaphane: possible role of Nrf2 upregulation and activation. *Oxid. Med. Cell. Longev.* 2012; 2012: 821936.

[58] Creager, M. A., Luscher, T. F., Cosentino, F., Beckman, J. A. Diabetes and vascular disease: pathophysiology, clinical consequences, and medical therapy: Part I. *Circulation* 2003; 108: 1527-32.

[59] Endemann, D. H., Schiffrin, E. L. Nitric oxide, oxidative excess, and vascular complications of diabetes mellitus. *Curr. Hypertens. Rep.* 2004; 6: 85-9.

[60] Evans, P. C. The influence of sulforaphane on vascular health and its relevance to nutritional approaches to prevent cardiovascular disease. *EPMA J.* 2011; 2: 9-14.

[61] Zakkar, M., Van der Heiden, K., Luong le, A. et al. Activation of Nrf2 in endothelial cells protects arteries from exhibiting a proinflammatory state. *Arterioscler. Thromb. Vasc. Biol.* 2009; 29: 1851-7.

[62] Miao, X., Bai, Y., Sun, W. et al. Sulforaphane prevention of diabetes-induced aortic damage was associated with the up-regulation of Nrf2 and its down-stream antioxidants. *Nutr. Metab.* (Lond.) 2012; 9: 84.

[63] Ha, H., Kim, K. H. Pathogenesis of diabetic nephropathy: the role of oxidative stress and protein kinase C. *Diabetes Res. Clin. Pract.* 1999; 45: 147-51.

[64] Li, B., Tian, S., Liu, X., He, C., Ding, Z., Shan, Y. Sulforaphane protected the injury of human vascular endothelial cell induced by LPC through up-regulating endogenous antioxidants and phase II enzymes. *Food Funct.* 2015; 6: 1984-91.

[65] Yoo, S. H., Lim, Y., Kim, S. J. et al. Sulforaphane inhibits PDGF-induced proliferation of rat aortic vascular smooth muscle cell by up-regulation of p53 leading to G1/S cell cycle arrest. *Vascul. Pharmacol.* 2013; 59: 44-51.

[66] Louis, S. F., Zahradka, P. Vascular smooth muscle cell motility: From migration to invasion. *Exp. Clin. Cardiol.* 2010; 15: e75-85.

[67] Kwon, J. S., Joung, H., Kim, Y. S. et al. Sulforaphane inhibits restenosis by suppressing inflammation and the proliferation of vascular smooth muscle cells. *Atherosclerosis* 2012; 225: 41-9.

[68] Zhou, X., Zhang, C., Wu, J., Zhang, G. Association between Helicobacter pylori infection and diabetes mellitus: a meta-analysis of observational studies. *Diabetes Res. Clin. Pract.* 2013; 99: 200-8.

[69] Demir, M., Gokturk, H. S., Ozturk, N. A., Kulaksizoglu, M., Serin, E., Yilmaz, U. Helicobacter pylori prevalence in diabetes mellitus patients with dyspeptic symptoms and its relationship to glycemic control and late complications. *Dig. Dis. Sci.* 2008; 53: 2646-9.

[70] Hamed, S. A., Amine, N. F., Galal, G. M. et al. Vascular risks and complications in diabetes mellitus: the role of helicobacter pylori infection. *J. Stroke Cerebrovasc. Dis.* 2008; 17: 86-94.

[71] Galan, M. V., Kishan, A. A., Silverman, A. L. Oral broccoli sprouts for the treatment of Helicobacter pylori infection: a preliminary report. *Dig. Dis. Sci.* 2004; 49: 1088-90.

[72] Yanaka, A., Fahey, J. W., Fukumoto, A. et al. Dietary sulforaphane-rich broccoli sprouts reduce colonization and attenuate gastritis in Helicobacter pylori-infected mice and humans. *Cancer Prev. Res.* (Phila.) 2009; 2: 353-60.

[73] Fahey, J. W., Stephenson, K. K., Wade, K. L., Talalay, P. Urease from Helicobacter pylori is inactivated by sulforaphane and other isothiocyanates. *Biochemical and biophysical research communications* 2013; 435: 1-7.

[74] Haristoy, X., Angioi-Duprez, K., Duprez, A., Lozniewski, A. Efficacy of sulforaphane in eradicating Helicobacter pylori in human gastric xenografts implanted in nude mice. *Antimicrobial agents and chemotherapy* 2003; 47: 3982-4.

[75] Bahadoran, Z., Mirmiran, P., Yeganeh, M. Z., Hosseinpanah, F., Zojaji, H., Azizi, F. Complementary and alternative medicinal effects of broccoli sprouts powder on Helicobacter pylori eradication rate in Type 2 diabetic patients: A randomized clinical trial. *Journal of Functional Foods* 2014; 7: 390-7.

In: Broccoli
Editor: Bernhard H. J. Juurlink

ISBN: 978-1-63484-313-3
© 2016 Nova Science Publishers, Inc.

Chapter 13

HUMAN CLINICAL STUDIES INVOLVING SULFORAPHANE/GLUCORAPHANIN

Bernhard H. J. Juurlink[*]
Department of Anatomy & Cell Biology, University of Saskatchewan,
Saskatoon, SK, Canada

ABSTRACT

Sulforaphane, the metabolite of glucoraphanin, activates the Nrf2 signalling system. Activation of the Nrf2 signalling system has been shown to positively affect a variety of disturbances in homeostasis, including disturbances in redox, in intermediary metabolism and mitochondrial function as well as disturbances in lipid metabolism. Such disturbances are present in many human diseases suggesting sulforaphane may have therapeutic effects. A number of studies of the effects of sulforaphane and/or glucoraphanin have been carried out in humans. This is a review of such studies to date. Studies reviewed include human pharmacological studies; effects on *Helicobacter pylori* infections; responses to allergens; effect on neurological disorders such as autism spectrum disorder and schizophrenia; effect on the cardiovascular disorders; and effect on prostate cancer.

Keywords: allergy, asthma, autism, clinical trial, glucoraphanin, peptic ulcers, pharmacokinetics, schizophrenia, sulforaphane

INTRODUCTION

Well over two thousand years ago Hippocrates stated "let food be your medicine and medicine your food," however, it is only recently that we have begun to understand how phytochemicals may influence cellular signalling pathways and, thereby, gene expression and health. This area of research has been called nutrigenomics and there has developed a great

---
[*] Corresponding author: Email: bernhard.juurlink@usask.ca.

interest in how such nutrigenomic knowledge may be used to positively influence health. Nutrigenomics along with proteomic and metabolomics technologies has initiated the third era of nutritional research where we are beginning to understand how certain molecules (mainly phytochemicals) we consume affect cell signalling and thereby gene expression [1]: the first era being devoted to understanding the roles of carbohydrates, lipids and proteins in nutrition with the second era being devoted to understanding the roles of metals and vitamins. A major driving force in the development of the third era of nutritional studies is the Talalay laboratory with their studies on how nutritional factors influence the probability of developing a variety of cancers, their honing in onto phase 2 enzyme inducers and subsequently onto other Nrf2 activators (see Chapter 1). The research of the Talalay lab was inspired by the research of Lee W. Wattenberg who spent decades examining how certain food constituents decreased the probability of developing cancer. It was the Watternberg lab that identified that induction of phase 2 enzymes is a major anti-cancer mechanism [2]. Dr Talalay and colleagues have also been the major driving force in translating basic nutrigenomic research into human medicine. Chapter 12 outlines the human clinical studies in the context of Type 2 diabetes. Below is a brief outline of other studies that have been carried out in humans by the Talalay laboratory as well as other laboratories on diets enriched in sulforaphane or glucoraphanin (sulforaphane glucosinolate).

HUMAN CLINICAL STUDIES

Pharmacological Studies

Glucosinolates are converted to isothiocyanates by enzymatic reaction, either by endogenous myrosinase (thioglucosidase) activity present within the crucifers or by enzymatic actions of gut flora [3]. Myrosinase is stored in a different cellular compartment than glucosinolates. One requires physical disruption of plant cells to allow myrosinase to access the glucosinolates. A number of studies have examined the effect of cooking, which destroys endogenous myrosinase activity, on the conversion of glucosinolates to isothiocyanates and subsequent uptake of the isothiocyanates. The conclusion of these studies is that the most effective means of delivering isothiocyanates such as sulforaphane to our tissues is to convert the glucosinolates to isothiocyanates in our oral cavities allowing effective exposure of the glucosinolates to myrosinase actions: this is 3-4 times more effective than relying upon gut bacterial enzymatic activities [4-6]. Exposure of glucosinolates to myrosinase action can occur, for example, by chewing the cruciferous vegetable. Once glucosinolates are hydrolyzed into the isothiocyanates they are rapidly absorbed with plasma levels peaking at 1 hr following ingestion, with a plasma half-life of 1.8 hr [7] to 2.5 hr [8] and with 60% excreted in the urine within 8 hours [7].

In a study on the safety of consuming high doses of Nrf2-activating isothiocyanates, human subjects were fed broccoli sprouts containing up to 100 μmol sulforaphane-equivalents plus a myrosinase source every eight hr for seven days and routine blood and urine analyses were performed as well as thyroid and liver function tests [9]. The conclusion of this study was: "No significant or consistent subjective or objective abnormal events (toxicities) associated with any of the sprout extract ingestions were observed."

The anti-carcinogen properties of isothiocyanates such as sulforaphane has been attributed to their being monofunctional inducers of phase 2 proteins and having inhibitory effects on the activities of phase 1 enzymes such as cytochrome P450 2E1 (CYP2E1) [10, 11]. Broccoli, however, contains a variety of phytochemicals including flavonoids such as quercetin and kaempferol (see Chapter 7) and, thus, these may influence the activities of specific cytochrome P450 enzymes. It is known that both quercetin and kaempferol are ligands for the aryl hydrocarbon receptor [12] - see Chapter 4 for a discussion on the aryl hydrocarbon receptor. Kali and colleagues have shown that consuming 500 g broccoli/day induces CYP1A2 and CYP2E1 [13]. Another study by Hakooz and Hamdan has shown that broccoli consumption increases the activities not only of CYP1A2 but also CYP2A6 [14].

Effect of Sulforaphane on Helicobacter Infections

In the mid 1980s a series of papers by Barry Marshall and colleagues set out the evidence that the majority of peptic ulcers were due to an infection by *Helicobacter (Campylobacter) pylori* [15-18]. Since that time the majority of patients with peptic ulcers have been cured through antibiotic treatment; however, a significant fraction of patients with peptic ulcers have antibiotic-resistant strains of *H. pylori* resulting in the presence of persistent peptic ulcers. *H. pylori* infection can result in ulceration of stomach mucosa in the short term and lead to the development of gastric cancer in the long term [19].

Based on some anecdotal evidence that consumption of broccoli sprouts ameliorated persistent peptic ulcers, *in vitro* studies were initiated on the effects of sulforaphane on *H. pylori* [20]. This research demonstrated that sulforaphane had a median minimal bacteriostatic effect on several strains of *H. pylori* at ~10 µM, including antibiotic-resistant strains, with a maximal bacteriocidal effect at 50 to 100 µM, depending upon strain. The bacteriocidal effect was seen for both extracellular and intracellular *H. pylori*. Although these are high concentrations, they can be achieved at the level of the stomach and duodenum through dietary intake. The *in vitro* studies were soon followed by a small clinical study where 9 patients with peptic ulcers were given broccoli sprouts in three dosages (containing 318 to 1271 µmoles glucosinolates) for each of seven days [21]. The outcomes held promise in that one-out-of-three patients in each dosage group became negative for *H. pylori*. The authors suggested that a larger group of patients be tested with broccoli consumption being extended beyond seven days.

A more recent publication demonstrated that consumption of an homogenate of broccoli sprouts high in sulforaphane (3 µmoles sulforaphane equivalent/day) attenuated mucosal infection by *H. pylori* in wild-type mice but not in Nrf2 knockout mice [22]. This suggests that a significant therapeutic effect is mediated via upregulation of the ability to cope with oxidative stress and not just via the bacteriostatic/bacteriocidal effects of sulforaphane. This same study also demonstrated that humans consuming broccoli sprouts containing 420 micromoles equivalent of sulforaphane glucosinolate daily for a period of 8 weeks decreased but did not eliminate *H. pylori* infections in humans. Thus, there is sufficient preliminary clinical evidence to warrant further larger clinical trials to determine the efficacy of consumption of broccoli high in sulforaphane glucosinolate in treating *H. pylori* infections. A very nice review on diet and *H. pylori* infections can be found in Fahey and colleagues [23].

Effect of Sulforaphane on Lipid Metabolism

Both genetic knockdown and Nrf2 activation studies in mice have shown that Nrf2 activation downregulates sterol regulatory element binding protein-1 and expression of associated genes whose protein products are involved in lipid synthesis while upregulating fatty acid oxidation [24] (see also Chapter 6). Sulforaphane also promotes lipolysis via hormone-sensitive lipase activity [25]. Further animal experiments have shown that Nrf2 promotes availability of mitochondrial substrates for oxidative phosphorylation [26]. It has been suggested that promotion of mitochondrial function by Nrf2 activation is mediated by better redox states ensuring decreased probability of oxidation of critical cysteine residues [27]. My laboratory has shown, in a dietary trial in mice examining the effects of an Nrf2 activator, that mice consuming tertiary butyl hydroxyanisole were more physically agile and gained far less weight as they aged (up to 18 months of age) than mice on control diet even though there were no differences in total food consumption in the two groups of mice [28]. These mice also had an increase of 30% in their lifespan (see Figure 9, Chapter 5). Thus, the animal experimental data suggest that human clinical trials on the effect of Nrf2 activators on lipid metabolism are warranted.

Murashima and colleagues [29] carried out a small phase 1 human clinical trial (6 male and 6 female) where they examined the effects of consumption of 100 g of fresh broccoli sprouts on a number of blood parameters. This study showed a significant decrease in total cholesterol and LDL-cholesterol in males and a significant increase in HDL-cholesterol in females. Furthermore, there was a decrease in a variety of plasma oxidative stress parameters, including decreases in phosphatidylcholine hydroperoxide, reduced levels of 8-isoprostane, reduced levels of 8-hydroxydeoxyguanosine and an increase in the ratio of reduced coenzyme Q10 relative to the oxidized form.

Significant decreases in total triglycerides and atherogenic index was seen in Type 2 diabetic patients following four weeks of consuming 10 g of a commercial broccoli sprout powder containing 225 µmoles of sulforaphane isothiocyanate equivalent with no significant effects seen with a dose of 112 µmoles sulforaphane equivalents [30].

Armah and colleagues [31] conducted a 12 week-long double-blinded two-arm parallel study where human subjects at mild to moderate risk of cardiovascular disease consumed either 400 g of high-glucoraphanin broccoli/week (45 subjects) or 400 g of standard broccoli/week (48 subjects). The broccoli was supplied frozen and steamed prior to consumption. This study found that the high-glucoraphanin broccoli significantly lowered plasma LDL-cholesterol but had no effect on total cholesterol nor on triglycerides. A previous small clinical trial by this group reported that high-glucoraphanin broccoli had a pronounced effect on normalizing β-oxidation of fatty acids by mitochondria in a population containing a variant of the PAPOLG (Poly[A] Polymerase Gamma) gene [32]. How PAPOLG protein product affects metabolism is currently not known. The fact that consuming Nrf2 activators normalizes fatty acid metabolism in a subset of people carrying the gene variant of PAPOLG is congruent with our own experiments in rats that indicate that consuming high-glucoraphanin broccoli sprouts tends to normalize many physiological parameters when these are abnormal prior to feeding but has little effect on normal physiology rats [33].

Effect of Sulforaphane on Responses to Air-Borne Components

A dose response study in humans showed that consumption of increasing amounts of sulforaphane delivered via a high-glucoraphanin broccoli sprout homogenate resulted in induction of phase 2 enzymes in nasal respiratory epithelial cells obtained through nasal lavage [34]. The subjects were dosed once daily for 3 days with the total amount of sulforaphane consumed varying from around 12.5 µmoles to about 100 µmoles - very large increases in phase 2 protein gene expression seen with the higher doses. Thus, sulforaphane intake allowed the epithelial cells to increase their anti-oxidant defenses. Since decreased oxidative stress decreases the likelihood of inflammatory responses (see 5) one might expect less inflammation of the respiratory epithelium under conditions that normally promote inflammatory responses.

Diesel exhaust particles are known to promote allergic inflammatory responses in the respiratory epithelium [35, 36], with asthmatics being more susceptible to such exhaust particles [37]. A small human study comprised of 29 participants who responded positively to cat allergens were tested for their inflammatory response to nasally-administered diesel exhaust particles before and after they consumed a broccoli sprout extract 4 times per day for 4 days in a row [38]. The extract contained 100 µmoles sulforaphane, thus, subjects consumed 400 µmoles sulforaphane/day. The inflammatory response examined was the increase in white blood cells at 6 and 24 hr following exposure as determined by a nasal lavage. Diesel particle exposure significantly increased white blood cell counts both at 6 and 24 hr under control conditions. Intake of sulforaphane abrogated this increase in white blood cells following exposure to diesel particles. This study also examined plasma sulforaphane and metabolites to ensure patients complied.

Another small human study (50 subjects) involved a cross-over pilot trial to examine the efficacy of sulforaphane/glucoraphanin to counter the effects of air pollution. The subjects consumed a broccoli extract containing 800 µmoles glucoraphanin daily for a period of 7 days [39]. The endpoint being examined was the excretion of mercapturic acid metabolites of air pollutants such as benzene, a known carcinogen [39]. This was followed with a wash-out period of 5 days and then consumption for an additional 7 days of 150 µmoles of sulforaphane. The conclusion drawn from this research was that both 800 µmoles glucoraphanin intake daily as well as 150 µmoles sulforaphane increased the excretion of mercapturic acid metabolites of benzene, acrolein, crotonaldehyde and ethylene oxide by 20-50%. A second larger (267 subjects) study by this group examined the effect of consuming 600 µmoles glucoraphanin plus 40 µmoles sulforaphane daily on the ability to detoxify air pollutants [40]. Subjects were randomly assigned to the control group who drank a placebo drink or to the experimental group who drank a fluid containing glucoraphanin and sulforaphane. Control and experimental drinks were consumed daily for a 12-week period. Overnight urine samples were collected before and after the 12-week period in both control and experimental subjects. This study demonstrated a significantly increased excretion of mercapturic acid derivatives of benzene and acrolein in the experimental group.

These studies support the concept that sulforaphane intake decreases the probability of developing a variety of cancers due to environmental carcinogens.

Effects of Sulforaphane on Neurological Disorders

Sulforaphane administration has been shown to normalize a number of CNS functions in animal models of CNS disorders [41-43]. This is perhaps not too surprising since such CNS disorders often have an oxidative stress and mitochondrial dysfunction components to the disease processes. As mentioned elsewhere sulforaphane administration through activation of the Nrf2 signalling pathway will tend to normalize redox states and mitochondrial function (e.g., Chapter 6); hence, it is not too surprising that clinical trials have been initiated to examine the ability of sulforaphane to ameliorate CNS disorders.

Autism Spectrum Disorder

Autism spectrum disorder (ASD) is characterized by oxidative stress [44, 45] and mitochondrial dysfunction [45-47]. This is the rationale for conducting a double-blinded sulforaphane dietary clinical trial in 40 subjects diagnosed with autism as published recently [48].

In this clinical trial, 26 subjects consumed capsules containing sulforaphane (50 to 150 moles depending upon weight) and 14 subjects consumed the placebo capsule for either 4 weeks or 18 weeks. Subjects were initially assessed using the Ohio Autism Clinical Global Impression Severity Scale (CGI-I) to ensure that the placebo and experimental groups were well matched. The subjects were scored using the Adverse Behavioral Checklist (ABC) and the Social Responsiveness Scale (SRS) prior to the intervention as well as 4 weeks and 14 weeks following the intervention. Subjects consuming sulforaphane significantly improved in these care-giver assigned scores. Clinical staff were blinded to the treatment and scored subjects using the CGI-I scale. Analyses of these data showed that 40% of subjects who consumed sulforaphane were much or very much improved on the following functions: social interactions (46%), aberrant behaviours (54%) and verbal communication (42%). Placebo consuming subjects showed no improvement. Four weeks after treatment all subjects who were in the sulforphane treatment group reverted back to the original baseline.

This study has been criticized for an uncommon use of common outcome measures [49]. For a response to these criticisms see Talalay and Zimmerman [50]. It seems clear that more research is warranted to examine the effects of normalizing redox states on individuals diagnosed with the autism spectrum disorder. The subjects in the study by Singh et al. ranged in age from 13 to 27 with a median age of 17. It would be of interest to see if normalizing redox in early childhood would have a more pronounced positive outcome.

Schizophrenia

Schizophrenia is another neurological disorder where there is considerable evidence that there are disturbances in the redox states of cells and extracellular fluids [51]. For additional references please see Issue 7 of Volume 15 of the journal 'Antioxidants & Redox Signalling.' This was the rationale for a small open label clinical trial of 10 subjects with ages ranging from 20 to 65, with 3 subjects withdrawing before the completion of the trial. Subjects consumed 169 µmoles sulforaphane daily for a period of 8 weeks and were then tested for cognitive function using CogState battery of tests and evaluated for psychiatric symptoms using the Positive and Negative Syndrome Scale. Only one of the battery of tests in the CogState scale significantly improved (the one-card learning test) and no changes were seen in the Positive and Negative Syndrome Scale in this study. The caveat to this study is that it was a very small open label study and there may have been bias in the evaluators. Furthermore, the positive effect on the one CogState parameter may be a placebo effect since there was no placebo component to this trial.

Schizophrenia is associated with abnormal cytosine methylation patterns reflecting a change in the epigenetics and, thus, gene regulation. We have previously shown that DNA of the kidneys in hypertensive rats is aberrantly methylated and that normalizing the renal redox state through sulforaphane administration from weaning until adulthood normalizes the total DNA cytosine methylation state [52]. It may well be that an early intervention with sulforaphane in schizophrenics may result not only in normalization of tissue redox states but also normalization of the methyl epigenome, possibly resulting in better outcomes. The evidence for oxidative stress in schizophrenics warrants further studies examining the therapeutic effect of sulforaphane, especially in young people newly diagnosed with schizophrenia.

Effect of Sulforaphane Administration on the Cardiovascular System

A study on stroke-prone spontaneously hypertensive rats demonstrated that intake of 5.5 µmoles of sulforaphane-equivalents in the form of dried broccoli sprouts from weaning to adulthood resulted in a greatly reduced increase in blood pressure that was associated with a more normal redox state and better endothelial function [33]. This animal study formed the basis of a human clinical trial where hypertensive subjects were placed on a daily diet containing dried broccoli sprouts that contained 485 µmoles of glucosinolates of which half was in the form of glucoraphanin [53]. No effect of the 4-week dietary intervention was seen in endothelial function nor in blood pressure. The authors suggest that the differences with the animal results may be due to the fact that the animal studies was a study from weaning until adulthood whereas the human clinical trial was done on adults. On the other hand, the investigators could find no evidence of isothiocyanates in the blood of the participants suggesting that very little of the glucosinolates had been converted to isothiocyanates. Clearly more human studies are required.

Sulforaphane and Prostate Cancer

Sulforaphane, at high concentrations, has been shown to cause a variety of cancer cells, including prostate cancer, to undergo apoptosis [54, 55]. Sulforaphane appears to act upon cell cycle regulators [56] and, as well, in prostate cancer destabilizes the androgen receptor [57] – the androgen receptor is a major driver of prostate cancer cell proliferation. These observations were the basis for carrying out a small open label clinical trial examining the effect of sulforaphane on prostate cancer [8]. Sixteen patients completed the trial where they consumed 200 µmoles of sulforaphane daily for a period of 20 weeks. Sulforaphane and metabolites were measured in plasma with sulforaphane half-life determined to be 2.5 hr. Prostate-specific antigen (PSA) was the major outcome being measured with a 50% decline considered to be evidence of therapeutic effect. Only one patient had such a 50% decline with the average PSA increased by 57% over the trial period, which was significantly less than the expected doubling. Clearly more studies are required to determine whether sulforaphane has any effect on the progression of prostate cancer.

CONCLUSION

Clearly more clinical trials are required examining the effects of Nrf2 activators in a variety of conditions associated with disturbed homeostasis. A major problem with such studies is finding a funding source. Unfortunately, the major paradigm for funding clinical trials is the pharmaceutical company sponsored trial. Pharmaceutical companies have no interest in funding trials where they have no vested intellectual property rights. Since so many the diseases associated with aging involve disturbances of homeostasis (e.g., see Chapter 5), it behooves public funding agencies to increase investment in such nutritional clinical trials before aging-related diseases become too burdensome for the economy to bear.

REFERENCES

[1] Juurlink, BHJ. The beginning of the nutri-geno-proteo-metabolo-mics era of nutritional studies. *National Research Council of Canada PBI Bulletin*, 2003, 1, 9-13.

[2] Wattenberg, LW. Chemoprevention of cancer. *Cancer Res*, 1985, 45, 1-8.

[3] Angelino, D; Jeffery, E. Glucosinolate hydrolysis and bioavailability of resulting isothiocyanates: Focus on glucoraphanin. *J Func Foods*, 2014, 7, 67-76.

[4] Shapiro, TA; Fahey, JW; Wade, KL; Stephenson, KK; Talalay, P. Human metabolism and excretion of cancer chemoprotective glucosinolates and isothiocyanates of cruciferous vegetables. *Cancer Epidemiol Biomarkers Prev*, 1998, 7, 1091-100.

[5] Conaway, CC; Getahun, SM; Liebes, LL; et al. Disposition of glucosinolates and sulforaphane in humans after ingestion of steamed and fresh broccoli. *Nutr Cancer*, 2000, 38, 168-78.

[6] Shapiro, TA; Fahey, JW; Wade, KL; Stephenson, KK; Talalay, P. Chemoprotective glucosinolates and isothiocyanates of broccoli sprouts: metabolism and excretion in humans. *Cancer Epidemiol Biomarkers Prev*, 2001, 10, 501-8.

[7] Ye, L; Dinkova-Kostova, AT; Wade, KL; Zhang, Y; Shapiro, TA; Talalay, P. Quantitative determination of dithiocarbamates in human plasma, serum, erythrocytes and urine: pharmacokinetics of broccoli sprout isothiocyanates in humans. *Clin Chim Acta*, 2002, 316, 43-53.

[8] Alumkal, JJ; Slottke, R; Schwartzman, J; et al. A phase II study of sulforaphane-rich broccoli sprout extracts in men with recurrent prostate cancer. *Invest New Drugs*, 2015, 33, 480-9.

[9] Shapiro, TA; Fahey, JW; Dinkova-Kostova, AT; et al. Safety, tolerance, and metabolism of broccoli sprout glucosinolates and isothiocyanates: a clinical phase I study. *Nutr Cancer*, 2006, 55, 53-62.

[10] Zhang, Y; Talalay, P. Anticarcinogenic activities of organic isothiocyanates: chemistry and mechanisms. *Cancer Res*, 1994, 54, 1976s-81s.

[11] Zhang, Y; Talalay, P; Cho, CG; Posner, GH. A major inducer of anticarcinogenic protective enzymes from broccoli: isolation and elucidation of structure. *Proc Natl Acad Sci U S A*, 1992, 89, 2399-403.

[12] Rahden-Staron, I; Czeczot, H; Szumilo, M. *Induction of rat liver cytochrome P450 isoenzymes CYP 1A and CYP 2B by different fungicides, nitrofurans, and quercetin.* Mutat Res, 2001, 498, 57-66.

[13] Kall, MA; Vang, O; Clausen, J. Effects of dietary broccoli on human in vivo drug metabolizing enzymes: evaluation of caffeine, oestrone and chlorzoxazone metabolism. *Carcinogenesis*, 1996, 17, 793-9.

[14] Hakooz, N; Hamdan, I. Effects of dietary broccoli on human in vivo caffeine metabolism: a pilot study on a group of Jordanian volunteers. *Curr Drug Metab*, 2007, 8, 9-15.

[15] Marshall, BJ; Warren, JR. Unidentified curved bacilli in the stomach of patients with gastritis and peptic ulceration. *Lancet*, 1984, 1, 1311-5.

[16] Marshall, BJ; Armstrong, JA; McGechie, DB; Glancy, RJ. Attempt to fulfil Koch's postulates for pyloric Campylobacter. *Med J Aust*, 1985, 142, 436-9.

[17] Marshall, BJ; McGechie, DB; Rogers, PA; Glancy, RJ. Pyloric Campylobacter infection and gastroduodenal disease. *Med J Aust*, 1985, 142, 439-44.

[18] Goodwin, CS; Armstrong, JA; Marshall, BJ. Campylobacter pyloridis, gastritis, and peptic ulceration. *J Clin Pathol*, 1986, 39, 353-65.

[19] Ishaq, S; Nunn, L. Helicobacter pylori and gastric cancer: a state of the art review. *Gastroenterol Hepatol Bed Bench*, 2015, 8, S6-S14.

[20] Fahey, JW; Haristoy, X; Dolan, PM; et al. Sulforaphane inhibits extracellular, intracellular, and antibiotic-resistant strains of Helicobacter pylori and prevents benzo[a]pyrene-induced stomach tumors. *Proc Natl Acad Sci U S A*, 2002, 99, 7610-5.

[21] Galan, MV; Kishan, AA; Silverman, AL. Oral broccoli sprouts for the treatment of Helicobacter pylori infection: a preliminary report. *Dig Dis Sci*, 2004, 49, 1088-90.

[22] Yanaka, A; Fahey, JW; Fukumoto, A; et al. Dietary sulforaphane-rich broccoli sprouts reduce colonization and attenuate gastritis in Helicobacter pylori-infected mice and humans. *Cancer Prev Res (Phila)*, 2009, 2, 353-60.

[23] Fahey, JW; Stephenson, KK; Wallace, AJ. Dietary amelioration of Helicobacter infection. *Nutr Res*, 2015, 35, 461-73.

[24] Yates, MS; Tran, QT; Dolan, PM; et al. Genetic versus chemoprotective activation of Nrf2 signalling: overlapping yet distinct gene expression profiles between Keap1 knockout and triterpenoid-treated mice. *Carcinogenesis*, 2009, 30, 1024-31.

[25] Lee, JH; Moon, MH; Jeong, JK; et al. Sulforaphane induced adipolysis via hormone sensitive lipase activation, regulated by AMPK signalling pathway. *Biochem Biophys Res Commun*, 2012, 426, 492-7.

[26] Holmstrom, KM; Baird, L; Zhang, Y; et al. Nrf2 impacts cellular bioenergetics by controlling substrate availability for mitochondrial respiration. *Biol Open*, 2013, 2, 761-70.

[27] Hayes, JD; Dinkova-Kostova, AT. The Nrf2 regulatory network provides an interface between redox and intermediary metabolism. *Trends Biochem Sci*, 2014, 39, 199-218.

[28] Noyan-Ashraf, MH; Sadeghinejad,; Davies, GF; et al. Phase 2 protein inducers in the diet promote healthier aging. *J Gerontol A Biol Sci Med Sci*, 2008, 63, 1168-76.

[29] Murashima, M; Watanabe, S; Zhuo, XG; Uehara, M; Kurashige, A. Phase 1 study of multiple biomarkers for metabolism and oxidative stress after one-week intake of broccoli sprouts. *Biofactors*, 2004, 22, 271-5.

[30] Bahadoran, Z; Mirmiran, P; Hosseinpanah, F; Rajab, A; Asghari, G; Azizi, F. Broccoli sprouts powder could improve serum triglyceride and oxidized LDL/LDL-cholesterol ratio in Type 2 diabetic patients: a randomized double-blind placebo-controlled clinical trial. *Diabetes Res Clin Pract*, 2012, 96, 348-54.

[31] Armah, CN; Derdemezis, C; Traka, MH; et al. Diet rich in high glucoraphanin broccoli reduces plasma LDL cholesterol: Evidence from randomised controlled trials. *Mol Nutr Food Res*, 2015, 59, 918-26.

[32] Armah, CN; Traka, MH; Dainty, JR; et al. A diet rich in high-glucoraphanin broccoli interacts with genotype to reduce discordance in plasma metabolite profiles by modulating mitochondrial function. *Am J Clin Nutr*, 2013, 98, 712-22.

[33] Wu, L; Noyan Ashraf, MH; Facci, M; et al. Dietary approach to attenuate oxidative stress, hypertension, and inflammation in the cardiovascular system. *Proc Natl Acad Sci U S A*, 2004, 101, 7094-9.

[34] Riedl, MA; Saxon, A; Diaz-Sanchez, D. Oral sulforaphane increases Phase II antioxidant enzymes in the human upper airway. *Clin Immunol*, 2009, 130, 244-51.

[35] Ring, J; Eberlein-Koenig, B; Behrendt, H. Environmental pollution and allergy. *Ann Allergy Asthma Immunol*, 2001, 87, 2-6.

[36] Takano, H; Yanagisawa, R; Inoue, K. Components of diesel exhaust particles diversely enhance a variety of respiratory diseases related to infection or allergy: extracted organic chemicals and the residual particles after extraction differently affect respiratory diseases. *J Clin Biochem Nutr*, 2007, 40, 101-7.

[37] Brandt, EB; Biagini Myers, JM; Acciani, TH; et al. Exposure to allergen and diesel exhaust particles potentiates secondary allergen-specific memory responses, promoting asthma susceptibility. *J Allergy Clin Immunol*, 2015, 136, 295-303 e7.

[38] Heber, D; Li, Z; Garcia-Lloret, M; et al. Sulforaphane-rich broccoli sprout extract attenuates nasal allergic response to diesel exhaust particles. *Food Funct*, 2014, 5, 35-41.

[39] Kensler, TW; Ng, D; Carmella, SG; et al. Modulation of the metabolism of airborne pollutants by glucoraphanin-rich and sulforaphane-rich broccoli sprout beverages in Qidong, China. *Carcinogenesis*, 2012, 33, 101-7.

[40] Egner, PA; Chen, JG; Zarth, AT; et al. Rapid and sustainable detoxication of airborne pollutants by broccoli sprout beverage: results of a randomized clinical trial in China. *Cancer Prev Res (Phila)*, 2014, 7, 813-23.

[41] Lavich, IC; de Freitas, B; Kist, LW; et al. Sulforaphane rescues memory dysfunction and synaptic and mitochondrial alterations induced by brain iron accumulation. *Neuroscience*, 2015, 301, 542-52.

[42] Zhang, R; Miao, QW; Zhu, CX; et al. Sulforaphane ameliorates neurobehavioral deficits and protects the brain from amyloid beta deposits and peroxidation in mice with Alzheimer-like lesions. *Am J Alzheimers Dis Other Demen*, 2015, 30, 183-91.

[43] Zhang, R; Zhang, J; Fang, L; et al. Neuroprotective effects of sulforaphane on cholinergic neurons in mice with Alzheimer's disease-like lesions. *Int J Mol Sci*, 2014, 15, 14396-410.

[44] James, SJ; Cutler, P; Melnyk, S; et al. Metabolic biomarkers of increased oxidative stress and impaired methylation capacity in children with autism. *Am J Clin Nutr*, 2004, 80, 1611-7.

[45] Rossignol, DA; Frye, RE. Evidence linking oxidative stress, mitochondrial dysfunction, and inflammation in the brain of individuals with autism. *Front Physiol*, 2014, 5, 150.

[46] Giulivi, C; Zhang, YF; Omanska-Klusek, A; et al. Mitochondrial dysfunction in autism. *JAMA*, 2010, 304, 2389-96.

[47] Yui, K; Sato, A; Imataka, G. Mitochondrial dysfunction and its relationship with mTOR signalling and oxidative damage in Autism Spectrum Disorders. *Mini Rev Med Chem*, 2015, 15, 373-89.

[48] Singh, K; Connors, SL; Macklin, EA; et al. Sulforaphane treatment of autism spectrum disorder (ASD). *Proc Natl Acad Sci U S A*, 2014, 111, 15550-5.

[49] Scahill, L. Uncommon use of common measures in sulforaphane trial. *Proc Natl Acad Sci U S A*, 2015, 112, E349.

[50] Talalay, P; Zimmerman, AW. Reply to Scahill: Behavioral outcome measures in autism. *Proc Natl Acad Sci U S A*, 2015, 112, E350.

[51] Yao, JK; Reddy, R. Oxidative stress in schizophrenia: pathogenetic and therapeutic implications. *Antioxid Redox Signal*, 2011, 15, 1999-2002.

[52] Senanayake, GV; Banigesh, A; Wu, L; Lee, P; Juurlink, BH. The dietary phase 2 protein inducer sulforaphane can normalize the kidney epigenome and improve blood pressure in hypertensive rats. *Am J Hypertens*, 2012, 25, 229-35.

[53] Christiansen, B; Bellostas Muguerza, N; Petersen, AM; et al. Ingestion of broccoli sprouts does not improve endothelial function in humans with hypertension. *PLoS One*, 2010, 5, e12461.

[54] Choi, S; Lew, KL; Xiao, H; et al. D,L-Sulforaphane-induced cell death in human prostate cancer cells is regulated by inhibitor of apoptosis family proteins and Apaf-1. *Carcinogenesis*, 2007, 28, 151-62.

[55] Singh, SV; Srivastava, SK; Choi, S; et al. Sulforaphane-induced cell death in human prostate cancer cells is initiated by reactive oxygen species. *J Biol Chem*, 2005, 280, 19911-24.

[56] Wang, L; Liu, D; Ahmed, T; Chung, FL; Conaway, C; Chiao, JW. Targeting cell cycle machinery as a molecular mechanism of sulforaphane in prostate cancer prevention. *Int J Oncol*, 2004, 24, 187-92.

[57] Gibbs, A; Schwartzman, J; Deng, V; Alumkal, J. Sulforaphane destabilizes the androgen receptor in prostate cancer cells by inactivating histone deacetylase 6. *Proc Natl Acad Sci U S A*, 2009, 106, 16663-8.

In: Broccoli
Editor: Bernhard H. J. Juurlink

ISBN: 978-1-63484-313-3
© 2016 Nova Science Publishers, Inc.

Chapter 14

BROCCOLI CULTIVATION IN WARMER CLIMATES

Karistsapol Nooprom
Program in Agricultural Technology, Faculty of Agricultural Technology,
Songkla Rajabhat University, Muang, Songkhla, Thailand

ABSTRACT

Broccoli (Brassica oleracea var. italica) is one of the most popular vegetable crops grown in many countries around the world due to its high nutritional value. It has the most specific climate and an agricultural requirement, which limits its commercial cultivation to a few favored locations around the globe, due to the fact that it is the best suited to countries or areas with a cooler climate.

Broccoli cultivation has been expanding in recent years, especially in tropical countries like Thailand. For the best cultivation results, broccoli has to be planted in the north of Thailand where the climate is cooler, to ensure maximum cultivation results, or in the North-east during the winter season. As you progress further down to the south of Thailand, the climate becomes increasingly more tropical because of the high light intensity and higher climate conditions during the dry season. High rain fall during the raining season also results in the low growth of broccoli and therefore results into small cultivation units and causes broccoli cultivation to come to a halt.

Therefore it is pivotal to select suitable broccoli cultivars, planting dates, and planting methods for each season to ensure successful broccoli cultivation in tropical climates.

Keywords: calabrese, tropical climate, heat tolerance, cultivars, southern Thailand

INTRODUCTION

Broccoli is a member of the Brassicaceae family (a wild form of this family) (Decoteau, 2000). Other members of the family include cauliflower, cabbage, Chinese cabbage, Brussels sprouts, and Kohlrabi (Gad and Abd El-Moez, 2011). Broccoli is an Italian vegetable, native to the Mediterranean region, first cultivated in Italy during ancient Roman times and also in

England around 1720. On the other hand, it made its first appearance in the United States of America in 1806, but the commercial cultivation of broccoli only started around 1923 (Nooprom and Santipracha, 2013a; Ouda and Mahadeen, 2008).

Broccoli is one of the most important and popular vegetable crops in many countries around the world (AVRDC, 2007) such as Australia, New Zealand, Japan, Canada, Germany, Netherlands, and the United States of America (Tan, 1999). In the United States of America broccoli was one of the top vegetable exports of the country. Broccoli for the fresh produce market was a $1,786.66 million industry in 2013. This was up from $1,357.23 in 2012. The broccoli for the processing market is considerably smaller than that of the fresh produce market, with a production value of $18.21 and $40.30 million in 2012 and 2013, respectively as shown in Table 1 (National Agricultural Statistics Service, 2015).

Broccoli has become widespread in Asia in recent decades because of its organoleptic properties and high nutritional value (Sermenli et al. 2011). Tilaar et al. (2012) reported that broccoli is rich in nutrients such as vitamins and minerals. In addition, it has also high antioxidant compounds that reduce the risk associated with several cancers and neurodegenerative diseases.

Broccoli is a cool season crop. It is generally considered hardy in cold temperatures. Optimum temperatures for successful broccoli growth are between 60° and 68°F (Decoteau, 2002). The yield of broccoli is strictly determined by temperatures (KałuŻewicz, et al. 2012). High temperatures more than 80°F for even relatively short periods of time and warm temperatures more than 75°F for extended periods of time may cause the broccoli head to be rough with an uneven flower bud sizes and thus; deemed as commercially unacceptable (Barham et al. 2001).

In the tropics, broccoli production has some setbacks in regard to unsuitable environments for sufficient broccoli growth. In the dry season, there are high light intensity and high temperature conditions. While in rainy season, there is continuous heavy rainfall. These conditions affect the growth, and yield quality of broccoli (Santipracha, 2007).

Table 1. The production value of broccoli for fresh produce and processing market in the United States of America

Broccoli	Value of production (1,000 dollars)	
	2012	2013
Fresh market	1,357,236	1,786,669
Processing market	18,216	4,0368

Source: Adapted from National Agricultural Statistics Service (2015)

CULTIVAR SELECTION

Broccoli cultivars differ in days of maturity. They are classified as early, medium, and late cultivars. These cultivars respond to the time of planting (Nooprom, 2014). The early cultivars are adapted for planting to the period from late winter to early summer for harvest from late spring to early fall. The medium cultivars are seeded in the summer and early fall for harvest in the late fall and early winter.

Table 2. Horticultural characters of four broccoli cultivars

Cultivars	Harvest rate (%)	Maturity (day)	Heads Mean weight (g)	Thickness (cm)
KY-29A	75.00[b]	75.00[a]	225.90[a]	14.30[a]
NB-32	93.80[a]	64.00[c]	202.80[ab]	13.80[ab]
Green King 553	89.60[a]	71.00[b]	192.70[b]	12.90[b]
Green Bao	95.80[a]	72.00[b]	151.70[c]	10.90[c]
F-test	*	*	*	*
C.V. (%)	6.20	1.30	7.98	6.31

Source: Adapted from Jiyong (1999)

Mean in each column followed by the same letter are not significantly different at 5% level by DMRT.

Table 3. Yield of four broccoli cultivars

Cultivars	Yields (t.ha^{-1}) Marketable	Nonmarketable
KY-29A	5.80[a]	2.60[c]
NB-32	5.00[ab]	3.00[ab]
Green King 553	4.80[b]	1.80[bc]
Green Bao	1.40[c]	4.10[a]
F-test	**	**
C.V. (%)	4.40	35.20

Source: Adapted from Jiyong (1999)

Mean in each column followed by the same letter are not significantly different at 5% level by DMRT.

Table 4. Yield after trimming of seven early cultivars of broccoli

Cultivars	Yield (t.ha^{-1})
Green Queen	13.10[a]
Green King	9.10[b]
KY-29A	10.20[b]
Top Green	10.40[b]
Yok Kheo	14.00[a]
Big Green	1.40[c]
Special	9.40[b]
F-test	*
C.V. (%)	15.50

Source: Adapted from Nooprom and Santipracha (2011)

Mean in each column followed by the same letter are not significantly different at 5% level by DMRT.

The cultivars of late maturity are adapted to areas where broccoli can be grown throughout the winter and then be harvested in the late winter and early spring (Thompson and Kelly, 2002). Thailand has a tropical climate which is unsuitable for the growth of general broccoli cultivars, but suitable for the heat tolerant broccoli cultivars (Nooprom and

Santipracha, 2013b) because they will produce commercially acceptable broccoli heads under warm weather with heat stressed growing conditions (Barham et al. 2001). Jiyong (1999) did a study on the broccoli cultivar trial at the Asian Regional Center, Asian Vegetable Research and Development Center (ARC-AVRDC) in Kamphaeng Saen, Nakhon Pathom, Thailand during 1997-1998. It was found that KY-29A had the highest marketable head yield of 5.80 t.ha^{-1}, which means that the head weight is at 225.90 g, and means that the head has a thickness of 14.30 cm, making it a good cultivar for heat tolerance. NB-32 was considered as a good heat tolerant cultivar due to its early maturity, high harvest rate, and high marketable head yield. Table 2 and 3 shows the horticultural characteristics of four broccoli cultivars and yield of four broccoli cultivars, respectively.

Nooprom and Santipracha (2011) showed the research results about growth and yield of seven early cultivars of broccoli in Songkhla province, southern Thailand from 28 October 2012 to 7 January 2013. It was found out that the seven early cultivars of broccoli exhibited good performance, such as early growth and yield but, not for Big Green. Yok Kheo gave the highest yield of 14.00 t.ha^{-1} not significantly different from Green Queen which gave the yield of 13.10 t.ha^{-1}. Top Green, KY-29A, Special, and Green King were the second highest yielding cultivars which gave a yield of 10.40, 10.20, 9.40, and 9.10 t.ha^{-1}, respectively. Yok Kheo and Green Queen are interesting new hybrid cultivars because they gave a yield higher than Top Green and KY-29A. Besides, Green Queen can be harvested 10 days earlier than the Top Green and the Yok Kheo (Table 4).

PLANTING DATE SELECTION

The planting dates are an important factor for the yield of a crop (Shapla et al. 2014). Many experiments regarding planting dates are being conducted in different parts of the world which reveal that the total yield of the crop is remarkably influenced by different planting dates (Ahmed and Siddique, 2004).

The planting date is a limiting factor for broccoli production in southern Thailand which has a tropical climate. Thus, suitable planting dates for broccoli production in this area are highly important. For example, Nooprom and Santipracha (2014a) studied the growth and yield of broccoli planted all year round in Songkhla province, southern Thailand from January, 2011 to January, 2012. The design was a split-plot in a randomized complete block with four replications.

The main plots were planted in the months of: January, February, March, April, May, June, July, August, September, October, November, and December with sub-plots being early cultivars of broccoli: Top Green, Green Queen, Yok Kheo, and Special. The results showed that broccoli planted in the all months had a high survival rate of seedlings of 78.90-98.24%. They provided high plant height of 49.58-51.71 cm when planted in January, February, March, July, and December. Broccoli planted in January, February and March, had a 50% earlier flowering rate of 33-36 days after transplanting.

These results were consistent with the time of harvest compared with other planting dates. The highest total yield was obtained from broccoli planted in January of 9.36 t.ha^{-1}, followed by March of 7.58 t.ha^{-1} while broccoli planted in September had the lowest total yield of 1.68 t.ha^{-1} as shown in Figure 1.

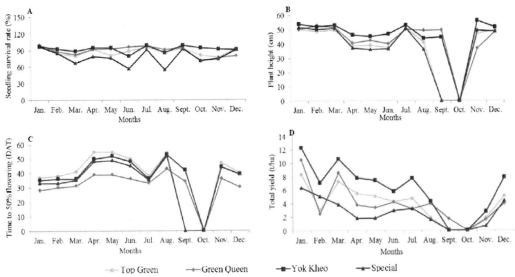

Source: Adapted from Nooprom and Santipracha (2014a)

Figure 1. Interactions of planting dates and cultivars on seedling survival rate (A), plant height (B), time to 50% flowering (C), and total yield (D) of four early cultivars of broccoli.

Table 5. Effect of planting dates on growth and yield of broccoli

Planting dates	Plant height (cm)	Leaf length (cm)	Diameter of head (cm)	Weight of head (cm)
20th April	24.81[b]	42.56[ab]	10.34[c]	171.49[c]
5th May	30.79[a]	47.31[a]	14.97[a]	200.65[a]
20th May	28.75[a]	44.25[a]	12.70[b]	184.33[b]
4th June	22.12[c]	39.31[bc]	8.46[d]	146.44[d]

Source: Adapted from Ahmed and Siddiuqe (2004)
Mean sharing same letters are not significant.

The growth responses showed that broccoli planted in March, June, August, October, and November had low seedling survival rates and plant heights, due to the fact that it had been planted during a period of continuous rain fall and high temperatures of 87-93°F. These factors contributed to the decreasing survival rate in the seedling stage. The high temperatures in the range of 86-104°F caused decreasing broccoli growths which affected yield losses (Kałużewicz et al. 2009). This result confirmed by Nooprom et al. (2013a) proved that high temperatures affected broccoli growth and resulted in yield losses.

In addition, Ahmed and Siddiuqe (2004) revealed that the research results indicated the effect of planting dates on growth and yield of broccoli under Rawalakot conditions of Pakistan which lies in this temperature zone. Broccoli seedlings were transplanted on four different planting dates: 20th April, 5th May, 20th May, and 4th June during the year 2002. This study showed that broccoli planted on the 5th of May had a higher plant height, leaf length, diameter of head, and weight of head than the other planting dates (Table 5).

BROCCOLI CULTIVATION IN THE DRY SEASON

In the tropical regions, high light intensity and high temperatures are contributing problems for various vegetable crop productions. Broccoli production in these areas was affected in growth, low seedling survival rate, and yield quality (Nooprom, 2014).

The shading technique is an important way to create the suitable environment for higher growth and yield of broccoli and other vegetable crops. Nooprom et al. (2013b) studied the shading technique to improve the growth and yield of broccoli during the dry season in southern Thailand from April to June, 2012. The experimental design was split-plot in a randomized complete block design (RCBD).

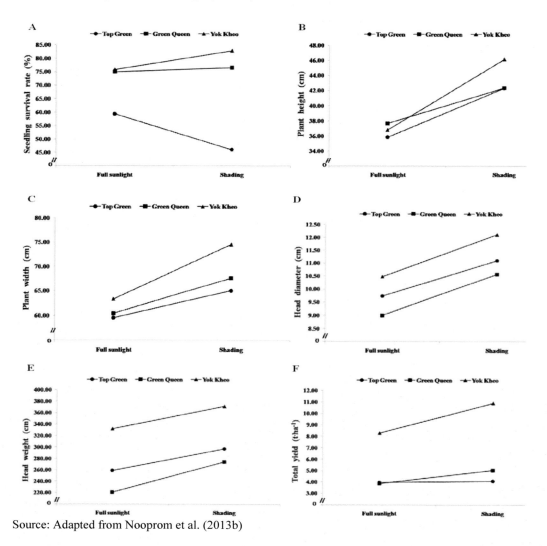

Source: Adapted from Nooprom et al. (2013b)

Figure 2. Interactions of shading and cultivars on seedling survival rate (A), plant height (B), plant width (C), head diameter (D), head weight (E), and total yield (F) of three early cultivars of broccoli.

The plot was split into main two plots with two different treatments. One plot was exposed to full sunlight and the other was covered by shade. Both plots were planted with different cultivars of broccoli such as Top Green, Green Queen and Yok Kheo.

The results showed that light intensity and temperatures under the shading were lower than that of the plot exposed to full sunlight, whereas the relative humidity of the air under shading was higher than full sunlight. These factors would support the increasing growth and yield of broccoli. They could adapt better due to the shading and increase seedling survival rate, plant height and plant width (Figure 2A, 2B, and 2C, respectively). Consequently, the broccoli under the shading had the highest in head diameter, head weight and total yield (Figure 2D, 2E, and 2F, respectively which was significantly better than full sunlight.

There was a positive impact of the shading technique on yield and the yield attributes of the three cultivars of broccoli used in the experiment. The highest total yield was obtained from the Yok Kheo under both full sunlight and shade resulting in 10.92 and 8.29 t.ha^{-1}, respectively, followed by the Green Queen under the shading of 6.21 t.ha^{-1}. The best suited broccoli cultivar on growing during dry season in southern Thailand was the Yok Kheo and Green Queen because their growth rate and yield were higher than that of the Top Green and they also had a bigger size and higher quality of head, particularly those grown under the shading because of the decreased light intensity and lowered temperature and the increased humidity compared to the yield exposed to full sunlight. These factors would support the increasing growth and yield of broccoli.

BROCCOLI CULTIVATION IN THE RAINING SEASON

Continuous and heavy rainfall is a contributing problem for broccoli production in humid tropical weather. The broccoli plant can become infected with head rot from the impact of raindrops (Nooprom et al. 2013), and be destroyed by the bacterium *Erwinia carotovora* ssp. *carotovora* that causes soft rot disease (Bhat et al. 2010). Nooprom et al. (2013c) studied the impact of using different rain protectors and cultivars on growth and yield of broccoli during the rainy season in southern Thailand. This study was carried out in a research field at Prince of Songkla University, Hat Yai, Songkhla province, Thailand from 28 October 2012 to 7 January 2013 using split-plots within a randomized complete block design. The main plots had three different types of rain protection: open field (control), under a green shade net and under a plastic sheet (5% UV polyethylene film with thickness of 200 μm) with subplots hosting cultivars of Top Green, Green Queen and Yok Kheo.

The results showed that broccoli grown under the green shade net and the plastic sheet had a higher growth and yield compared with those grown in the open field. The average highest total yields were cultivated from the broccoli cultivars grown under the plastic sheeting of 11.10 t.ha^{-1}. The yield rates for broccoli grown under the green shade net and in the open field were 7.54 and 5.61 t.ha^{-1}, respectively as shown in Table 6.

The average highest yields of broccoli were obtained from Yok Kheo of 10.22 t.ha^{-1}, followed by Green Queen and Top Green of 7.56 and 6.46 t.ha^{-1}, respectively. Broccoli plants grown under the plastic sheet could be harvested earlier than those grown in the open field and under green shade net. The cultivars grown under the plastic sheeting had an increase in growth of 13.25 and 2.50 days after transplanting, respectively.

Table 6. The effect of different rain protectors on different broccoli cultivars in regards to head diameter, head weight, and total yield of broccoli

Treatments	Cultivars			Mean
	Top Green	Green Queen	Yok Kheo	
Harvested plant (%)				
Open field	82.75^{ab}	85.37^{ab}	92.15^{ab}	86.75^{A}
Under green shade net	49.36^{c}	73.88^{b}	75.40^{b}	66.22^{B}
Under plastic sheet	96.48^{ab}	98.24^{ab}	100.00^{a}	98.24^{A}
Mean	76.20^{A}	85.83^{A}	89.19^{A}	
Head diameter (cm)				
Open field	9.30^{g}	8.70^{h}	10.05^{f}	9.36^{C}
Under green shade net	10.69^{e}	10.42^{e}	12.71^{b}	11.27^{B}
Under plastic sheet	12.24^{c}	11.72^{d}	13.04^{a}	12.33^{A}
Mean	10.74^{B}	10.29^{C}	11.93^{A}	
Head weight per plant (g)				
Open field	264.38^{e}	234.81^{f}	322.86^{cd}	274.21^{C}
Under green shade net	336.90^{c}	295.56^{d}	391.70^{b}	341.39^{B}
Under plastic sheet	345.46^{c}	306.52^{d}	434.13^{a}	362.04^{A}
Mean	315.58^{B}	278.96^{C}	382.90^{A}	
Total yield (t.ha^{-1})				
Open field	3.94^{e}	5.35^{d}	7.52^{c}	5.60^{C}
Under green shade net	5.05^{d}	7.88^{c}	9.67^{b}	7.53^{B}
Under plastic sheet	10.30^{b}	9.44^{b}	13.48^{a}	11.10^{A}
Mean	6.46^{C}	7.56^{B}	10.22^{A}	

Source: Nooprom et al. (2013c)
Values sharing the same superscript letters are not significantly different (P≤0.05) by DMRT.

The results indicated that broccoli should be grown under a plastic sheet or a green shade net to achieve higher yields than from plants grown in the open field. The Yok Kheo and Green Queen cultivars are recommended for Songkhla province and the surrounding area as shown Table 6. Moreover, broccoli growing under plastic sheet and green shade net had a lower incidence of soft rot disease (1.62 and 3.75%, respectively) than those grown in open field (13.33%) while their growing under plastic sheet (1.50%) had a lower incidence of black rot disease than those grown under green shade net and open field (18.75 and 32.88%, respectively). All broccoli cultivars were found to be statistically different in their response towards soft rot and black rot diseases. However, the Top Green had the highest disease incidence (8.33 and 21.08%, respectively) while the Yok Kheo had the lowest disease incidence (4.62 and 0.00%, respectively).

The highest total yield was obtained from the Yok Kheo when grown under the plastic sheeting (13.48 t.ha^{-1}) while the Top Green had lowest yield when grown in an open field (3.94 t.ha^{-1}) (Nooprom and Santipracha, 2014b) as shown in Table 7.

In addition, Chootummatouch et al. (2000) made a study about the yield of broccoli grown under nylon net compared with plants not covered by nylon net during raining season in Songkhla province, southern Thailand. The results showed that broccoli planted under nylon net had a higher yield, and that the percentage of yields lost from soft rot disease was lower than the broccoli not covered by the nylon net.

Table 7. The effect of different rain protectors on different cultivars in regards to soft rot and black rot diseases

Treatments	Cultivars			Mean
	Top Green	Green Queen	Yok Kheo	
Soft rot disease (%)				
Open field	38.15^a	31.67^b	28.83^b	32.88^A
Under green shade net	22.34^c	31.01^c	12.92^d	18.75^B
Under plastic sheet	2.75^e	1.75^e	0.00^e	1.50^C
Mean	21.08^A	18.14^B	13.91^C	
Black rot disease (%)				
Open field	28.01^e	25.93^f	31.03^c	28.32^C
Under green shade net	34.08^b	29.63^d	38.59^a	34.10^A
Under plastic sheet	29.43^d	27.00^f	35.14^b	30.52^B
Mean	30.51^B	27.52^C	34.92^A	

Source: Adapted from Nooprom and Santipracha (2014b)
Values sharing the same superscript letters are not significantly different (P≤0.05) by DMRT.

CONCLUSION

Broccoli production in tropical countries has its challenges in regards to the unsuitable environmental factors that influence the growth of this vegetable, such as high light intensity and high temperatures in the dry season continuous heavy rainfall during the rainy season. These factors have an enormous impact on the growth and yield quality of broccoli. However, the selection of heat tolerant broccoli cultivars, suitable planting dates, suitable planting techniques like green shading net coverings in dry season, and planting under plastic sheeting in raining season are crucial for successful broccoli cultivation in tropical climates.

ACKNOWLEDGMENTS

I would like to thank Assoc. Prof. Dr. Quanchit Santipracha and Asst. Prof. Dr. Ruamjit Nokkoul for providing me with useful commentary in order to write this chapter. Finally, I would like to mention my appreciation for the support, love and patience from my parents and my friends during the period of this chapter.

REFERENCES

Ahmed M. J. & W. Siddique, (2004). Effect of sowing dates on growth and yield of broccoli (*Brassica oleracea* L.) under Rawalakot condition. *Asian J. Sci.*, 3: 167-169.
AVRDC, (2007). AVRDC Report 2004. Shanhua: AVRDC-The World Vegetable Center.
Barham, R. & D. Joynt, (2001). Heat Tolerant Broccoli. Gilroy: R & D AG ,Incorporation.

Bhat, K. A., D. Masood, N. A. Bhat, M. A. Bhat, S. M. Razvi, M. R. Mir, A. Sabina, N. Wani & M. Habib, (2010). Current status of post harvest soft rot in vegetables: a review. *Asian J. Plant Sci.*, 9: 200-208.

Chootummatouch, W., P. Maneenit, C. Chaikwang & W. Kunchara Na Ayuttaya, (2000). Yield trial of broccoli and cabbage grown as hygienic fresh vegetables during rainy season in Songkhla. *Thai Agricultural Research Journal,* 18: 31-42

Decoteau, D. R., (2000). Vegetable Crops. New Jersey: Prentice-Hall ,Incorporation.

Gad, N. & M. R. Abd El-Moez, (2011). Broccoli growth, yield quantity and quality as affected by cobalt nutrition. *Agric. Biol. J. Am.*, 2: 116-231.

Jiyong, Y., (1999). Cultivar perfotmance In: AVRDC (eds) ARC training report 1998, Asian Vegetable Research and Development Center, Tainan, pp 5-9.

Kałużewicz, A., W. Krzesiński & M. Knaflewski. (2009). Effect of temperature on yield and quality of broccoli heads. *Vegetable Crops Research Bulletin,* 71: 51-56.

Kałużewicz, A., W. Krzesiński, M. Knaflewski, J. Lisiecka, T. SpiŻewski & Fraszczak, (2012). Effect of temperature on the growth of broccoli (*Brassica oleracea* L. var. *italica* Plenck) cv. Fiesta. *Vegetable Crops Research Bulletin,* 77: 129-141.

National Agricultural Statistics Service, (2015). Vegetables 2014 Summary (January 2015). [Online] 2015 March, 9. Available from: http://www.nass.usda.gov/Publications/Todays_Reports/reports/vgan0115.pdf.

Nooprom, K., (2011). Planting dates and production of off-season broccoli in Songkhla. Ph.D. Thesis, Prince of Songkla University.

Nooprom, K. & Q. Santipracha, (2011). Growth and yield of 7 early varieties of broccoli in Songkhla province. *King Mongkut's Agric. J.,* 8: 357-361.

Nooprom, K. & Q. Santipracha, (2013a). Effects of planting dates and varieties on growth and yield of broccoli during rainy season. *AJABS,* 19: 54-61.

Nooprom, K. & Q. Santipracha, (2013b). Planting times and varieties on incidence of bacterial disease and yield quality of broccoli during rainy season in southern Thailand. *MAS,* 7: 9-14.

Nooprom, K. & Q. Santipracha, (2014a). Incidence of bacterial disease and yield of broccoli as influenced by different rain protectors and varieties during the rainy season in southern Thailand. *Res. J. Appl. Sci. Eng. Technol.,* 7: 2687-2692.

Nooprom, K. & Q. Santipracha, (2014b). Growth and yield of broccoli planted year round in Songkhla province, Thailand. *AJABS,* 7: 4157-4161.

Nooprom, K., Q. Santipracha & S. Te-chato, (2013a). Effect of planting time on incidence of bacterial disease and yield of broccoli during dry season in southern Thailand. *Res. J. Environ. Earth Sci.,* 5: 457-461.

Nooprom, K., Q. Santipracha & S. Te-chato, (2013b). Effect of shading and variety on the growth and yield of broccoli during dry season in southern Thailand. *IJPAES,* 3: 111-115.

Nooprom, K., Q. Santipracha & S. Te-chato, (2013c). Growth and yield of broccoli under different rain protectors during the rainy season in Songkhla province, southern Thailand. *Kasetsart J. (Nat. Sci)* 5: 457-461.

Ouda, B. A. & A. Y. Mahadeen, (2008). Effect of fertilizers on growth, yield, yield components, quality and certain nutrient content in broccoli (*Brassica oleracea*). *IJAB,* 10: 627-632.

Santipracha, Q., (2007). *Vegetable Crop* Variety and Growing Season of Southern Thailand. Bangkok: Text Journal Publication.

Sermenli, T., K. Mavi & S. Yilmaz, (2011). Determination of transplanting dates of broccoli (*Brassica oleracea* L. var. *italica*) under Antakya condition. *J. Anim. Plant Sci.*, 21: 638-641.

Shapla, S. A., M. A. Hussain, M. S. H. Mandal, H. Mehraj & A. F. M. Jamal Uddin, (2014). Growth and yield of broccoli (*Brassica oleracea* var. *italica* L.) to different planting times. *IJBSSR*, 2: 95-99.

Thompson, H. C. & W. C. Kelly, (2002). Vegetable Crops. Danville: Interstate Publishers, Incorporation.

Tilaar, W., S. Ashair, B. Yanuwiadi, J. Polii-Mandang F. h. Tomasowa, (2012). Shoot induction from broccoli explants hypocotyls and biosynthesis of sulforaphane. *IJBAS*, 12: 44-48.

In: Broccoli
Editor: Bernhard H. J. Juurlink

ISBN: 978-1-63484-313-3
© 2016 Nova Science Publishers, Inc.

Chapter 15

BROCCOLI: AGRICULTURAL CHARACTERISTICS, HEALTH BENEFITS AND POST-HARVEST PROCESSING ON GLUCOSINOLATE CONTENT

Olga Nydia Campas-Baypoli[*], *Ernesto Uriel Cantú-Soto*
and José Antonio Rivera-Jacobo
Departamento de Biotecnología y Ciencias Alimentarias.
Instituto Tecnológico de Sonora. Cd. Obregón, Sonora, México

ABSTRACT

This chapter outlines some of the cultivation characteristics of broccoli as well as the nutrient composition of broccoli, including trace elements, vitamins, fatty acids and phytochemicals with a particular emphasis on glucosinolate profiles. A review of the recent history of world production of broccoli is given. Of the glucosinolates, the focus of this chapter is on glucoraphanin and its hydrolysis metabolite sulforaphane. Glucosinolate/sulforaphane content of some different cultivars and different portions of the plant (florets, stalks, leaves and seeds) is reviewed. The effect of growth conditions are also examined, including soil nutrients, temperature and photoperiod as well as post-harvest processing and cooking on glucosinolate profiles. Sulforaphane absorption and metabolism is briefly considered as well as the mechanisms whereby sulforaphane inhibits tumor development. Finally, a brief consideration is given to methods being researched to improve the stability of sulforaphane.

1. INTRODUCTION

Broccoli is a vegetable of great interest due to its nutritional contributions, which are a rich source of fiber, proteins, lipids, vitamins and minerals. Additionally positive effects for the human health are attributed to the plant because of its high content of phytochemicals,

---

[*] Email: olga.campas@itson.edu.mx.

such as flavonoids and glucosinolates. The products of the glucosinolates hydrolysis are the isothiocyanates, which have antimicrobial, chemoprotective and anticarcinogenic properties. Glucoraphanin is the major glucosinolate in broccoli, whose hydrolysis product with biological activity is the sulforaphane isothiocyanate. Our investigation group has studied the content of this compound in the seed, the freshly harvested vegetable, leaves and stems. Also the effect of the processing in the content of sulforaphane, such as drying, fermented, germination and some storage conditions has been evaluated.

2. BROCCOLI (*BRASSICA OLERACEA L. VAR. ITALICA*)

2.1. Botanical Characteristics

The plants of the *Brassicales* order and the *Cruciferae* or *Brassicaceae* family cover around 350 genera with a total of around 2000 species, among which some plants of commercial interest are included such as the cabbage, cauliflower, Brussels sprouts and broccoli [1]. Broccoli originated through a selection process of the wild cabbage in the Southern Europe and Asia Minor [2]. The word broccoli is derived of the Italian *brocco* and the Latin *brachium*, which mean branch or arm. Broccoli is a plural word, and it refers to its numerous sprouts in inflorescence shape (Figure 1). The plant develops an erect stem, pulpy and thick with limp and spaced leaves. Those stems emerge with leaf axils creating inflorescences; generally a central one of higher size and others laterals. The central inflorescence measure between 7.5 and 20 cm of diameter, and the height average in the plant is 30-60 cm. Because of its edible quality the part of the plant with commercial interest is the thick inflorescence, which is formed by a group of flower buds with its pulpy stems but, unlike the cauliflower, can produce others of small size that grow on the principal stem leaf axils [1, 3, 4].

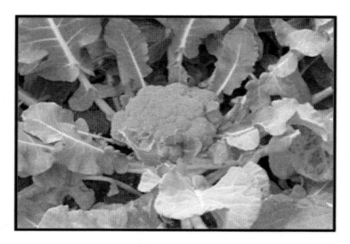

Figure 1. Inflorescence of the broccoli plant.

2.2. Agricultural Characteristics

Broccoli is a cold season crop that is sowed in a great diversity of soils. However, the best results are obtained on loamy, deep soils with a large content of organic matter and pH between 5.5 and 6.5. In order to establish a hectare, a seedbed of approximately 150 m^2 is made using 250 and 300 grams of seed [4]. Broccoli seed can germinate between 4 and 35°C, but the optimal growth is reached when temperatures are between 16 and 18°C. The seedlings are transplanted between 30 and 45 days. In commercial sowings of broccoli under optimal conditions large and leafy plants are obtained that produce compact inflorescences with a large and branched stem [5]. The consumption of fresh broccoli implies a simple chain of cold or a fast freezing process. Industrially broccoli is used in the production of pickles [4]. In Mexico, the inflorescences with commercial quality are harvested manually off the field and packed in boxes (Figure 2), and then transported to the plant to make disinfection and fast cooling.

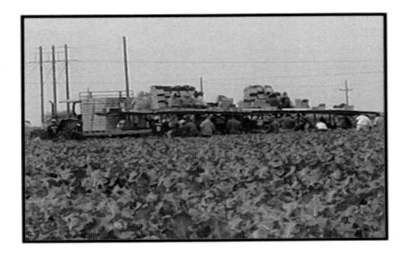

Figure 2. Harvesting of broccoli on the field.

Afterwards, the boxes of fresh broccoli are stored in low temperatures for a short period of time to immediately transport it to its final destination. A summary of the general characteristics of the broccoli is presented in Table 1.

2.3. Chemical Composition

Crucifer family vegetables provide nutrients such as vitamin C, folic acid, calcium, potassium, fiber and low fat content [6]. Broccoli has been rated as the vegetable that contains a greater quantity of nutrients and less calories per unit of weight of edible product; this vegetable contributes around 3 g of proteins, 2.6 of dietary fiber and only 34 kcal each per 100 g of fresh product. Some authors emphasize that its medicinal and nutritional value reside mainly in its high content of vitamins A, B2 and C, carbohydrates, proteins and chemoprotective substances as glucosinolates and flavonoids [7, 8]. It is recommended that broccoli be consumed fresh and of recent harvest since this vegetable undergoes a fast senescence, which is characterized by the change of color in the vegetable head (yellow inflorescence), loss of texture, unpleasant odors and reduction of the nutritional value [9]. Complex factors are involved in the senescence process such as ethylene biosynthesis, temperature and the vegetal respiration process [10]. The chemical composition of the fresh broccoli per edible portion reported by the USDA [11] is shown in Table 2.

Table 1. Technical specifications of broccoli

Common name	Broccoli, Bróculi, Brécol, Brécoles
Scientific name	*Brassica oleracea L. var itálica*
Order	*Brassicales*
Family	*Cruciferae, Brassicaceae*
Origin	Southern Europe and Asia Minor
Cultivation	It requires loamy and deep soils. Optimal temperatures of growth are low (18°C). It is recommended that broccoli is cultivated in rotation with other vegetables.
Plants	The plants of broccoli are vigorous and leafy with deep roots.
Varieties	Precocious or early cultivars whose harvesting time is under 90 days after the sowing. Intermediate cultivars that are harvested between 90 and 110 days after the sowing. Late cultivars that take more than 110 days to achieve the adequate development.
Collection	The harvest begins when the inflorescences have achieved a decent development, diameter greater than 13 cm and before flower buds are open.
Uses	Generally it is consumed fresh in salads, cooked in soups, dressings.

Source: FAO [4]

Table 2. Chemical composition of broccoli raw (value per 100 g)

Nutrient	Florets	Leaves	Stalks
Proximates			
Water (g)	89.30	90.69	90.69
Energy (kcal)	34	28	28
Protein (g)	2.82	2.98	2.98
Total lipid (g)	0.37	0.35	0.35
Carbohydrated, by difference (g)	6.64	5.24	5.24
Fiber, total dietary (g)	2.6	----	----
Minerals			
Ca (mg)	47	48	48
Fe (mg)	0.73	0.88	0.88
Mg (mg)	21	25	25
P (mg)	66	66	66
K (mg)	316	325	325
Na (mg)	33	27	27
Zn (mg)	0.41	0.40	0.40
Vitamins			
Vitamin C (mg)	89.2	93.2	93.2
Thiamin (mg)	0.071	0.065	0.065
Riboflavin (mg)	0.117	0.119	0.119
Niacin (mg)	0.639	0.638	0.638

Nutrient	Florets	Leaves	Stalks
Vitamin B-6 (mg)	0.175	0.159	0.159
Folate (µg)	63	71	71
Vitamin A (IU)	623	16000	400
Vitamin E (mg)	0.78	----	----
Vitamin K (µg)	101.6	----	----
Lipids			
Fatty acids, total saturated (g)	0.039	0.054	0.062
Fatty acids, total monounsaturated (g)	0.011	0.024	0.027
Fatty acids, total polyunsaturated (g)	0.038	0.167	0.190

Source: USDA [11]

Table 3 shows the approximate composition, the total phenolic compounds content, total isothiocyanates and antioxidant capacity of the inflorescence of the commercial quality broccoli analyzed in our laboratory.

Table 3. Proximate composition, total polyphenols, total isothiocyanates and antioxidant capacity of broccoli raw

Analysis	Florets
Proximates (value per 100 g).	
Water (g)	89.47
Protein (g)	3.12
Total lipid (g)	0.88
Total ash (g)	0.5
Fiber, total dietary (g)	6.1
Polyphenols	
Total polyphenols (mg GAE/g dry matter)	17.21
Isothiocyanates (mg/g dry matter)	
Total isothiocyanates	31.93
Antioxidant capacity (mmol TE/g dry matter)	
DPPH Radical scavenging capacity	112
ABTS Radical scavenging capacity	123

Data expressed as the mean ± standard deviation of three assays (in triplicate).
GAE, Gallic acid equivalent
TE, trolox equivalent

2.4. Production

During recent years the vegetables demand of the *Brassica* genus has been increased, particularly broccoli and cauliflower, because its frequent consumption promotes numerous health benefits. This has generated in the international context, a constant increase of its production in the last 25 years (Figure 3). Currently, China, India, Italy, Mexico, France, Poland, and the United States of America are the seven worldwide major producers of cauliflower and broccoli (Figure 4) [12].

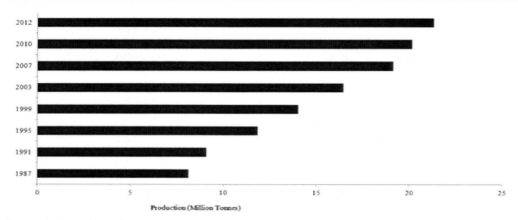

Source: FAOSTAT [12]

Figure 3. World production of cauliflower and broccoli.

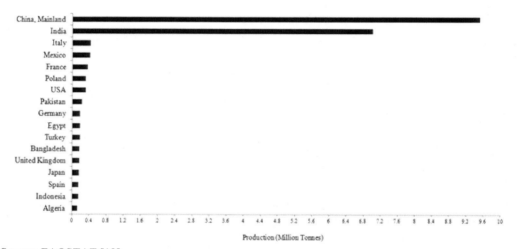

Source: FAOSTAT [12]

Figure 4. Major producer's countries of cauliflower and broccoli worldwide in 2012.

3. GLUCOSINOLATES

3.1. Chemical Nature

A characteristic of cruciferous plants is the synthesis of sulfur-rich compounds, such as glucosinolates [13]. The *Brassicas*, and a few other edible plants drawn from the order Capparales are the source of all glucosinolates in the human diet. Around 100 different compounds have been identified, which are distributed throughout the plant, although its concentration varies between tissues [14]. Glucosinolates are synthesized and stored in plants as relatively stable precursors of isothiocyanates.

Glucosinolates are water soluble, anionic, non-volatile, and heat-stable, they do not possess direct biological activity. These are located within the vacuole of plant cell [15]. Glucosinolates are classified as S-glycosides (Figure 5), because they are the result of binding a reducing sugar and sulfur in a molecule that has a carbohydrate character (known as aglycone) [16]. The glucose molecule, which imparts hydrophilic characteristics to glucosinolates, is unlike isothiocyanates that has hydrophobic properties [17].

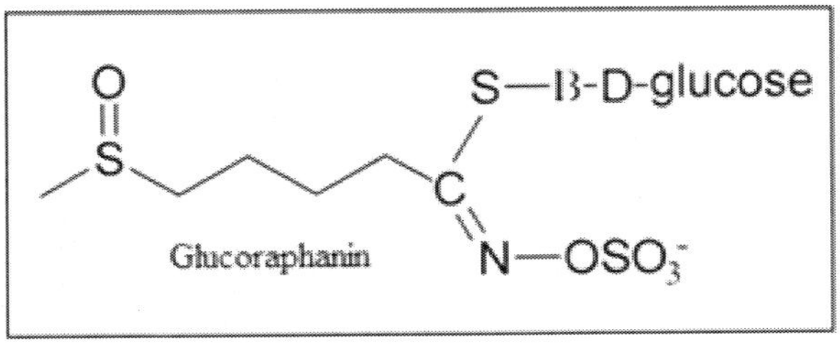

Source: Bones & Rossiter [18].

Figure 5. Chemical structure of glucoraphanin.

Glucosinolates are synthesized by the Shikimic Acid Pathway, whose precursors are the three amino acids: phenylalanine, tryptophan and tyrosine. These three amino acids provide the carbon atoms for the production of glucosinolates in the family *Brassicaceae* [16]. Furthermore, hybrids can be obtained with high glucoraphanin (sulforaphane precursor) by implanting genome segments from the wild ancestor of *Brassica villosa* [19]. Some glucosinolates present in broccoli are shown in Table 4.

Table 4. Major glucosinolates found in broccoli

Glucosinolates (GLS)	Chemical name	Trivial names
Aliphatic-GLS	4-Metyl-sulphinyl-3-butenyl-glucosinolate	Glucoraphanin
	2(R)-Hidroxy-3-butenyl-glucosinolate	Progoitrin
	3-Metyl-sulphinyl-propyl-glucosinolate	Glucoiberin
	5-Metyl-sulphinyl-pentenyl-glucosinolate	Glucoalyssin
	3-Butenyl-glucosinolate	Gluconapin
	2-Propenyl-glucosinolate	Sinigrin
	2-Hidroxy-4-pentenyl-glucosinolate	Napoleiferin
Indole-GLS	4-Hydroxy-3-indolyl-methyl-glucosinolate	4-Hydroxy-Glucobrassicin
	3-Indolyl-methyl-glucosinolate	Glucobrassicin
	4-Methoxy-3-indolyl-methyl-glucosinolate	4-Methoxy-Glucobrassicin
	1-Methoxy-3-indolyl-methyl-glucosinolate	Neoglucobrassicin
Phenyl-GLS	2-Phenyll-ethyl-glucosinolate	Gluconasturtiin

Source: Baik et al. [20]; Delaquis & Mazza [7].

3.2. Hydrolysis

Glucosinolates are chemically stable in tissues and normal cells. However when the tissue and plant cells are damaged (chopped or chewed) glucosinolates are hydrolyzed (Figure 6) by a group of enzymes thioglucosidases (E.C. 3.2.3.1.) or myrosinases. These enzymes are contacted with the substrate and release glucose molecules, bisulfate and the corresponding aglycone (Thiohydroximate-O-sulphonate), which then undergoes an intramolecular (Lossen) arrangement that generates isothiocyanates, nitriles, methylisothiocyanates, methylnitriles and thiocyanates (all of low molecular weight), which are responsible for the typical odor and flavor of these products [15, 18, 21, 22]. The reaction conditions at 40°C and neutral pH are necessary for efficient conversion of sulforaphane from glucoraphanin. The isothiocyanates formed are insoluble in water, but easily soluble in organic solvents such as methanol, dichloromethane, acetonitrile and ethyl acetate [15].

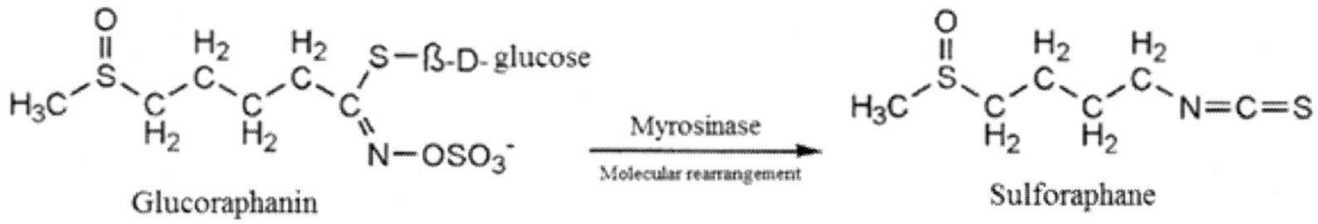

Source: Vermeulen et al. [23].

Figure 6. Reaction of hydrolysis of glucoraphanin to sulforaphane.

The type of products generated during the enzymatic hydrolysis of glucosinolates will depend on the pH conditions in which to carry out the reaction, the presence of metal ions (such as Fe^{2+} ions) and other protein elements (ESP, epithiospecifier protein) [18]. Glucosinolates with consistent aliphatic chain on a β-hydroxyl group spontaneously form isothiocyanates, which cyclize to form oxazolidine-2-thiones; these compounds and their hydrolysis products are known for their toxic effects (mainly as goitrogenic, see also Chapter 2) in man and animals in high doses, in contrast to low doses that act as chemoprotective agents [24]. Intact glucosinolates have limited biological activity, but increase their activity when hydrolyzed to isothiocyanates [13].

Farming practices, storage conditions, and food preparation conditions have a potential impact on the hydrolysis of glucosinolates. The system glucosinolate-myrosinase present in cruciferous vegetables has a significant variability due to the myrosinase activity and the concentration of cofactors [25]. Table 5 shows the bioactive compounds (isothiocyanates) of great importance in broccoli, which result from the hydrolysis of glucosinolates.

3.3. Effect of Growth Conditions

During evolutionary and cultivation processes brassica plants may have developed typical profiles of glucosinolates, which are involved in defense mechanisms against insects and phytopathogens [28]. Genetic factors and environmental factors contribute significantly to the variation in levels of glucosinolates in brassica plants. Other factors that can influence this variation include growing sites, soil type, sulphate and nitrate fertilization, climate and date of harvest [29]. Growing broccoli under optimal temperatures will produce broccoli with higher nutritive and bioactivity values through activated glucosinolates biosynthesis [30]. Sulfur fertilization will accelerate the biosynthesis of aliphathic glucosinolates and nitrogen fertilization enhanced indolic glucosinolates [31]. Specifically, the application of $ZnSO_4$ as a sulphur (S)-source enhanced glucoraphanin content in broccoli sprouts [32]. Mølmann et al. [33] found that both temperature and light can influence sensory and phytochemical contents of broccoli florets. Low temperature and long photoperiod seem to produce the highest aliphatic glucosinolate content, while the indolic glucosinolate content seems to favor a short photoperiod and high temperature.

Table 5. Major isothiocyanates found in broccoli

Glucosinolate (precursor)	Isothiocyanates (hydrolysis products of glusosinolates)	
	Chemical name	Trivial name
Glucoraphanin	1-isothiocyanate-4-(methylsulphinyl)butane	Sulforaphane
Progoitrin	1-cyano-2-hydroxy-3-butene	Crambene
Glucoiberin	1-isothiocyanate-3-methylsulphinylpropane	Iberin
Sinigrin	3-isothiocyanate-1-propene	Allyl-isothiocyanate
Glucobrassicin	Indole-3-carbinol	I3C

Source: Moreno et al. [26]; Van Eylen et al. [27]

3.4. Post-Harvest Stability

Hydrolysis of glucosinolates can take place during harvest and storage caused by senescence. Domestic and commercial treatments including chopping, blanching, cooking, steaming, microwaving and freezing have wide impact on glucosinolates content [29]. The postharvest process that has the most effect on glucosinolate content is the cooking. In general microwaving and boiling resulted in the largest losses of glucosinolates, and steaming minimizes the loss of glucosinolates. Moreover, the leaching of glucosinolates into of cooking water is a major cause of loss [34]. According to Cieślik et al. [35] the blanching of cruciferous vegetables results in significant decreases in total glucosinolates ranging from 2.7% to 30%. Nevertheless, boiling leads to higher losses of total glucosinolates compared to blanching, ranging from 35.3% to 72.4%. Glucobrassicin content in broccoli and cauliflower was not affected (even increased) by steam cooking. However, boiling treatment during 5, 10 and 20 minutes showed a slight decrease, but pickling and fermentation treatments showed a significant decrease in the concentration of this glucosinolate [36].

On the other hand, some authors have studied the effect of the storage conditions in the content of glucosinolates in broccoli. According to Vallejo et al. [37], during storage at 1°C over 7 days, over 3 days at 15°C, the degraded quantity of glucosinolates was in the range of 71 to 80%. In another study, during broccoli storage the effect of postharvest treatments and packaging in the content of glucoraphanin was evaluated. It was determined that at 20°C, the concentration of glucoraphanin decreased by 55% the third day after being stored in open boxes. Moreover, a loss of 56% in broccoli stored in plastic bags at was found at 7 days. The glucoraphanin concentration fluctuated slightly during 25 days while stored in controlled atmospheres (1.5% O_2 + 6% de CO_2) with air at 4°C. Also, it was found that broccoli heads, stored without packing at 4°C, last a week without important losses in glucoraphanin concentration [38]. Cooling and controlled atmosphere treatments (21% O_2 + 10% CO_2 at 5°C) maintain the glucosinolates content of the broccoli florets for 20 days [39]. Moreover, packaging of broccoli florets in a polyethylene film (4 µm thick, 20 cm x 30 cm) without holes is a simple, economical and effective method for maintaining the visual quality and chemopreventive glucosinolates content [40].

4. SULFORAPHANE

4.1. Chemical Nature

Sulforaphane has a molecular weight of 177.29 and a molecular formula $C_6H_{11}NOS_2$. Its chemical structure (Figure 7) has a sulfoxide group wherein the sulfur is a chiral center with four different groups around the sulfur: oxygen, a four-carbon chain terminating in an isothiocyanate, a methyl group and the electron pair solitary [41]. Because of this, the isothiocyanates are strongly electrophilic compounds that can react with nucleophilic groups such as thiol, hydroxyl, and amino groups to form dithiocarbamates, thiourea derivatives or thiocarbamates [42]. In addition, broccoli is the primary natural source of sulforaphane precursor glucoraphanin and its isothiocyanate that constitutes between 50% and 80% of total glucosinolates present in this vegetable [27, 43].

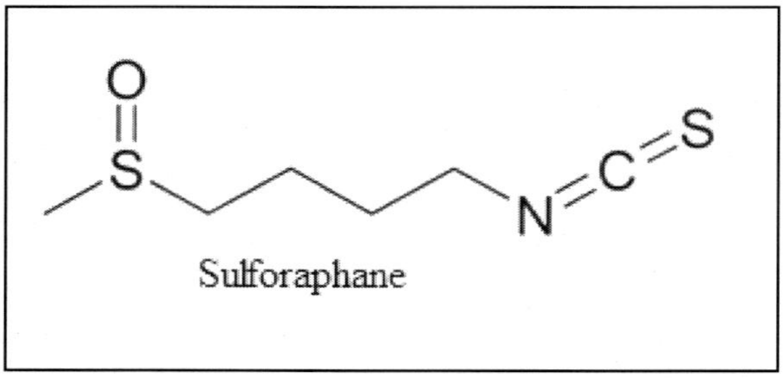

Figure 7. Chemical structure of sulforaphane.

4.2. Metabolism and Bioavailability

Sulforaphane is absorbed in the intestinal epithelium, enters the circulatory system and is subsequently conjugated with glutathione and eventually excreted in the urine as the corresponding conjugate of N-acetylcysteine or as mercapturic acids [25]. Glutathione-sulforaphane conjugates are the means of transport of this bioactive compound through the human body.

Sulforaphane that passes into the small intestine is absorbed by passive diffusion. Within epithelial cells sulforaphane can bind to glutathione (GSH + SFN) or in its simplest form, can be excreted into the intestinal lumen by active transport through P-glycoprotein (Pgp-1) or resistant protein multiple drugs (MRP-1) and discarded in feces together with unabsorbed fraction. Sulforaphane and SFN+GSH that is not excreted from epithelial cells pass via passive diffusion into the bloodstream. Within the enterocytes, sulforaphane can spontaneously bind to glutathione or N-acetylcysteine, and is transported to the tissues subsequently processed in the metabolic pathway of the mercapturic acids and subsequently excreted in the urine [44].

The FDA [45] has defined the term bioavailability as the rate and extent to which active substances or therapeutic moieties contained in a drug are absorbed and becomes available at the site of action. The absorption and bioavailability of sulforaphane is affected by multiple factors. The first factor involves the hydrolysis of glucoraphanin to sulforaphane through myrosinase activity. This first step is critical because only the correct form of ITC is biologically active and has the desired properties against cancer. It is noteworthy that mammalian cells have no endogenous myrosinase activity. Myrosinases are found in the plant. However, myrosinase is heat labile and therefore cooking procedures inactivate the enzyme and can significantly reduce the bioavailability of sulforaphane up to three times. Another source of myrosinase activity is the intestinal microbial flora. Studies indicate that glucoraphanin can be converted to sulforaphane by the colonic flora [46, 47, 48].

In human studies [49] it has been found that the concentration of total isothiocyanates (this includes sulforaphane) in blood plasma begins to increase from 30 minutes after consumption, and reaching a peak between 1.5 to 3 hours, depending on the source of sulforaphane and food with which it is accompanied. After being absorbed and metabolized most of the ingested sulforaphane (around 60-65%) is excreted in urine as N-acetylcysteine+Sulforaphane (SFN-NAC) within 24 hours. In experiments performed in rodents it has been found that sulforaphane after being transported through the bloodstream is distributed in virtually all tissues of the body. In most cases a peak concentration is reached between 4 and 6 hours after consumption and becomes almost undetectable after 24 hours, except in prostate tissue [50].

4.3. Distribution and Postharvest Stability

The content of sulforaphane in broccoli has been widely studied for its biological activity. The concentration of the precursor of sulforaphane (glucoraphanin) varies greatly depending on the genotype, maturity of tissues and postharvest treatment. It is also important to mention that the chemical conditions (such as pH, presence of metal ions, the activity of the enzyme myrosinase and its cofactors) where the conversion of glucoraphanin to sulforaphane takes place are crucial to its final concentration [25]. In the mature plant, the inflorescence has the largest concentration. However sprouts and seeds have higher contents of sulforaphane compared to mature broccoli [51]. Furthermore, it is noteworthy that the processing of the vegetable has a significant effect on the content of sulforaphane, some data obtained in our laboratory show that the sulforaphane content decreases by 50% on the third day in fresh broccoli kept at room temperature. Furthermore broccoli frozen and refrigerated for 7 days had a sulforaphane loss of 14 and 29%, respectively [52]. Sulforaphane was not detected in broccoli flour obtained by convection drying at 60°C [53]. Moreover, during the lactic acid fermentation process of pickling broccoli it was not possible to detect quantifiable sulforaphane. In addition we found that blanching broccoli at 60°C for 3 minutes increases the conversion efficiency of glucoraphanin to sulforaphane. Table 6 shows the results of sulforaphane content broccoli parts reported by different authors.

Table 6. Sulforaphane content in the broccoli plant

Sample	Sulforaphane content (µg/g dry matter)	Reference
Broccoli florets (Autolyzed samples)	17.99	Bertelli et al. [54]
Broccoli florets (Autolyzed samples)	12.69	
Broccoli florets (pH 3 hydrolysis)	31.82	
Broccoli florets (pH 3 hydrolysis)	49.28	
Broccoli stalks (pH 3 hydrolysis)	17.45	
Broccoli leaves (pH 3 hydrolysis)	110.03	
Broccoli commercial: Cultivar Brigadier	335	Matusheski et al. [55]
Cultivar Brigadier +	603	
Broccoli seeds: Zhongqing II	4748	Liang et al. [21]
Greenshirt	4548	
Greenyu	2036	
Broccoli 70	1619	
Greenball	1349	
Greenwave	2746	
Mature broccoli (supermarket) A: Florent	1713	Nakagawa et al. [56]
Stem	893	
Mature broccoli (supermarket) B: Florent	691	
Stem	443	
Mature broccoli (supermarket): Florent	585	Campas-Baypoli et al. [52]
Leaves	420	
Stalks	229	

The method to quantify sulforaphane used in our laboratory, consist in four phases, the first is the conversion of glucoraphanin to sulforaphane, the second is the extraction with dichloromethane, the third is purification in column of the solid phase extraction (SPE) and last the chromatography quantification HPLC-DAD [52]. Figure 8 shows the variation in the content of sulforaphane for different types of samples.

Although sulforaphane has been demonstrated to have great promise as a chemopreventive agent, its potential for clinical use is limited by the number of factors that can affect its bioavailability including the food matrix and the instability under normal storage conditions [57], due to its a sensitive compound to the oxidants, pH, temperature and heating time, favoring its degradation after exposure to these factors [58, 59].

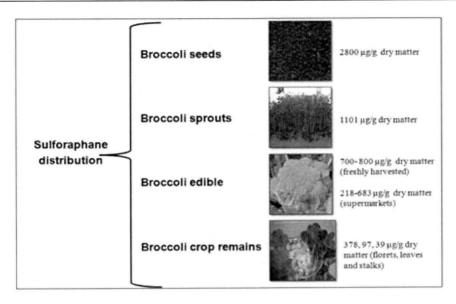

Figure 8. Sulforaphane concentration in seeds, sprouts, florets and crop remains of broccoli.

4.4. Beneficial Effects in Health

A balanced alimentation is essential for an adequate nutrition and health. The discovery of bioactive (phytochemicals) in food suggests the possibility to improve public health through the diet. Even so, the content of those phytochemicals in edible plants is very variable, which make the quality control and food intake recommendations really problematic. The variations depend on environmental and genetic factors, growing conditions, harvest, storage, processing, and preparation of food [60]. As some authors mention [61, 62, 63], fruit and vegetable consumption is not a guarantee of reduction in breast cancer. However, there exists sufficient evidence to state that the *Brassica* genus has a potential effect in the prevention of this type of cancer. Also, the isothiocyanate levels in urine in Asia populations have been correlated with a reduction in breast cancer risk in pre- and post-menopausal women [64].

The biotransformation process consists in the chemical conjugation that increases the solubility of the potentially toxic substances with the goal to facilitate excretion (see Chapter 4), this effect is called generally detoxication [65]. Sulforaphane is considered a powerful inducer of the phase II enzymes (e.g., glutathione-S-transferase, quinone reductase) [66, 67] that inactivate potential carcinogens. Sulforaphane acts as an indirect antioxidant. This has been shown in *in vivo* (animals) and in *in vitro* (cell culture) experimental models that reduce the incidence of some tumors [54]. Another benefit to health is its *in vitro* antimicrobial activity against *Helicobacter pylori* [68] (see Chapter 13). Furthermore, recent studies have shown that the topical application of broccoli sprout extract rich in sulforaphane protects against ultraviolet rays on animals and humans [69] (see Chapter 10).

A variety of *in vitro* and *in vivo* studies indicate that sulforaphane has high anticarcinogenic activity against breast, prostate, lung, stomach, skin and others types of cancer [69, 70, 71, 72]. Some of the proposed mechanisms about the chemopreventive and anticarcinogenic mechanisms include: **a)** the detoxification of potentially carcinogenic substances by the induced phase II enzymes (e.g., glutathione-S-transferase, quinone reductase) [66, 67]. Sulforaphane forms a bond with Keap1-Nrf2 complex by direct reaction with the sulfhydryl groups of the cysteine residues of Keap1 [70], thereby activating the nuclear factor Nrf2 signalling pathway, which induces enzymes that repair some of the damages caused by the free radicals is induced [73]; **b)** through modulation of the phase I cytochrome P-450 (CYP) enzymes that are important in the normal metabolic processing of numerous endogenous and exogenous compounds, but can also activate certain chemical carcinogens [74]; **c)** by the induction of the apoptosis and cell cycle arrest, in tumor cells. It has been reported that sulforaphane can activate a variety of programmed cell death mechanisms including the mitochondria-mediated apoptosis, the death receptor mediated apoptosis, death cell by autophagy and the arrest of cell in phase G2/M of the cell cycle; **d)** by the inhibition of the angiogenesis and metastasis through inhibition of vascular endothelial cell growth factor thus inhibiting new blood vessels formation in tumors [70].

5. PERSPECTIVES ON SULFORAPHANE RESEARCH

The chemopreventive and anticarcinogenic capacity of the sulforaphane has been widely documented in a great quantity of *in vitro* and *in vivo* studies. A growing interest exist in the activity of sulforaphane against cancer has developed. This is why there has been, in the last years, a great amount of research to establish the main mechanisms of action of sulforaphane, both *in vivo* and *in vitro,* and the development of markers to monitor sulforaphane intake. We have discovered that the main disadvantage of sulforaphane is its rapid degradation in the food matrix as well as in the purified extracts. This is the reason why a variety of strategies are being studied to improve its chemical stability and effectiveness, for example the creation of encapsulates using micro-spheres with bovine serum albumin [75], with polymers such as poly-lactid acid/poli-glycolic acid [76], liposomes [75] and inclusion complex formation with β-cyclodextrin [59]. Currently, our investigation group is working to determine the bioavailability of natural sulforaphane extracts in different biological matrices, as well as in the research of alternatives to improve its stability through the microencapsulation process.

REFERENCES

[1] Oronoz M, Roaro D, Rodríguez I. Tratado elemental de Botánica. 15ta ed.: Ed. ECLALSA; 1983. México DF p. 663-664.
[2] Schery RW. Plantas útiles al hombre. Colección Agrícola Salvat, Barcelona, España. 1956. p 756.
[3] Sánchez S. La flora del valle de México. 6ª. Edición. 1980. México, D.F. pp. 150.
[4] FAO, Organización de las Naciones Unidas para la Agricultura y la Alimentación. 2006. Ficha técnica del brócoli. Available in: http://www.fao.org/inpho/content/documents/vlibrary/ae620s/Pfrescos/BROCOLI.HTM.
[5] LeStrange M,. Mayberry KS, Koyke ST, Valencia J. La Producción de Brócoli en California. Centro de Información e Investigación de Hortalizas Serie de Producción de

Hortalizas. 2003. University of California – Division of Agriculture and Natural Resources Publication 7211-Spanish.

[6] West LG, Meyer KA, Balch BA, Rossi FJ, Schultz MR, Haas GW. Glucoraphanin and 4-Hydroxyglucobrassicin Contents in Seeds of 59 Cultivars of Broccoli, Raab, Kohlrabi, Radish, Cauliflower, Brussels Sprouts, Kale, and Cabbage. *J Agric Food Chem* 2004; 52(4): 916-926.

[7] Delaquis P, Mazza G. Productos funcionales en las verduras. En: Mazza, G. Alimentos funcionales aspectos bioquímicos y de procesado. 2nd ed. Zaragoza, España: Acribia SA; 2000. p. 200-204.

[8] Arala LH, Clavijo RC, Herrera C. Capacidad antioxidante de frutas y verduras cultivados en Chile. *Arch Latinoam Nutr* 2006; 56(4): 361-365.

[9] Carvalho PT, Clemente E. The influence of the Broccoli (*Brassica oleracea var. Itálica*) fill weight on postharvest quality. Ciência e Tecnologia de Alimentos, Campinas 2004; 24(4): 646-651.

[10] Chen Y, Chen LO, Shaw J. Senescence-associated genes in harvested broccoli florets. Plant Sci 2008; 175: 137-144.

[11] U.S. Department of Agriculture, Agricultural Research Service. 2014. USDA National Nutrient Database for Standard Reference, Release 27. Nutrient Data Laboratory Home Page, http://www.ars.usda.gov/ba/ bhnrc/ndl.

[12] FAOSTAT. Organización de las Naciones Unidas para la Agricultura y la Alimentación Estadísticas. 2014. Índices de producción. Available in: http://faostat.fao.org/site/ 612/default.aspx#ancor.

[13] Nafisi M, Sonderby IE, Hansen BG, Geu-Flores F, Nour-Eldin HH, Norholm MHH, Jensen NB, Li J, Halkier BA. Cytrochromes P450 in the biosinthesis of glucosinolates and indole alkaloids. *Phytochem Rev* 2006; 5: 331-346.

[14] Pokorny J., Yanishlieva N., Gordon M. Antioxidantes de los alimentos, aplicaciones prácticas. Ed. ACRIBIA, S.A. España; 2001. p. 111-112.

[15] Gu Z, Guo Q, Gu Y. Factors influencing glucoraphanin and sulforaphane formation in Brassica plants: A review. *J Integr Agric.* 2012; 11(11): 1804-1816.

[16] Lampe, JW. Spicing up a vegetarian diet: chemopreventive effects of phytochemicals. *Am J Clin Nutr* 2003; 78 (suppl): 579S-583S.

[17] Fahey JW, Zhang Y, Talalay P. Broccoli sprouts: An exceptionally rich source of inducers of enzymes that protect against chemical carcinogens. *Proc Natl Acad Sci* 1997; 94: 10367-10372.

[18] Bones AM, Rossiter JT. The enzymic and chemically induced decomposition of glucosinolates. *Phytochemistry* 2006; 67(11): 1053–1067.

[19] Sarikamis G, Marquez J, MacCormack R, Bennett RN, Roberts J, Mithen R. High glucosinolate broccoli: a delivery system for sulforaphane. *Mol Breed* 2006; 18: 219–228.

[20] Baik HY, Juvic JA, Jeffery EH, Walling MA, Kushad M, Klein BP, Relating glucosinolate content and flavor of broccoli cultivars. *J Food Sci* 2003; 68(3):1043-1050.

[21] Liang H, Yuan QP, Xiao Q. Purification of sulforaphane from *Brassica oleracea* seed meal using low-pressure column chromatography. *J Chromatogr B* 2005; 828: 91–96.

[22] Valdés MSE. Hidratos de Carbono. En: Badui SD. Química de los Alimentos. 4ta ed. México D.F: Pearson Educación; 2006. pag. 41-46.

[23] Vermeulen M, Klöpping-Ketelaars IWAA, Van Denberg R, Vaes WHJ. Bioavailability and Kinetics of Sulforaphane in Humans after Consumption of Cooked versus Raw Broccoli. *J Agric Food Chem* 2008; 56(22): 10505-10509.

[24] Das S, Tyagi AK, Kaur H. Cancer modulation by glucosinolates: A review. *Curr Sci* 2000; 79(12): 1665–1671.

[25] Rungapamestry V, Duncan AJ, Fuller Z and Ratcliffe B. Effect of cooking brassica vegetables on the subsequent hydrolysis and metabolic fate of glucosinolates. *Proc Nutr Soc* 2007; 66 (1): 69–81.

[26] Moreno DA, Carvajal M, López-Berenguer C, García-Viguera C. Chemical and biological characterisation of nutraceutical compounds of broccoli. *J Pharm Biomed Anal* 2006; 41: 1508–1522.

[27] Van Eylen D, Bellostas N, Strobel BW, Oey I, Hendrickx M, Van Loey A, Sørensen H, Sørensen JC. Influence of pressure/temperature treatments on glucosinolate conversion in broccoli (Brassica oleraceae L. cv Italica) heads. *Food Chem* 2009; 112(3): 646-653.

[28] Meyer M, Adam ST. Comparison of glucosinolate levels in commercial and red cabbage from conventional and ecological farming. *Eur Food Res Technol* 2008; 226: 1429-1437.

[29] Dekker M, Verkerk R, Jongen MF. Predictive modeling of health aspects in the food production chain: a case study on glucosinolates in cabbage. *Trends Food Sci Technol* 2000; 11: 174–181.

[30] Pék Z, Daood H, Nagyné MG, Neményi A, Helyes L. Effect of environmental conditions and water status on the bioactive compounds of broccoli. *Cent Eur J Biol* 2013; 8(8): 777-787.

[31] Falk KL, Tokuhisa JG, Gershenzon J. The effect of sulfur nutrition on plant glucosinolate content: physiology and molecular mechanisms. *Plant Biol* 2007; 9: 573-581.

[32] Yang R, Guo L, Jin X, Shen C, Zhou Y, Gu Z. Enhancement of glucosinolates and sulforaphane formation of broccoli sprouts by zinc sulphate via its stress effect. *J Funct Foods* 2015; 13: 345-349.

[33] Mølmann JAB, Steindal ALH, Bengtsson GB, Seljåsen R, Lea P, Skaret J, Johansen TJ. Effects of temperature and photoperiod on sensory quality and contents of glucosinolates, flavonols and vitamin C in broccoli florets. *Food Chem* 2015; 172: 47–55.

[34] Jones RB, Frisina CL, Winkler S, Imsic M, Tomkins RB. Cooking method significantly effects glucosinolate content and sulforaphane production in broccoli florets. *Food Chem* 2010; 123: 237-242.

[35] Cieślik E, Leszczyńska T, Filipiak-Florkiewicz ES, Pisulewski PM. Effects of some technological processes on glucosinolate contents in cruciferous vegetables. *Food Chem* 2007; 105: 976-981.

[36] Sosińska E, Obiedziński MW. Effect of processing on the content of glucobrassicin and its degradation products in broccoli and cauliflower. *Food control* 2011; 22: 1348-1356.

[37] Vallejo F, Tomás-Barberán F, García-Viguera C. Health-Promoting Compounds in Broccoli as Influenced by Refrigerated Transport and Retail Sale Period. *J Agric Food Chem* 2003; 51: 3029-3034.

[38] Rangkadilok N, Tomkins B, Nicolas ME, Premier RR, Bennett RN, Eagling DR, Taylor PW. The Effect of Post-Harvest and Packaging Treatments on Glucoraphanin Concentration in Broccoli (*Brassica oleracea var. italica*). *J Agric Food Chem* 2002; 50: 7383-7391.

[39] Xu C, Guo D, Yuan J, Yuan G, Wang Q. Changes in glucoraphanin content and quinone reductase activity in broccoli (Brassica oleracea var. italica) florets during cooling and controlled atmosphere storage. *Postharvest Biol Technol* 2006, 43: 175-184.

[40] Jia C, Xu C, Wei J, Yuang J, Yuang G, Wang B, Wang Q. Effect of modified atmosphere packaging on visual quality and glucosinolates of broccoli florets. *Food Chem* 2009; 114: 28-37.

[41] Whitesell JK, Fox MA. Química orgánica. Segunda edición. Editorial Addison Wesley Longman S.A. de C.V. ISBN: 968-444-335-8, 2000, pag 268.

[42] Song D, Liang H, Kuang P, Tang P, Hu G, Yuang Q. Instability and structural change of 4-methiylsulfinyl-3-butenyl isotiocyanate in the hydrolitic process. *J Agric Food Chem* 2013; 61: 5097-5102.

[43] Borowski J, Szajdek A, Borowska EJ, Ciska E, Zieliński H. Content of selected bioactive components and antioxidant properties of broccoli (*Brassica oleracea L.*). *Eur Food Res Technol* 2008; 226: 459–465.

[44] Jhonson IT. Phytochemicals and cancer. *Proc Nutr Soc* 2007; 66: 207-215.

[45] Food and Drug Administration (FDA). 2014. Code of Federal Regulation. Title 21- Food and drugs, Chapter I, Volume 5, part 320. Available in: http://www.accessdata.fda.gov, cite: 21CFR320.

[46] Conaway CC, Getahun SM, Liebes LL, Pusateri DJ, Topham DKW, Botero-Omary M, Fung-Lung C. Disposition of Glucosinolates and Sulforaphane in Humans After Ingestion of Steamed and Fresh Broccoli. *Nutr Cancer* 2000; 38(2): 168-178.

[47] Clarke JD, Dashwood RH, Ho E. Multi-targeted prevention of cancer by sulforaphane. *Cancer Lett* 2008; 269(2): 291-304.

[48] Boddupalli S, Mein JR, Lakkanna S, James DR. Induction of phase 2 antioxidant enzymes by broccoli sulforaphane: perspectives in maintaining the antioxidant activity of vitamins A,C y E. *Front Genet* 2012; 3(7): 1-15.

[49] Cramer J, Teran-Garcia M, Jeffery E. Enhancing suforaphane absortion and excretion in healthy men through the combined comsumption of fresh broccoli sprouts and a glucoraphanin-rich powder. *Br J Nutr* 2011; 10: 1–6.

[50] Clarke J., Hsu A., Williams D., Dashwood R., Stevens J., Yamamoto M., Ho E. Metabolism and tissue distribution of sulforaphane in Nrf2 Knockout and wild-type mice. *Pharm Res* 2011; 28: 3171–3179.

[51] López-Cervantes J, Tirado-Noriega LG, Sánchez-Machado DI, Campas-Baypoli ON, Cantú-Soto EU, Núñez-Gastélum JA. (2013): Biochemical composition of broccoli seeds and sprouts at different stages of seedling development. *Int J Food Sci Technol* 48: 2267-2275.

[52] Campas-Baypoli ON, Sánchez Machado DI, Bueno-Solano C, Ramírez-Wong B., López-Cervantes J. HPLC method validation for measurement of sulforaphane level in broccoli by-products. *Biomed Chromatogr* 2010; 24: 387-392.

[53] Campas-Baypoli ON, Sánchez-Machado DI, Bueno-Solano C, Núñez-Gastélum JA, Reyes-Moreno C, López-Cervantes J. Biochemical composition and physicochemical properties of broccoli flours. *Int J Food Sci Nutr* 2009; 60:1-11.

[54] Bertelli D, Plessi M, Braghiroli D, Monzani A. Separation by solid phase extraction and quantification by phase reverse HPLC of sulforaphane in broccoli. *Food Chem* 1998; 63(3): 417-421.

[55] Matusheski NV, Jeffery HE Comparison of the Bioactivity of Two Glucoraphanin Hydrolysis Products Found in Broccoli, Sulforaphane and Sulforaphane Nitrile. *J Agric Food Chem* 2001; 49: 5743-5749.

[56] Nakagawa K, Umeda T, Higuchi O, Tsuzuki T, Suzuki T, Miyazawa T. Evaporative light-scattering analysis of sulforaphane in broccoli samples: Quality of broccoli products regarding sulforaphane contents. *J Agric Food Chem* 2006; 54(7): 2479-2483.

[57] Van Eylen D, Oey I, Hendrickx M, Van Loey. Kinetics of the Stability of Broccoli (*Brassica oleracea Cv. Italica*) Myrosinase and Isothiocyanates in Broccoli Juice during Pressure/Temperature Treatments. *J Agric Food Chem* 2007; 55(6): 2163-2170.

[58] Wu H, Liang H, Yuan Q, Wang T, Yan X. Preparation and stability investigation of the inclusion complex of sulforaphane with hydroxypropyl-β.cyclodextrin. *Carbohydr Polym* 2010; 82(3): 613-617.

[59] Wu Y, Mao J, You Y, Liu S. Study on degradation kinetics of sulforaphane in broccoli extract. Food Chem 2014; 155: 235-239.

[60] Jeffery EH, Brown AF, Kurilich AC, Keck AS, Matusheski N, Klein BP, Juvic JA. Variation in content of bioactive components in broccoli. *J Food Compost Anal* 2003; 16: 323–330.

[61] Michels KB, Giovannucci E, Joshipura K J, Rosner BA, Stampfer MJ, Fuchs CS, Colditz GA, Speizer FE, Willett WC. Prospective Study of Fruit and Vegetable Consumption and Incidence of Colon and Rectal Cancers. *J Natl Cancer Inst* 2000; 92(21): 1740-1752.

[62] Flood A, Velie EM, Chaterjee N, Subar AF, Thompson FE, Lacey JV, Schairer C, Troisi R, Schatzkin A. Fruit and vegetable intakes and the risk of colorectal cancer in the

[63] Riboli E, Norat T. Epidemiologic evidence of the protective effect of fruit and vegetables on cancer risk. *Am J Clin Nutr* 2003; 78(3Suppl): 559S-569S.

[64] Fowke JH, Chung FL, Jin F, Qi D, Cai Q, Conaway C, Cheng J, Shu XO, Gao YT, Zheng W. Urinary Isothiocyanate Levels, Brassica, and Human Breast Cancer. *Cancer Res* 2003; 63:3980–3986.

[65] Mckee T, Mckee JR. Biochemistry: the molecular basis of life. Biotransformation Chapter Nineteen. The Mc Graw-Hill companies. 3rd edition. 2003: 559-566.

[66] Zhang Y, Callaway EC. High cellular accumulation of sulphoraphane, a dietary anticarcinogen, is followed by rapid transporter-mediated export as a glutathione conjugate. *Biochem J* 2002; 364: 301-307.

[67] Morimitsu Y, Nakagawa Y, Hayashi K, Fujii H, Kumagai T, Nakamura Y, Osawa T, Horio F, Itoh K, Lida K, Yamamoto M, Uchida K. A Sulforaphane Analogue that Potently Activates the Nrf2-dependent Detoxification Pathway. *J Biol Chem* 2002; 277(5): 3456–3463.

[68] Haristoy X, Angioi-Duprez K, Duprez A, Lozniewski A. Efficacy of Sulforaphane in Eradicating Helicobacter pylori in Human Gastric Xenografts Implanted in Nude Mice. *Antimicrob Agents and Chemother* 2003; 47(12): 3982-3984.

[69] Talalay P, Fahey JW, Healy ZR, Wehage SL, Benedict AL, Min C, Dinkova-Kostova AT. Sulforaphane mobilizes cellular defenses that protect skin against damage by UV radiation. *Proc Natl Acad Sci* 2007; 104(44): 17500-17505.

[70] Zhang Y, Tang L. Discovery and development of sulforaphane as a cancer chemopreventive phytochemical. *Acta Pharmacol Sin* 2007; 28(9): 1343-1354.

[71] Xu C, Shen G, Chen C, Gélinas C, Kong AT. Suppression of NF-κB-regulated gene expression by sulforaphane and PEITC through IκBα, IKK pathway in human prostate cancer PC-3 cells. *Oncogene* 2005, 24: 4486-4495.

[72] Pawlik A, Wiczk A, Kaczyńska A, Antosiewicz J, Herman-Antosiewicz A. Sulforaphane inhibits growth of phenotypically different breast cancer cells. *Eur J Nutr* 2013; 52: 1949-1958.

[73] Garber K. A radical treatment. *Nature,* 2012; 489: S4-S6.

[74] Yoxall V, Kentish P, Coldham N, Kuhnert N, Sauer MJ, Ioannides C. Modulation of hepatic cytochromes P450 and phase II enzymes by dietary doses of sulforaphane in rats: Implications for its chemopreventive activity. *Int J Cancer* 2005, 117: 356-362.

[75] Do DP, Pai SB, Rizvi SAA, D'Souza MJ. Development of sulforaphane-encapsulated microspheres for cancer epigenetic theraphy. *Int J Pharm* 2010; 386: 114-121.

[76] Ko J, Choi Y, Jeong G, Im G. Sulforaphane-PLGA microspheres for the intra-articular treatment of osteoarthritis. *Biomaterials* 2013; 34: 5359-5368.

[77] Narayanan N, Nargi D, Randolph C, Narayanan BA. Liposome encapsulation of curcumin and resveratrol in combination reduces prostate cancer incidence in PTEN knockout mice. *Int Journal Cancer* 2009; 125: 1-8

In: Broccoli
Editor: Bernhard H. J. Juurlink

ISBN: 978-1-63484-313-3
© 2016 Nova Science Publishers, Inc.

Chapter 16

BROCCOLI: NUTRITIONAL ASPECTS, HEALTH BENEFITS AND POSTHARVEST CONSERVATION

José Guilherme Prado Martin, Natalia Dallocca Berno and Marta Helena Fillet Spoto*

Fruits and Vegetables Laboratory, Agri-food Industry, Food and Nutrition Department, Luiz de Queiroz College of Agriculture, University of São Paulo (USP), Piracicaba/SP, Brazil

ABSTRACT

Broccoli (*Brassica oleracea* var. italica) is recognized as a vegetable rich in bioactive compounds that have different biological properties. There are a large number of scientific studies relating to the benefits of broccoli consumption. Less recognized is that one requires the application of proper conservation techniques for optimal retention of these bioactive compounds. In this chapter we discuss the main health benefits of broccoli, with reference to its nutritional content and biofunctionality of its components.

We also discuss the different post-harvest techniques necessary for preservation of these health-benefitting characteristics of broccoli.

HEALTH BENEFITS OF BROCCOLI

There are many studies relating certain compounds found in broccoli to biological activities such as antioxidant [1], anti-inflammatory [2], antimicrobial [3] and anti-proliferative activity [4], among others. We can highlight the glucosinolates, which are assigned as one of the major broccoli bioactive components. Some of the glucosinolate

---

* Corresponding author: Fruits and Vegetables Laboratory, Agri-food Industry, Food and Nutrition Department, Luiz de Queiroz College of Agriculture, University of São Paulo (USP). Av. Pádua Dias, 11, CEP 13418-900, Piracicaba/SP, Brazil. E-mail: jguilhermepm@usp.br.

bioactivity can be related to the ability of the human intestinal microbiota to perform the hydrolysis generating various bioactive compounds that are absorbed primarily in the human colon [5].

The release of glucosinolates occurs only through a physical procedure on the broccoli tissue structure, such as: processing, cutting, cooking, freezing and even during chewing [6, 7]. When such physical disruption occurs the glucosinolates are exposed to the action of myrosinase enzyme that is also presented in the plant. Myrosinase is responsible for hydrolyzing the glucosinolates to isothiocyanates, compounds with biological activity [8].

One of the most studied isothiocyanates is sulforaphane. Broccoli is recognized as one of the vegetables with the greatest amount of this component. Sulforaphane is of interest mainly due to its properties in preventing cancer and as is an inducer of nuclear factor erythroid 2-related factor 2 (Nrf2), the latter is responsible for the activation of endogenous defenses of the cell by activating specific cytoprotective genes [9].

In the next few sections we discuss the main biological activities of broccoli by presenting some scientific studies developed in recent years, especially broccoli's antioxidant, anti-proliferative, and nutritional properties.

Antioxidant and Anti-Proliferative Activity

Yuan et al. (2010) evaluated the antioxidant activity of extracts obtained from fresh broccoli according to various methodologies, such as DPPH radical assay, Superoxide anion radical assay and Hydroxyl radical assay. The authors point out a high antioxidant activity due to the presence of isothiocyanates; among the main compounds with antioxidant potential, sulforaphane has been identified as a major contributor to this activity. The amount of isothiocyanates present, however, is strongly influenced by temperature and storage conditions. This study demonstrated the potential use of broccoli as a source of isothiocyanates for food additives, in order to produce healthy foods in the future [1]. Kaulman et al. (2014) identified a high antioxidant activity in broccoli through FRAP and ABTS methodologies. Their antioxidant activity was mainly attributed to the presence of flavonoids, chlorogenic acid, anthocyanins, lutein, and vitamin C. Thus, vegetable consumption should prevent inflammatory diseases and oxidative stress related generally to chronic diseases [10].

An antioxidant activity was also investigated in fresh broccoli and in broccoli juice extract. The extracts based on methanol and acetone exhibited a higher amount of antioxidants compared to the aqueous extracts. However, there was no significant difference in the total phenolic content compared to the vegetable *in natura*. The antioxidant activity demonstrated a significant relationship with the flavonoid content found in plant tissue [11].

Jang et al. (2015) assessed the antioxidant capacity of fresh broccoli sprout extracts prepared by three different methods: distilled water, dichloromethane and lyophilization. All the extracts showed high antioxidant activity, especially freeze-dried extracts. The compound in the highest concentration identified by gas chromatography was 5-methylthiopentylnitrile, an isothiocyanate recognized as a great antioxidant. They also identified other antioxidants phenolic compounds such as 4-1-methylpropyl phenol, 4-methylphenol and 2-methoxy-4-vinylphenol. The authors emphasized the importance of broccoli as a major source of natural antioxidants [12].

Melo et al. (2014) also highlighted the presence of considerable amounts of phenolic compounds in unconventional edible parts of several vegetable crops, especially broccoli stalks, that showed the highest antioxidant activity among the samples analyzed [13]. Martin et al. (2012) also reported the presence of phenolic compounds with antioxidant potential in different agro-industrial wastes, including broccoli stalks, plant portions that are usually discarded during vegetable consumption, and that have, according to the authors, a potential for the extraction of antioxidants to be used as natural preservatives in food [14].

Some research has shown the possibility of applying broccoli extracts as natural antioxidants, more specifically in food, as viable alternatives to chemical additives used for this purpose. Banerjee et al. (2012) evaluated the antioxidant capacity of broccoli extract powder and its application in goat meat nuggets at different concentrations.

The results were similar to the activity of butylated hydroxytoluene (BHT), an antioxidant used by the food industry. Moreover, its application did not cause undesirable effects on the sensory characteristics of the nuggets, proving the extracts to be a viable alternative antioxidant in this type of food product [15].

Duthie et al. (2013) evaluated the effects of dried broccoli extracts on oxidative stability of turkey meat patties. Although to a lesser extent in comparison with other evaluated vegetables, broccoli extracts were able to improve the oxidative stability of the product, mainly because of the high concentration of phenolic compounds. Thus, the use of vegetable powders with chemical complexity offers an alternative to isolated antioxidants, and can help to increase the shelf-life of food of animal origin [16].

Several studies have linked the consumption of broccoli to a reduced risk of developing different types of cancer. It is known that the effect of the bioactive compounds in broccoli on the body is related to the reduction risk of lung, stomach, colon and rectal cancers, and to a lesser extent, prostate, endometrial and ovarian cancers [17].

Broccoli glucosinolates are able to reduce cancer risk by preventing the cancerous cell metabolism and inducing apoptosis. A significant inhibition of superoxide radical formation was observed using extracts of seeds, shoots, leaves and broccoli florets, with significant differences in the composition of glucosinolates isolated from these structures; florets showed the highest antioxidant activity [18].

Ambrosone et al. (2004) observed an inversely proportional association between the consumption of broccoli and the risk of breast cancer in women during menopause. The authors postulated that the consumption of this vegetable might play an important role in reducing breast cancer risk in women who are premenopausal [19].

Xu et al. (2015) demonstrated the antiproliferative power of purified polysaccharides extracted from broccoli in models of liver, cervical and breast carcinoma. The results obtained from the models studied reinforce the need for further research elucidating the mechanisms of action of these compounds that may in the future be used as additives in functional foods [20]. Bachiega et al. (2016) evaluated the effect of biofortification process during the broccoli maturation process on the phenolic compounds content and antioxidant capacity of the plant. The authors concluded that the biofortification process consists of a viable and effective technique to increase significantly the antioxidant capacity in broccoli and its cancer anti-proliferative effect as shown *in vitro* [4]. Some scientific surveys have shown the capacity of fortified fertilizer to contribute significantly to increase the levels of glucosinolates in broccoli. The application of sulfur, nitrogen and selenium during cultivation of broccoli favors the production of these components in plant tissue [21].

Source of Vitamins and Minerals

Broccoli plants are rich in vitamins, compounds essential for the normal development of the organism since they are precursors of important enzyme cofactors necessary for metabolic processes. Moreover, vitamins play important roles in the regulation of mineral metabolism of cells and tissues during growth and differentiation [22].

Ascorbic acid, for example, is regarded as a vitamin largely responsible for the antioxidant capacity of plant materials. Humans are unable to synthesize it and are therefore dependent on food sources for their supply. Vitamin C is essential to neutralize the action of free radicals involved in the aging process, assist in collagen synthesis, in addition to a role in the absorption of iron in the body [23].

A portion of 91 g of raw broccoli provides, in recommended daily amounts per person (diet based in 2000 kcal daily): about 11% of vitamin A, 116% of vitamin K and 135% of vitamin C (81.2 mg). The plant also provides significant quantities of folic acid (14%), vitamin B6 (8%), riboflavin (6%) and pantothenic acid (5%). Other important vitamins found are vitamin E (α-tocopherol) (4%), thiamine and niacin [24].

Among the mechanisms by which broccoli has a beneficial effect on health are the presence of high amounts of micronutrients such as folic acid and other vitamins. Therefore, broccoli presents itself as an important component for providing the basic vitamins necessary for maintenance of metabolism; thus, its daily intake becomes relevant in health promotion [25].

In relation to minerals, the same portion of raw vegetable provides 10% of daily recommended manganese intake, 8% of potassium, 6% of phosphorus, 5% of magnesium, 4% of calcium and phosphorus. Broccoli also provides selenium (5%), zinc (2%) and copper (2%). Noteworthy is the low concentration of sodium (1%), relevant in a scenario in which there is an increasing restriction to the daily intake of sodium in order to reduce the damage caused by high blood pressure, contributing in this way to the better life quality of the population [24].

Broccoli also provides significant amounts of dietary fiber (9%), 5% of protein and minimal amounts of fat: a portion of 91 g of raw broccoli contains only 0.3 g of total fat. It is, therefore, a healthy source of vitamins and minerals, since the energy input by its consumption is significantly reduced, contributing to healthier diets with reduced amounts of fat [24].

In addition to the plant, its seedlings also consist of important source of bioactive health promoters. Medina et al. (2015) evaluated the effect of the consumption of daily doses of broccoli sprouts (30 and 60 g) on urinary biomarkers in humans. The diet produced an increase in the concentration of metabolites for sulforaphane and vitamin C, both negatively associated with inflammation and vascular reactions, without exerting any significant influence on the oxidation of phospholipids in vivo. This research therefore showed the beneficial effect of broccoli sprouts against inflammation and cardiovascular problems in humans obtained from the daily intake of vegetable [2].

It is worth pointing out that the thermal processes generally used in the preparation of the plant for human consumption cause significant loss of these compounds of interest, as they degrade important enzymes in the process of release and availability of phytochemicals [8]. Thus, choosing the best method of cooking before consumption is essential to keep its beneficial nutritional characteristics.

Martinez et al. (2013) evaluated the effects of different heat treatments on the bioactive compounds of broccoli (see also Chapter 17). All the treatments caused significant losses in glucosinolate levels, highlighting boil and *sous-vide*, that accounted for reductions of around 80%. Regarding the ascorbic acid concentration, treatment with microwaves was the least harmful, demonstrating a loss of 21%, while the *sous-vide* caused a reduction of over 90% in the levels of vitamin C. In general, cooking in steam under low pressure (low pressure steaming) and microwave methods had the least effects on the content of bioactive compounds in broccoli [26].

The effects of different cooking processes of a broccoli-based product have been evaluated. The main health promoting compounds were significantly affected by the cooking methods used, such as cooking, frying, baking and microwave. No changes were observed in total phenolic content; however, the antioxidant activity was significantly impaired. The cooking processes, except for cooking and baking using steam, resulted in significant losses in chlorophylls, carotenoids and flavonoids, with approximate loss ranging from 15 to 60%. The concentration of glucosinolates decreased significantly during all the processes employed, except for the microwaving [27].

Hamausu and Zhang (2004) demonstrated the effects of heat treatment on the reduction of bioactive compounds broccoli florets and stems using conventional cooking and microwave. The authors observed that the concentrations of phenolic compounds after these processes were reduced to about 1/3 of the initial concentration for florets, and to about 1/2 for stems; the quantities of ascorbic acid was reduced to half of the initial concentration for both structures. The antioxidant activity suffered loss of about 2/3 for the samples submitted to the thermal process. The results demonstrate that great losses of antioxidant compounds occur during the cooking of the broccoli, and the authors suggest that these losses should be considered in intake calculating of these compounds from cooked broccoli [28].

Other Biological Activities

Researchers observed that the use of broccoli and fermented products made from this plant can suppress the differentiation of osteoclasts through the suppression of lipid peroxidation in serum in subjects consuming high-cholesterol diets, thus preventing bone loss thereby assisting in the prevention of osteoporosis [29].

Townsend et al. (2014) demonstrated that dietary interventions through the controlled intake of broccoli can reduce the oxidative stress and the glial reactivity responsible for the aging process. Thus, a high-broccoli diet can help prevent chronic degenerative diseases and to reduce the effects of natural senescence process that affects the proper functioning of the body [30].

Mueller et al. (2013) evaluated the protective and curative effect of broccoli extracts on process-induced colitis in rats through oral administration of the plant material during the experiment. The extracts were able to decrease the levels of mRNA for vascular cell adhesion molecule 1 (VCAM-1), molecules that play an important role in the early stages of the inflammatory response. Broccoli extracts, therefore, showed significant anti-inflammatory effects and promises to be an agent for the prevention of intestinal inflammatory diseases [31].

Antimicrobial activity of broccoli stems was observed against *Listeria monocytogenes*. The broccoli stem extract showed antimicrobial activity against this microorganism. Analysis by CG-MS allowed the identification of organic acids such as ascorbic and malic acids, and phenolic compounds such as sinapinic, ferulic and caffeic acids. The use of flow cytometry to evaluate the antimicrobial activity of the extracts was very suitable, enabling one to infer their mechanism of action. The authors reinforce the importance of new studies about the use of vegetal wastes as sources of natural preservatives in food and beverage industry [3].

Besides the importance of high levels of bioactive compounds in broccoli, its storage mode and postharvest treatment strongly influences the conservation of its biological properties. Therefore, the application of techniques to preserve its properties is fundamental in offering consumer products with considerable amounts of beneficial compounds. In the next section we present the main postharvest techniques and their relation to preservation of the bioactive compounds.

POST-HARVEST TECHNIQUES and Bioactive COMPOUNDS CONTENT IN BROCCOLI

Broccoli contains several chemical compounds of great importance to consumer health, particularly vitamin C and phytochemicals, such as glucosinolates, flavonoids and carotenoids. However, these benefits are only achieved if the vegetable presents the expected quality. With a short shelf-life, around three days at 20°C [32] or two days at 25°C [33], it is necessary to apply some techniques capable of extending its use but also maintaining the intrinsic quality of the broccoli, mainly the compounds of interest. These changes reinforce the importance of the post-harvest period in the product conservation.

Despite the impossibility to completely stop the reactions that occur in plants after harvest, these can be minimized. Some technologies used in post-harvest can reduce plant metabolism and visual or qualitative losses, thus increasing the shelf-life of the product [34, 35]. In this topic, we present the main technologies used in post-harvest and its effects on broccoli bioactive compounds.

Storage Temperature

The first and main technology used in post-harvest of fruits and vegetables conservation is the application of low temperatures during storage. It can be considered the most economical method for long-term storage of fruits and vegetables [34]. For broccoli, it is recommended a storage between 0 and 4°C and 98-100% relative humidity (RH). Under these conditions, the vegetable durability will be around 2 to 3 weeks [36].

The storage at low temperatures, concomitantly with increase of humidity environment, aims to reduce the biological activity, microorganism's growth and water loss. Thus, the metabolic rate of the product is kept to a minimum [34].

Several studies have shown that the storage temperature has a major influence on the content of vitamin C. Kaluzewicz et al. (2012) shown that storage at ambient temperature storage for 6 and 24 hours resulted in a great loss in the vitamin C content of broccoli 'Monterey' as contrasted to broccoli stored at recommended temperatures [37].

Likewise, Rybarczyk-Plonska et al. (2014) demonstrated that the vitamin C content of broccoli 'Marathon' was reduced 20% during the pre-storage at 0 and 4°C for 7 days and storage at 10°C and 18°C for three days [38].

The antioxidant capacity is also influenced by storage temperature. Kevers et al. (2007) demonstrated a decrease of more than 50% in antioxidant capacity (DPPH) of broccoli stored under 4°C for 27 days [39].

On the other hand, several studies have shown that flavonoid content is relatively stable to the storage temperature. Kaluzewicz et al. (2012) observed an increase in quercetin, kaempferol and total flavonoids content during storage at room temperature and a decrease in total flavonoids and kaempferol content at cold storage [37]. Other studies with broccoli chilled (4°C during 27 days) showed a transient increase in phenolic compounds content [39]. The broccoli 'Marathon' didn't present significant differences in glucoraphanin, quercetin and kaempferol content when it was stored at 1 and 4°C followed by three days at commercialization temperature (8, 15 or 20°C), although there was great loss in the visual quality [40].

Yuan et al. (2010) demonstrated that broccoli stored at 20°C for 5 days greatly lost some compounds such as total aliphatic and glucosinolates. Similarly, Xu et al. (2013) proved that total glucosinolate and sulforaphane content from broccoli stored at 15°C for 5 days is decreased considerably [41]. These compounds can be preserved using storage at lower temperatures, as demonstrated by Rangkadilok et al. (2002), who observed a decrease of 50% in glucoraphanin content in broccoli 'Marathon' after 7 days stored at 20°C, remaining stable at 4°C [42].

Thus, it was concluded that the temperature and the time of storage has no harmful effects on the level of flavonoids from broccoli, whose stability have been showed.

However, it cannot be extended to vitamin C, antioxidant capacity and components such as glucosinolates and sulforaphane, for which storage temperatures are very important.

Controlled and Modified Atmosphere (MAP)

The gas concentration in the atmosphere around the plant can be controlled when there is a strict control of the gas content within storage chambers, or it can be modified by the appliance of gas within the packaging. Regardless of how this change is achieved, its aim consists of reducing the oxygen and increasing the carbon dioxide concentration. The benefits of atmosphere modification consists of retarding the maturation and the senescence of vegetables, and to control certain biological processes such as microorganisms' growth and rot of the vegetable tissues. This technology has been widely studied for increasing the shelf-life of horticultural products during transportation, storage and marketing [34, 43, 44].

The application of oxygen around 10 kPa and CO_2 between 1 and 2 kPa already can reduce the respiration rate and sensitivity to ethylene and, as well, affect the maturation, development and senescence processes of vegetables. Furthermore, CO_2 concentrations above 10 kPa inhibit the growth of many microorganisms [45-47].

To prevent intrinsic physiological disorders for broccoli the recommended CO_2 and O_2 concentrations are around 5-10% and 1-2%, respectively, and temperatures around 0-5°C

(48). O_2 concentrations below 1% and CO_2 above 10% may cause the appearance of off flavor and anaerobic respiration, contributing to the degradation of the product [49].

Similarly, a condition of 100% of O_2 also becomes harmful, accelerating the aging process of broccoli [50]. A study using controlled atmosphere for conservation of broccoli showed that the concentration of 10% O_2 and 5% CO_2 under 1-2°C and 85-90% RH during 21 days was effective in maintaining the visual aspects and the health promoting compounds such as chlorophyll, carotenoids, phenolic compounds, phenolic acids, flavonols, glucosinolates and antioxidant capacity, as compared to broccoli under standard atmosphere. The same O_2 and CO_2 concentrations were more efficient in preserving quality, maintenance of bioactive compounds and extending shelf-life of 'Parthenon' broccoli than using 1-methylcyclopropene (1-MCP) at low temperatures [51].

Guo et al. (2013) observed that an environment with 40% O_2 and 60% CO_2 at 15°C was capable of extending the storage period, keeping the post-harvest quality and reducing oxidative stress and lipid peroxidation in broccoli 'Youxiu' [50].

Regarding the use of packaging, Serrano et al. (2006) studied the influence of different packaging (macro-perforated, micro-perforated and non-perforated) on the functional quality of broccoli 'Marathon' stored at 1°C and 90% RH for 28 days. The authors demonstrated that the containers were capable of maintaining a high antioxidant activity, reducing the loss of vitamin C and phenolic compounds, preserving visual aspects and extending the shelf-life of the vegetable [52]. Similarly, Carvalho and Clemente (2004) showed that the modified atmosphere is an effective technique for broccoli 'Legacy,' especially in relation to the preservation of fresh weight, turgor and vitamin C [53]. The use of minimal processing combined with the use of packaging resulted in a better retention of vitamins, moisture and color in florets of broccoli during post-harvest storage [54].

The low density polypropylene packaging also contributed to reduction in the loss of glucoraphanin in broccoli. While not-packaged broccoli lost 50% of these compounds, those stored under modified atmosphere conditions showed no change during 10 days [42].

Vallejo et al. (2003) found that broccoli stored in low density polyethylene containers (11 mm thick) showed a small variation in the content of vitamin C, both at 1°C for seven days as at 15°C for 3 days. However, since the change of gas concentrations inside the package was not significant, the content of flavonoids and glucosinolates suffered a great loss, caused by the natural aging process of the plant [55]. It is especially important to highlight that to improve this technology it is possible to use it combined with low temperatures [56]. Furthermore, the choice of the packaging material is very important, since the permeability of the material interferes with the gas concentration. Both techniques involved in the physiology and biochemistry of plants should be considered in post-harvest of these products.

Edible Coatings

Edible coatings are thin layers of material applied and adhered directly to the surface of a food product; this covering is considered as part of the final product.

The application of these coatings improves the product quality; protects them from physical damage, chemical and biological deterioration; reduces particle agglomeration; and improve the visual and tactile characteristics of the product surface. Edible coatings can also protect from moisture loss or gain, growth of microorganisms, changes induced by light and oxidation of nutrients. Moreover, it can be a carrier of antioxidants, antimicrobials, dyes and condiments [57-59].

The coatings can be manufactured from different types of materials, such as proteins, polysaccharides (starch and non-starch polysaccharides), lipids and biopolymers. The choice should be based on the specific food application and the major quality deterioration mechanisms. The use of coating may partially or totally replace the conventional packages [57, 59].

Some studies have shown that the use of chitosan and carboxymethylcellulose may reduce the loss of vitamin C and chlorophyll [60]. Other research has evaluated the application of chitosan films in the microbiological quality of minimally processed broccoli, but it is not yet clear what its influence on bioactive compounds is [61].

There are yet few studies about this technique. It is possible that the physical and physiological structure of broccoli (inflorescences) can be a complicating factor in the application of coatings.

1-Methylcyclopropene

The 1-methylcyclopropene (1-MCP) is a gaseous compound recognized as an efficient inhibitor of ethylene by blocking its sites of action [62, 63]. This molecule binds to hormone receptors located in the membranes of the endoplasmic reticulum of the plant cells, thereby blocking ethylene's action [64]. The treatment with MCP-1 inhibits the maturation and represses the expression of the majority of genes regulated directly or indirectly by ethylene [65]. The use of 1-MCP has been shown to be very promising in the maintenance of the quality of broccoli, mainly by reducing the degradation of chlorophyll and significantly increasing the useful life of the plant [66-68].

Xu et al. (2013) showed that the use of 1-MCP in broccoli 'Chaoda No 1' maintains a high activity of the antioxidant enzymes during storage at 15°C, while it increases the biosynthesis of glucosinolates and the formation of sulforaphane [41]. Likewise, Ku et al. (2013) studied broccoli 'Magic Green' stored at 4°C, and observed the efficiency of MCP-1 in maintain compounds of interest [69].

Yuan et al. (2010) also demonstrated that the use of 1-MCP can extend the useful life, preserving the visual quality while reducing the loss of ascorbic acid and compounds that promote health, especially glucosinolates [1].

All studies indicate that 1-MCP contributes to the maintenance of visual and nutritional quality of broccoli, especially when storing and marketing of these products are not under the ideal temperature, as observed in countries such as Brazil and China.

Other Techniques

Other different techniques have been applied for the preservation of broccoli postharvest quality. The use of ethanol vapor (500 uL/L) was studied by Xu et al. (2012), who showed that this technique is effective in reducing the degradation of chlorophyll and increasing the total content of phenolic compounds, glucosinolates and sulforaphane from broccoli 'Chaoda No. 1' [70]. Heat treatment has also been studied. Tian et al. (1997) showed that broccoli dipped in hot water (47°C for 7.5 minutes) caused a significant reduction of respiration, starch, sucrose and soluble protein contents during the first 24 hours after harvest [71].

Zapata et al. (2013) showed that heat treatment at 50°C for 15 minutes was effective in retarding the senescence of broccoli, without any detrimental effect on the phenolic content and antioxidant capacity [72].

Jin et al. (2015) demonstrated the effects of green LED lighting on broccoli, such as increase in the total phenolic content, glucosinolates and antioxidant capacity (DPPH). This technology was capable of extending broccoli's shelf-life and maintaining the visual quality [73]. Other LED colors were used by Ma et al. (2014) that showed that irradiation with red light LED was effective in retarding senescence in broccoli after harvesting. With modified white LED there was a retardation in the decrease of ascorbate content and a reduction in the ethylene production process [74].

Lemoine et al. (2010) studied a combined treatment with hot air and UV-C radiation in broccoli minimally processed on the antioxidant system during storage at 20°C. The authors found that combination treatments increased by approximately 13% the total antioxidant levels immediately following the treatment, and also during storage. Moreover, the methodology contributed to the increment of phenolic compounds, ascorbic acid and activity of enzymes involved in the removal of reactive oxygen species [75].

Alternative technologies have shown satisfactory results in preserving the nutritional quality of broccoli, reinforcing the requirement for further studies in this area.

CONCLUSION

Scientific studies about benefits of broccoli consumption have been developed in recent years. Among broccoli's main health properties are providing some vitamins and minerals essential for metabolism. Other components promote health by slowing oxidative stress thus delaying aging, preventing inflammation, and preventing various types of cancer.

We can, however, highlight that many of these nutrients and bioactive compounds are lost during the post-harvest period. It is not yet entirely clear what technology is more efficient maintaining the biochemical compounds of interest in broccoli longer and in greater amounts, although it is known that their use helps considerably in the maintenance of the visual and nutritional quality of these products. Although many technologies have been discussed in this chapter, it is worth noting that the development of new research is necessary for a better understanding of the various technologies effects on the phytochemical content of broccoli.

REFERENCES

[1] Yuan, H., Yao, S., You, Y., Xiao, G., You, Q. Antioxidant Activity of Isothiocyanate Extracts from Broccoli. *Chinese Journal of Chemical Engineering*. 2010;18(2):312-21.

[2] Medina, S., Domínguez-Perles, R., Moreno, D. A., García-Viguera, C., Ferreres, F., Gil, J. I. et al. The intake of broccoli sprouts modulates the inflammatory and vascular

prostanoids but not the oxidative stress-related isoprostanes in healthy humans. *Food Chemistry.* 2015;173:1187-94.

[3] Correa, C. B., Correa, C. B., Martin, J. G. P., Alencar, S. M., Porto, E. Antilisterial activity of broccoli stems (*Brassica oleracea*) by flow cytometry. *International Food Research Journal.* 2014;21(1).

[4] Bachiega, P., Salgado, J. M., de Carvalho, J. E., Ruiz, A. L. T. G., Schwarz, K., Tezotto, T. et al. Antioxidant and antiproliferative activities in different maturation stages of broccoli (Brassica oleracea Italica) biofortified with selenium. *Food Chemistry.* 2016;190:771-6.

[5] Glade, M. J., Meguid, M. M. A Glance at... Broccoli, glucoraphanin, and sulforaphane. *Nutrition.* 2015;31(9):1175-8.

[6] Getahun, S. M., Chung, F.-L. Conversion of Glucosinolates to Isothiocyanates in Humans after Ingestion of Cooked Watercress. *Cancer Epidemiology Biomarkers and Prevention.* 1999;8(5):447-51.

[7] Shapiro, T. A., Fahey, J. W., Wade, K. L., Stephenson, K. K., Talalay, P. Chemoprotective glucosinolates and isothiocyanates of broccoli sprouts: metabolism and excretion in humans. *Cancer Epidemiol. Biomarkers Prev.* 2001;10(5):501-8.

[8] Angelino, D., Jeffery, E. Glucosinolate hydrolysis and bioavailability of resulting isothiocyanates: Focus on glucoraphanin. *Journal of Functional Foods.* 2014;7:67-76.

[9] Houghton, C. A., Fassett, R. G., Coombes, J. S. Sulforaphane: translational research from laboratory bench to clinic. *Nutrition Reviews.* 2013;71(11):709-26.

[10] Kaulmann, A., Jonville, M.-C., Schneider, Y.-J., Hoffmann, L., Bohn, T. Carotenoids, polyphenols and micronutrient profiles of Brassica oleraceae and plum varieties and their contribution to measures of total antioxidant capacity. *Food Chemistry.* 2014;155(0):240-50.

[11] Sun, T., Powers, J. R., Tang, J. Evaluation of the antioxidant activity of asparagus, broccoli and their juices. *Food Chemistry.* 2007;105(1):101-6.

[12] Jang, H. W., Moon, J.-K., Shibamoto, T. Analysis and Antioxidant Activity of Extracts from Broccoli (Brassica oleracea L.) Sprouts. *Journal of Agricultural and Food Chemistry.* 2015;63.

[13] Melo, C. M. T., Faria, J. V. Composição centesimal, compostos fenólicos e atividade antioxidante em partes comestíveis não-convencionais de seis olerícolas. *Bioscience Journal.* 2014;30(1).

[14] Martin, J. G. P., Porto, E., Corrêa, C. B., Alencar, S. M., Gloria, E. M., Cabral, I. S. R. et al. Antimicrobial potential and chemical composition of agro-industrial wastes. *Journal of Natural Products.* 2012;5:27-36.

[15] Banerjee, R., Verma, A. K., Das, A. K., Rajkumar, V., Shewalkar, A. A., Narkhede, H. P. Antioxidant effects of broccoli powder extract in goat meat nuggets. *Meat Science.* 2012;91(2):179-84.

[16] Duthie, G., Campbell, F., Bestwick, C., Stephen, S., Russell, W. Antioxidant Effectiveness of Vegetable Powders on the Lipid and Protein Oxidative Stability of Cooked Turkey Meat Patties: Implications for Health. *Nutrients.* 2013;5(4).

[17] Verhoeven, D. T., Goldbohm, R. A., van Poppel, G., Verhagen, H., van den Brandt, P. A. Epidemiological studies on brassica vegetables and cancer risk. *Cancer Epidemiology Biomarkers and Prevention.* 1996;5(9):733-48.

[18] Chaudhary, A., Sharma, U., Vig, A. P., Singh, B., Arora, S. Free radical scavenging, antiproliferative activities and profiling of variations in the level of phytochemicals in different parts of broccoli (Brassica oleracea italica). *Food Chemistry.* 2014;148:373-80.

[19] Ambrosone, C. B., McCann, S. E., Freudenheim, J. L., Marshall, J. R., Zhang, Y., Shields, P. G. Breast cancer risk in premenopausal women is inversely associated with consumption of broccoli, a source of isothiocyanates, but is not modified by GST genotype. *J. Nutr.* 2004;134(5):1134-8.

[20] Xu, L., Cao, J., Chen, W. Structural characterization of a broccoli polysaccharide and evaluation of anti-cancer cell proliferation effects. *Carbohydr. Polym.* 2015;126:179-84.

[21] Verkerk, R., Schreiner, M., Krumbein, A., Ciska, E., Holst, B., Rowland, I. et al. Glucosinolates in Brassica vegetables: the influence of the food supply chain on intake, bioavailability and human health. *Mol. Nutr. Food Res.* 2009;53 Suppl. 2:S219.

[22] Ares, A. M., Bernal, J., Nozal, M. J., Turner, C., Plaza, M. Fast determination of intact glucosinolates in broccoli leaf by pressurized liquid extraction and ultra high performance liquid chromatography coupled to quadrupole time-of-flight mass spectrometry. *Food Research International.* 2015;76, Part 3:498-505.

[23] Davey, M. W., Montagu, M. V., Inzé, D., Sanmartin, M., Kanellis, A., Smirnoff, N. et al. Plant L-ascorbic acid: chemistry, function, metabolism, bioavailability and effects of processing. *Journal of the Science of Food and Agriculture.* 2000;80(7):825-60.

[24] *NutritionData.* SelfNutrionData - Raw Broccoli http://nutritiondata.self.com/facts/vegetables-and-vegetable-products/2356/22015 [cited 2015 22/08/15].

[25] Berenbaum, F. Does broccoli protect from osteoarthritis? *Joint Bone Spine.* 2014;81(4):284-6.

[26] Martinez-Hernandez, G. B., Formica, A. C., Falagan, N., Artes, F., Artes-Hernandez, F., Gomez, P. A. et al. Extending the Shelf Life of the New Bimi (R) Broccoli by Controlled Atmosphere Storage. *Vii International Postharvest Symposium.* 2013;1012: 925-32.

[27] Barakat, H., Rohn, S. Effect of different cooking methods on bioactive compounds in vegetarian, broccoli-based bars. *Journal of Functional Foods.* 2014;11:407-16.

[28] Zhang, D., Hamauzu, Y. Phenolics, ascorbic acid, carotenoids and antioxidant activity of broccoli and their changes during conventional and microwave cooking. *Food Chemistry.* 2004;88(4):503-9.

[29] Tomofuji, T., Ekuni, D., Azuma, T., Irie, K., Endo, Y., Yamamoto, T. et al. Supplementation of broccoli or Bifidobacterium longum-fermented broccoli suppresses serum lipid peroxidation and osteoclast differentiation on alveolar bone surface in rats fed a high-cholesterol diet. *Nutr. Res.* 2012;32(4):301-7.

[30] Townsend, B. E., Chen, Y.-J., Jeffery, E. H., Johnson, R. W. Dietary broccoli mildly improves neuroinflammation in aged mice but does not reduce lipopolysaccharide-induced sickness behavior. *Nutrition Research.* 2014;34(11):990-9.

[31] Mueller, K., Blum, N. M., Mueller, A. S. Examination of the Anti-Inflammatory, Antioxidant, and Xenobiotic-Inducing Potential of Broccoli Extract and Various Essential Oils during a Mild DSS-Induced Colitis in Rats. *ISRN Gastroenterol.* 2013; 2013:710856.

[32] Wang, C. Y. Effect of aminoethoxy analog of rhizobitoxine and sodium benzoate on senescence of broccoli. *Hortscience*. 1977;12(1):54-6.

[33] Finger, F. L., Endres, L., Mosquim, P. R., Puiatti, M. Physiological changes during postharvest senescence of broccoli. *Pesquisa Agropecuária Brasileira*. 1999;34:1565-9.

[34] Chitarra, M. F. I., Chitarra, A. B. Pós-colheita de frutas e hortaliças: fisiologia e manuseio. *revisada e ampliada*. 2 rev. e ampl. Lavras: Universidade Federal de Lavras, 2005. p. 785.

[35] Kader, A. A. *Postharvest technology for horticultural crops*. UCANR Publications, 2002.

[36] Toivonen, P. M. A., Forney, C. Broccoli. In: USDA A., editor. The commercial storage of fruits, vegetables, and florist and nursery stocks. *Agriculture Handbook Number 66 (HB-66)*. Washington, DC.: USDA, ARS; 2004.

[37] Kaluzewicz, A., Gliszczynska-Swiglo, A., Klimczak, I., Lisiecka, J., Tyrakowska, B., Knaflewski, M. The Influence of Short-Term Storage on the Content of Flavonoids and Vitamin C in Broccoli. *European Journal of Horticultural Science*. 2012;77(3):137-43.

[38] Rybarczyk-Plonska, A., Hansen, M. K., Wold, A.-B., Hagen, S. F., Borge, G. I. A., Bengtsson, G. B. Vitamin C in broccoli (Brassica oleracea L. var. italica) flower buds as affected by postharvest light, UV-B irradiation and temperature. *Postharvest Biology and Technology*. 2014;98:82-9.

[39] Kevers, C., Falkowski, M., Tabart, J., Defraigne, J.-O., Dommes, J., Pincemail, J. Evolution of Antioxidant Capacity during Storage of Selected Fruits and Vegetables. *Journal of Agricultural and Food Chemistry*. 2007;55(21):8596-603.

[40] Winkler, S., Faragher, J., Franz, P., Imsic, M., Jones, R. Glucoraphanin and flavonoid levels remain stable during simulated transport and marketing of broccoli (Brassica oleracea var. italica) heads. *Postharvest Biology and Technology*. 2007;43(1):89-94.

[41] Xu, F., Chen, X., Yang, Z., Jin, P., Wang, K., Shang, H. et al. Maintaining quality and bioactive compounds of broccoli by combined treatment with 1-methylcyclopropene and 6-benzylaminopurine. *Journal of the Science of Food and Agriculture*. 2013;93(5):1156-61.

[42] Rangkadilok, N., Tomkins, B., Nicolas, M. E., Premier, R. R., Bennett, R. N., Eagling, D. R. et al. The Effect of Post-Harvest and Packaging Treatments on Glucoraphanin Concentration in Broccoli (Brassica oleracea var. italica). *Journal of Agricultural and Food Chemistry*. 2002;50(25):7386-91.

[43] Floros, J. D., Matsos, K. I. Introduction to modified atmosphere packaging. In: Han, J. H. (Ed.). *Innovations in Food Packaging*. London: Academic Press, 2005. chap. 10, pp. 159-172.

[44] Yahia, E. M. Introduction. In: Yahia, E. M. (Ed.). *Modified and controlled atmospheres for the storage, transportation, and packaging of horticultural commodities*. Boca Raton, Florida: CRC Press, 2009. chap. 1, pp. 1-16.

[45] Fonseca, S. C., Oliveira, F. A. R., Brecht, J. K. Modelling respiration rate of fresh fruits and vegetables for modified atmosphere packages: a review. *Journal of Food Engineering*. 2002;52(2):99-119.

[46] Lencki, R. W. Modified atmosphere packaging for minimaly processed foods. In: Sun, D. W. (Ed.). *Emerging technology for food processing*. London: Elsevier Academic Press, 2005. chap. 28, pp. 733-756.

[47] Brandenburg, J. S., Zagory, D. Modified and controlled atmospheres packaging technology and applications. In: Yahia, E. M. (Ed.). *Modified and controlled atmospheres for the storage, transportation, and packaging of horticultural commodities*. Boca Raton, Florida: CRC Press, 2009. chap. 4, pp. 73-92.

[48] Cantwell, M., Suslow, T. Broccoli: recommendations for maintaining postharvest quality: Postharvest Technology, UCDavis; 1999 [12 January 2015]. Available from: http://postharvest.ucdavis.edu/pfvegetable/Broccoli/.

[49] Ballantyne, A., Stark, R., Selman, J. D. Modified atmosphere packaging of broccoli florets. *International Journal of Food Science and Technology*. 1988;23(4):353-60.

[50] Guo, Y., Gao, Z., Li, L., Wang, Y., Zhao, H., Hu, M. et al. Effect of controlled atmospheres with varying O-2/CO2 levels on the postharvest senescence and quality of broccoli (Brassica oleracea L. var. italica) florets. *European Food Research and Technology*. 2013;237(6):943-50.

[51] Fernandez-Leon, M. F., Fernandez-Leon, A. M., Lozano, M., Ayuso, M. C., Gonzalez-Gomez, D. Altered commercial controlled atmosphere storage conditions for 'Parhenon' broccoli plants (Brassica oleracea L. var. italica). Influence on the outer quality parameters and on the health-promoting compounds. *Lwt-Food Science and Technology*. 2013;50(2):665-72.

[52] Serrano, M., Martinez-Romero, D., Guillén, F., Castillo, S., Valero, D. Maintenance of broccoli quality and functional properties during cold storage as affected by modified atmosphere packaging. *Postharvest Biology and Technology*. 2006;39(1):61-8.

[53] Carvalho, P. d. T., Clemente, E. The influence of the broccoli (Brassica oleracea var. itálica) fill weigth on postharvest quality. *Food Science and Technology (Campinas)*. 2004;24(4):646-51.

[54] Barth, M. M., Zhuang, H. Packaging design affects antioxidant vitamin retention and quality of broccoli florets during postharvest storage. *Postharvest Biology and Technology*. 1996;9(2):141-50.

[55] Vallejo, F., Tomás-Barberán, F., García-Viguera, C. Health-Promoting Compounds in Broccoli as Influenced by Refrigerated Transport and Retail Sale Period. *Journal of Agricultural and Food Chemistry*. 2003;51(10):3029-34.

[56] Nath, A., Bagchi, B., Misra, L. K., C. Deka B. Changes in post-harvest phytochemical qualities of broccoli florets during ambient and refrigerated storage. *Food Chemistry*. 2011;127(4):1510-4.

[57] Han, J. H., Gennadios, A. Edible films and coatings: a review. In: Han, J. H. (Ed.). *Innovations in Food Packaging*. London: Academic Press, 2005. chap. 15, pp. 239-262.

[58] Lacroix, M., Le Tien, C. Edible films and coatings from nonstarch polysaccharides. In: Han, J. H. (Ed.). *Innovations in Food Packaging*. London: Academic Press, 2005. chap. 20, pp. 338-361.

[59] Pavlath, A. E., Orts, W. Edible films and coatings: why, what, and how. In: Embuscado, M. E. e Huber, K. C. (Ed.). *Edible films and coatings for food applications*. New York: Springer, 2009. chap. 1, pp. 1-24.

[60] Ansorena, M. R., Marcovich, N. E., Roura, S. I. Impact of edible coatings and mild heat shocks on quality of minimally processed broccoli (Brassica oleracea L.) during refrigerated storage. *Postharvest Biology and Technology*. 2011;59(1):53-63.

[61] Alvarez, M. V., Ponce, A. G., Moreira, M. d. R. Antimicrobial efficiency of chitosan coating enriched with bioactive compounds to improve the safety of fresh cut broccoli. *Lwt-Food Science and Technology*. 2013;50(1):78-87.

[62] Serek, M., Sisler, E., Reid, M. 1-Methylcyclopropene, a novel gaseous inhibitor of ethylene action, improves the life of fruits, cut flowers and potted plants. *Plant Bioregulators in Horticulture*, n. 394, pp. 337-346, 1994.

[63] Blankenship, S. M., Dole, J. M. 1-Methylcyclopropene: a review. *Postharvest Biology and Technology*. 2003;28(1):1-25.

[64] Sisler, E., Serek, M. Inhibitors of ethylene responses in plants at the receptor level: recent developments. *Physiologia Plantarum*, v. 100, n. 3, pp. 577-582, 1997.

[65] Gupta, S., Sharma, H., Burman, S. Anti diabetic activity of Brassica oleraceae var. italica extract in type II diabetes mellitus. *PharmaNutrition*. 2014;2(3):116.

[66] Gong, Y. P., Mattheis, J. P. Effect of ethylene and 1-methylcyclopropene on chlorophyll catabolism of broccoli florets. *Plant Growth Regulation*. 2003;40(1):33-8.

[67] Jones, R. B., Faragher, J. D., Winkler, S. A review of the influence of postharvest treatments on quality and glucosinolate content in broccoli (Brassica oleracea var. italica) heads. *Postharvest Biology and Technology*. 2006;41(1):1-8.

[68] Gomez-Lobato, M. E., Mansilla, S. A., Civello, P. M., Martinez, G. A. Expression of Stay-Green encoding gene (BoSGR) during postharvest senescence of broccoli. *Postharvest Biology and Technology*. 2014;95:88-94.

[69] Ku, K. M., Choi, J. H., Kim, H. S., Kushad, M. M., Jeffery, E. H., Juvik, J. A. Methyl Jasmonate and 1-Methylcyclopropene Treatment Effects on Quinone Reductase Inducing Activity and Post-Harvest Quality of Broccoli. *Plos One*. 2013;8(10).

[70] Xu, F., Chen, X., Jin, P., Wang, X., Wang, J., Zheng, Y. Effect of ethanol treatment on quality and antioxidant activity in postharvest broccoli florets. *European Food Research and Technology*. 2012;235(5):793-800.

[71] Tian, M. S., Islam, T., Stevenson, D. G., Irving, D. E. Color, ethylene production, respiration, and compositional changes in broccoli dipped in hot water. *Journal of the American Society for Horticultural Science*. 1997;122(1):112-6.

[72] Zapata, P. J., Tucker, G. A., Valero, D., Serrano, M. Quality parameters and antioxidant properties in organic and conventionally grown broccoli after pre-storage hot water treatment. *Journal of the Science of Food and Agriculture*. 2013;93(5):1140-6.

[73] Jin, P., Yao, D., Xu, F., Wang, H., Zheng, Y. Effect of light on quality and bioactive compounds in postharvest broccoli florets. *Food Chemistry*. 2015;172:705-9.

[74] Ma, G., Zhang, L., Setiawan, C. K., Yamawaki, K., Asai, T., Nishikawa, F. et al. Effect of red and blue LED light irradiation on ascorbate content and expression of genes related to ascorbate metabolism in postharvest broccoli. *Postharvest Biology and Technology*. 2014;94:97-103.

[75] Lemoine, M. L., Chaves, A. R., Martinez, G. A. Influence of combined hot air and UV-C treatment on the antioxidant system of minimally processed broccoli (Brassica oleracea L. var. Italica). *Lwt-Food Science and Technology*. 2010;43(9):1313-9.

In: Broccoli
Editor: Bernhard H. J. Juurlink

ISBN: 978-1-63484-313-3
© 2016 Nova Science Publishers, Inc.

Chapter 17

INNOVATIVE INDUSTRIAL COOKING OF BROCCOLI FOR IMPROVING HEALTH-PROMOTING COMPOUNDS

Ginés Benito Martínez–Hernández[1,2], Perla A. Gómez[2], Francisco Artés–Hernández[1,2] and Francisco Artés[1,2,*]

[1]Postharvest and Refrigeration Group,
Food Engineering Department,
Technical University of Cartagena (UPCT),
Murcia, Spain
[2]Food and Health Unit.
Institute of Plant Biotechnology-UPCT

ABSTRACT

Broccoli has been described as an extraordinary health promoting Brassica specie. There are a great number of epidemiological trials and laboratory studies supporting this statement. Broccoli consumption has shown numerous beneficial properties such as having chemopreventive, antioxidant, antitumor, antimutagenicity, anti–inflammatory, antimicrobial, antiviral properties as well as resulting in reduction of coronary heart disease risks. These properties are mainly related to its high content of phenolics compounds, glucosinolates (isothiocyanates), carotenoids, vitamins, unsaturated fatty acids, dietary fibre, minerals, etc. However, cooking treatments, like the ones used by the industry for preparation of Fifth Range products, may induce reductions of such bioactive compounds. For that reason, several studies have recently focused determining the effects of conventional and innovative cooking treatments on these biocompounds in order to establish the best processing conditions for better maintenance of the health-promoting properties of this vegetable.

---

[*] Corresponding author: E–mail: fr.artes@upct.es. Web site: www.upct.es/gpostref.

1. INTRODUCTION

1.1. Broccoli and Kailan-Hybrid Broccoli

Broccoli (*Brassica oleracea*, Italica group) is a vegetable of the *Brassicaceae* family. The word *broccoli* comes from the Italian plural of *broccolo*, diminutive of *brocco* (shoot), based on the Latin word *brocchus* (projecting). Broccoli has a high content of many health-promoting compounds but its particular flavor makes some consumers still reticent to choose it for their market basket. Accordingly, new broccoli varieties with milder flavor are being developed in order to promote its consumption [1]. Kailan-hybrid broccoli is a new natural hybrid between conventional broccoli (*Brassica oleracea* Italica group) and Chinese broccoli or kailan (*B. oleracea*, Alboglabra group). This hybrid was firstly developed by Sakata Seed Company (Yokohama, Japan) and registered as Bimi®. Other companies have developed different commercial kailan–hybrid varieties with registered trademarks: Asparation® (Sakata Seed America), Bellaverde® (Seminis Vegetable Seeds), Broccolini® (Mann Packaging Company), Tenderstem® (Marks and Spencer Plc.), etc. This hybrid has a long stem, similarly to an asparagus, with a small floret (Figure 1). In addition, it has more pleasant sensory characteristics (especially taste and aroma) than those of conventional cultivars (cvs) of broccoli. Furthermore, kailan-hybrid broccoli has excellent physicochemical properties that point this vegetable as a just the right raw material to be developed and marketed as a new cooked product, especially for the Fifth Range industry.

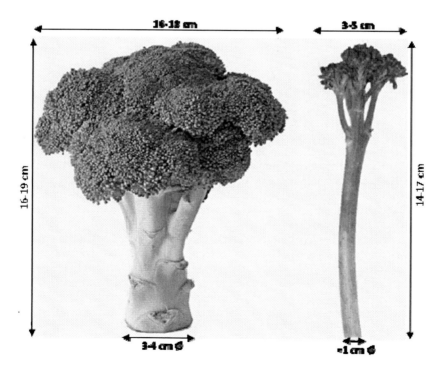

Figure 1. Conventional broccoli Parthenon cv (left) and Kailan–hybrid broccoli (right).

Because of its delicate physical properties, kailan–hybrid broccoli is hand harvested every day early in the morning. A primary packaging, including body icing precooling, is made on the field for minimizing handling, and extending shelf life. Due to its mild sensory characteristics regarding the conventional broccoli cv., it can be eaten either raw (i.e., in vegetable salads) or cooked. Mild cooking procedures can be used due to its tenderness, small size and, consequently, with high heat transmission during cooking. This represents a great advantage that drastically reduces the unavoidable nutritional losses during cooking treatments, commonly used for the consumption of the conventional broccoli cvs due to their slightly bitter and astringent flavor characteristics.

In Europe, the production of kailan-hybrid broccoli is concentrated from October to June in warm areas like Spain or Italy, while in summer it is produced in northern locations as UK, The Netherlands, etc. However, commercial production is mainly located in Africa (mainly South Africa), where it is assured all year around by intensive farming production systems. Spain is the main European kailan-hybrid producer with a cultivated surface (mainly concentrated in the south-east Mediterranean area) of about 120 ha and a production of about 1000 t in the 2014/15 campaign (data supplied by Sakata Seed Ibérica). Kailan–hybrid consumption has already begun in Belgium, UK, France, Germany, the Netherlands, Spain and the Scandinavian countries.

1.2. Main Bioactive and Nutritional Compounds of Conventional Broccoli and Kailan-Hybrid Broccoli

Gathering high quality products with a healthy diet, safety, and convenience is something to which consumers look forward. In addition to the commercial value of the fresh vegetable market, growing interest on the produce bioactive value has risen in growers and processors to specifically reach a health-oriented market. The relationship between dietary habits and health has been analyzed in several epidemiological studies showing that plant–derived foods, fruit and vegetables in a great extent, have a direct impact on preventing diseases [2]. These health–promoting properties of fruit and vegetables have been mainly associated with bioactive compounds, such as phenolics, glucosinolates, carotenoids, chlorophylls, fatty acids and antioxidant enzymes, among others. Over the last two decades, crops in the Brassicaceae have been the focus of intense research based on their health benefits [3]. The main nutritional compounds of broccoli are listed in Table 1 and described in the following paragraphs. The information data concerning the bioactive and nutritional compounds of kailan–hybrid broccoli are very scarce.

1.2.1. Dietary Fibre and proteins

The dietary fibre is mainly composed of macromolecules such as cellulose, hemicellulose, pectins, lignin, resistant starch and non–digestible oligosaccharides [7]. Broccoli is a rich source of dietary fibre with around 3 g 100 g^{-1} fw [4]. However, the dietary fibre content can greatly vary among different broccoli cvs.

Generally, the protein content of fruit and vegetables is less than 1 g 100 g^{-1} fw. However, broccoli is an excellent protein source of proteins with quantities between 1 and 4 g 100 g^{-1} fw, depending on the cv. [4, 8].

Table 1. Main constituents of conventional broccoli (Parthenon cv) and kailan–hybrid broccoli [4, 5, 6]

Constituents (per 100 g fw*)	Broccoli	Kailan-hybrid
Energy	28 kcal	29 kcal
Water	89.2 g	90.3 g
Protein (N x 6.25)	3.5 g	3.5 g
Fat	0.20 g	0.30 g
Carbohydrates	2.7 g	5.1 g
Total dietary fibre	3.0 g	3.2 g
Total minerals	6.32 g	8.27 g
Vitamin C	100 mg	411 mg
Vitamin A	373.8 µg	177.0 µg
Vitamin B$_1$	99 µg	
Vitamin B$_2$	178 µg	
Vitamin B$_5$	1.3 mg	
Vitamin B$_6$	280 µg	
Vitamin E	621 µg	
Vitamin K	154 µg	
Vitamin PP	1.0 mg	
Folic acid	114 µg	120 µg

*fw = fresh weight

1.2.2. Minerals

Conventional broccoli and kailan-hybrid broccoli are good sources of all macro elements and some important microelements, such as Fe, Zn, Mn and Cu [6] (Table 2). However, mineral composition varies among cvs and is also influenced by several preharvest factors such as climate conditions, cultural practices, etc. [9].

1.2.3. Vitamin C

Among different vitamins found in broccoli (C, B1, B2, B5, B6, E, K, etc.), vitamin C is the most abundant. The majority of vertebrates are able to synthesize vitamin C (L-ascorbic acid, L–AA), except a few mammalian species including humans; this deficiency is related to a lack of the terminal, flavo–enzyme, L–gulono–1,4–lactone oxidase [10]. L–AA (the AA isomer that occurs in nature) is stable when dry, but solutions readily oxidize, especially in the presence of trace amounts of Cu and alkali, leading to the dehydroascorbic (DHA) formation. DHA is unstable itself and undergoes irreversible hydrolytic ring cleavage to 2,3–diketogulonic acid (2, 3–DKG) that has no antiscorbutic activity, in aqueous solution. Factors such as concentration, temperature, light, pH, etc. influence the L–AA oxidation and DHA hydrolysis. The 2, 3–DKG and D–isoascorbic acid (AA stereoisomer) have little, if any, antiscorbutic activity [10]. Generally, three types of biological activity can be defined for L–AA: it is an enzyme cofactor, a radical scavenger and a donor/acceptor in the electron transport either at the plasma membrane or the chloroplasts [10]. The L–AA dietary needs are a minimum intake of 60 mg day^{-1}, with a recommendation to be increased to 75 mg day^{-1} for women and 90 mg day^{-1} for men [11].

Table 2. Mineral content of conventional broccoli (Parthenon cv.) and kailan–hybrid broccoli (extracted from [6])

Mineral nutrients[a]	Whole Parthenon	Whole Kalian-hybrid	Floret Parthenon	Floret Kalian-hybrid	Stem Parthenon	Stem Kalian-hybrid
P	11.1	8.0	11.1	10.0	7.6	6.4
S	13.9	10.0	13.9	14.2	9.8	6.9
Na	4.0	2.1	4.0	1.1	3.9	3.0
K	40.9	31.2	40.9	26.6	75.4	36.6
Ca	6.6	6.9	6.6	11.3	7.7	3.9
Mg	3.2	2.7	3.2	3.4	2.9	1.9
Cl	2.4	2.0	2.4	0.7	8.9	3.3
Mineral traces[b]						
Fe	122.0	37.2	122.0	124.5	57.0	59.6
Mn	43.8	40.2	43.8	71.3	19.0	16.0
Zn	64.0	42.5	64.0	70.1	32.0	24.2
Al	160.0	7.0	160.0	16.5	110.0	65.0
Si	199.0	53.0	199.0	85.0	140.0	51.0
Cu	5.0	5.0	5.0	6.3	5.0	3.5
Ni	ND	5.7	ND	8.6	ND	4.0

[a] g kg^{-1} dry weight [b] mg kg^{-1} dry weight

Among vegetables, broccoli and kailan-hybrid are considered as excellent L–AA sources. Many broccoli cvs have shown concentrations between 432 and 1,463 mg kg^{-1} fw [12]. Kailan-hybrid also registered high L–AA content, with around 1,737 mg kg^{-1} fw [5].

1.2.4. Fatty Acids

Essential fatty acids are those which must be ingested by humans and other animals, due to the incapacity to synthesize them, in order to meet body metabolic requirements. The ω–3 fatty acids can prevent cardiovascular inflammation and protect, or even enhance, the effect of medical treatments on diseases such as Alzheimer, multiple sclerosis and certain types of cancers [13]. A balanced intake of ω–6 and ω–3 fatty acids, with a ratio of 1–4:1, are recommended in order to achieve their health beneficial effects in the control of chronic diseases [14].

The major fatty acids reported in broccoli are the two unsaturated fatty acids α–linolenic [(C18:3, $\Delta^{9,12,15}$) (53% v/v) (ω–3)] and linoleic [(C18:2, $\Delta^{9,12}$) (18% v/v) (ω–6)], and the saturated palmitic (C16:0, 16% v/v). Broccoli also has small amounts of other unsaturated fatty acids (C16:1, C16:2, C16:3 and C18:1) and the saturated stearic acid (C18:0) according to Page et al. [15]. The total fatty acids content in the conventional Marathon broccoli was 34.2 µmol g^{-1} fw, with α–linolenic and linoleic acids (the main polyunsaturated fatty acids of broccoli) being approximately 19% and 53%, respectively, of the total fatty acids [15]. Similarly, Zhuang et al. [8] reported that the total polyunsaturated acid content of conventional Iron Duke broccoli represented 68% of the total fatty acids content. The linoleic, palmitic and stearic acid contents of kailan-hybrid broccoli were 8.4, 3.4 and 0.5 µmol g^{-1} fw, respectively [16].

1.2.5. Phenolic Compounds

The phenolic compounds contribute to the flavor and color of the plants. Furthermore, these compounds have many bioactive properties such as antimicrobial, antiviral, anti-inflammatory, antitumor, anticancer, antimutagenic, antioxidant potential and reduction in coronary heart disease risk [17].

The most widespread and diverse group of polyphenols in broccoli and kailan-hybrid broccoli are the hydroxycinnamic acids, flavonols and anthocyanins (Table 3). Redovniković et al. [18] studied the phenolic content of 13 different broccoli cvs, reporting data ranges for total phenolic, and sinapic and caffeic acid derivates of 15.5–26.9, 4.2–7.9 and 0.4–3.2 mg g^{-1} dw respectively. Furthermore, broccoli has been reported as one of the main dietary sources of lignans, comprising coumestans, the main group in this *Brassica* [19].

Table 3. Phenolic compounds found in broccoli and kailan-hybrid broccoli - marked as *x* - [20, 21, 22]

Phenolic Compounds	Broccoli	Kailan	Kailan-hybrid
Hydroxycinnamic acids			
3–*p*–coumaroyl quinic acid	x	x	
5–*p*–coumaroyl quinic acid		x	
5–feruloyl quinic acid		x	
Caffeic acid		x	
3–caffeoyl quinic acid (chlorogenic acid)	x	x	x
4–caffeoyl quinic acid		x	
5–caffeoyl quinic acid (neochlorogenic acid)	x	x	x
Sinapic acid		x	
1,2–disinapoylgentiobiose	x	x	x
1,2–diferuloylgentibiose	x	x	x
1–sinapoyl–2–feruloylgentiobiose	x	x	x
1–sinapoyl–2,2'–diferuloylgentiobiose	x	x	x
1–disinapoyl–2–feruloylgentiobiose		x	
1,2,2'–trisinapoylgentiobiose	x	x	x
1,2'–disinapoyl–2–feruloylgentiobiose	x	x	x
Isorhamnetin (I) derivates			
I–*O*–3–sophorotrioside–7–glucoside	x		
I–*O*–3–sophorotrioside–7–sophoroside	x		
I–*O*–3,7–di–*O*–glucoside	x		
I–*O*–diglucoside		x	
I–*O*–glucoside		x	
Quercetin (Q) derivatives			
Q–3–*O*–sophorotrioside–7–*O*–sophoroside	x		
Q–3–*O*–sophorotrioside–7–*O*–glucoside	x		
Q–3–O–sophoroside–7–*O*–glucoside	x		
Q–3,7–di–*O*–glucoside	x	x	
Q–3–*O*–sophoroside	x		

Phenolic Compounds	Broccoli	Kailan	Kailan-hybrid
Q–3–O–glucoside	x		
Q–3–O–glucoside–7–O–sophoroside	x		
Q–3–O–diglucoside		x	
Q–3–O–(caffeoyl)–sophorotrioside–7–O–glucoside	x		
Q–3–O–(caffeoyl)–diglucoside–7–O–glucoside		x	
Q–3–O–(sinapoyl)–sophorotrioside–7–O–glucoside	x		
Q–3–O–(sinapoyl)–sinapoyldiglucoside		x	
Q–3–O–(feruloyl)–sophorotrioside–7–O–glucoside	x		
Q–3–O–(p–coumaroyl)–sophorotrioside–7–Oglucoside	x		
Q–3–O–(feruloyl)–diglucoside–7–O–glucoside		x	
Q–3–O–(caffeoyl)–sophoroside–7–O–glucoside	x		
Q–3–O–(p–coumaroyl)–sophoroside–7–O–glucoside	x		
Q–3–O–(feruloyl)–sophoroside	x		
Kaempferol (K) derivatives			
K–3–O–tetraglucoside–7–O–sophoroside			
K–3–O–(hydroxyferuloyl)–diglucoside–7–O–glucoside		x	
K–3–O–(caffeoyl)–diglucoside–7–O–glucoside		x	
K–3–O–sinapoyltriglucoside–7–O–diglucoside		x	
K–3–O–sinapoyldiglucoside–7–O–glucoside		x	
K–3–O–sophorotrioside–7–O–sophoroside	x		
K–3–O–sohorotrioside–7–O–glucoside	x		
K–3–O–sophoroside–7–O–diglucoside	x		
K–3–O–sophoroside–7–O–glucoside	x		
K–3–O–sophoroside–7–O–sophoroside	x		
K–3,7–di–O–glucoside	x		
K–3–O–sophoroside	x		
K–3–O–triglucoside–7–O–diglucoside		x	
K–3–O–glucoside	x		
K–3–O–glucoside–7–O–sophoroside	x		
K–3–O–(caffeoyl)–sophorotrioside–7–Osophoroside	x		
K–3–O–(methoxycaffeoyl)–sophorotrioside–7–Osophoroside	x		
K–O–(sinapoyl)–sophorotrioside–7–O–sophoroside	x		
Kaempferol (K) derivatives (continuation)			
K–O–(feruloyl)–sophorotrioside–7–O–sophoroside	x		

Table 3. (Continued)

Phenolic Compounds	Broccoli	Kailan	Kailan-hybrid
K–3–O–(sinapoylhydroxyferuloyl)–triglucoside–7–O–diglucoside		x	
K–3–O–(feruloylhydroxyferuloyl)–triglucoside–7–O–diglucoside		x	
K–3–O–(p–coumaroyl)–diglucoside–7–O–glucoside		x	
K–3–O–(feruloyl)–triglucoside–7–O–glucoside		x	
K–3–O–(diferuloyl)–triglucoside–7–O–diglucoside		x	
K–3–O–(feruloyl)–diglucoside–7–O–glucoside		x	
K–3–O–(p–coumaroyl)–sophorotrioside–7–O–sophoroside	x		
K–3–O–(p–coumaroyl)–glucoside–7–O–sophoroside		x	
K–3–O–(caffeoyl)–sophorotrioside–7–O–glucoside	x		
K–3–O–(methoxycaffeoyl)–sophorotrioside–7–O–glucoside	x		
K–O–(sinapoyl)–sophorotrioside–7–O–glucoside	x		
K–O–(feruloyl)–sophorotrioside–7–O–glucoside	x		
K–3–O–(caffeoyl)sophoroside–7–O–glucoside	x		
K–3–O–(methoxycaffeoyl)–sophoroside	x		
K–3–O–(sinapoyl)–diglucoside		x	
K–3–O–(disinapoyl)–triglucoside–7–O–diglucoside		x	
K–3–O–(feruloyl)–diglucoside		x	

1.2.6. Glucosinolates

The glucosinolates (previously known as mustard oils) are sulphur–containing compounds mainly found in the *Brassicaceae* Family (see also Chapters 2 and 3). Four types of glucosinolates can be found in *Brassicas*: aromatic (derived from phenylalanine), aliphatic, alkenyl (the last two derived from methionine), and indoles glucosinolates (derived from tryptophan) [23]. Myrosinase (thioglucoside glucohydrolase; EC 3.2.3.1) is largely stored in separate cell compartments from the glucosinolates. When plant cells are damaged (i.e., during food preparation, mastication or mechanical injuries caused during harvesting and handling or by predators, such as insects), glucosinolates come into contact with the myrosinase. Then, this enzyme catalyzes the glucosinolates conversion to isothiocyanates (ITC) by several reactions (Figure 2). Other products of the glucosinolate hydrolysis can be thiocyanates and nitriles, both without bioactive properties, depending on the pH or the presence of metal ions [24]. Glucosinolates are water soluble, anionic, non–volatile and heat–stable compounds. It is believed that these molecules have no significant biological activity [25]. Contrary to them, ITC are biologically active, typically lipophilic, highly reactive, volatile, malodorous and bitter [24].

Glucosinolates profiles may vary among *Brassica* species and, in turn, the glucosinolate content differs among cvs. This content is highly influenced by genetics, but their concentrations can also be significantly altered by the environment on which the crop is grown [26]. The main glucosinolates found in broccoli and kailan are glucoraphanin, glucobrassicin, gluconapin and proigoitrin (Table 4).

The most bioactive ITC found in broccoli are sulforaphane (derived from glucoraphanin), allyl isothiocyanate (derived from sinigrin) and indole–3–carbinol (derived from glucobrassicin) according to Jones et al. [27]. ITC have antibacterial and antifungal activities in plants, and provide important protection from insect and herbivore attack [28]. A range of ITC, such as sulforaphane, inhibit Phase I enzymes, responsible for the activation of carcinogens, and induce Phase II detoxification enzyme systems, thereby increasing the cancer defence mechanisms of the human body, as it has been reported *in vitro* [29-31]. ITC have also been implicated in the inhibition of cancer cell proliferation and induction of apoptosis [32-34], as well as inhibition of *Helicobacter pylori*, the bacteria responsible for stomach ulcers [35]. Furthermore, sulforaphane derived from broccoli sprouts has been linked to prevention of cardiovascular disease in rats [36].

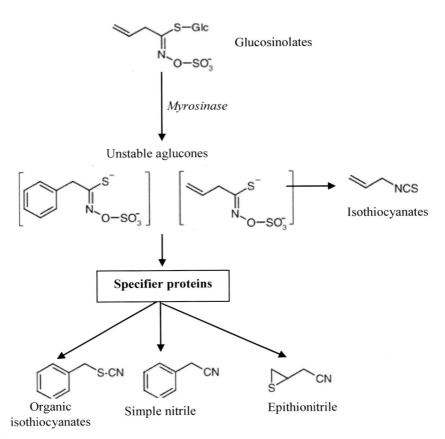

Figure 2. Enzymatic conversion of glucosinolates to isothiocyanates by plant myrosinase and non-isothiocyanate products.

Table 4. Main glucosinolates of broccoli (Emperor, Shogun, Marathon and Viola cvs) and kailan-hybrid broccoli (data from [37, 38])

Trivial name	Systematic name	Class	Content mg 100 g^{-1} fw (% relative abundance) Broccoli	Kailan-hybrid
Glucoraphanin	4–Methylsulphinylbutyl	Aliphatic	6.6–33.9 (27.6–52.3)	47.5 (27.3)
Glucobrassicin	3–Indolylmethyl	Indolyl	6.9–12.1 (11.9–42.6)	65.2 (37.4)
Gluconapin	3–Butenyl	Alkenyl	1.0 (1.6)	0.7 (0.4)
Proigoitrin	(2R) 2–Hydroxy–3–butenyl	Alkenyl	0.6–10.3 (3.7–15.8)	
4–Methoxyglucobrassicin	4–Methoxy–3–indolylmethyl	Indolyl	0.4–1.3 (1.4–3.9)	23.8 (13.7)
4–Hydroxyglucobrassicin	4–Hydroxy–3–indolylmethyl	Indolyl	0.06–0.36 (0.4–1.0)	3.4 (2.0)
Neoglucobrassicin	N–Methoxy–3–indolylmethyl	Indolyl	0.9–6.3 (3.1–9.1)	8.2 (4.7)
Sinigrin	2–Propenyl	Alkenyl	0.9 (1.5)	-
Glucoiberin	3–Methylsulphinylpropyl	Aliphatic	0.3–3.8 (1.6–14.8)	-
Glucobrassicanapin	4-Pentenyl	Aliphatic	-	19.9 (11.4)
Gluconasturtiin	2-Penylethil	Aromatic	-	5.6 (3.2)

1.2.7. Chlorophylls

There is a wide range of chlorophylls content reported in florets of conventional broccoli cvs, from 260 to 970 mg kg^{-1} fw, with chlorophyll *a* content around 3–fold higher than chlorophyll *b* [39, 40]. In contrast, whole (floret plus stem) kailan-hybrid broccoli has a 2–fold higher chlorophyll *b* content than *a* with a total chlorophyll content of about 100 mg kg^{-1} fw [22].

Chlorophylls have been associated with many health benefits, such as anti–inflammatory, antioxidant, anticancer properties and kidney stones prevention [41-44].

1.2.8. Carotenoids

Carotenoids play a very important role as protectors of chlorophyll and the photosynthetic apparatus in general, by blocking reactive forms of triplet chlorophylls (^{3}Chl) and singlet oxygen (^{1}O$_2$) formed during the capture of light energy. They also take an active part in the plant's photoprotective and antioxidant action [45]. Xanthophylls contain O$_2$ in their structure while carotenes are purely hydrocarbons, which do not have O$_2$. The xanthophyll group includes, among others, lutein, zeaxanthin, neoxanthin, violaxanthin, and *α*– and *β*–cryptoxanthin. The *α*–, *β*– and *γ*–carotenes are the main carotene types, that are very important as precursors of vitamin A [46]. *β*–carotene, *β*–cryptoxanthin, *α*–carotene, lycopene, lutein and zeaxanthin represent more than 95% of total blood carotenoids in humans. Lutein, zeaxanthin and other xanthophylls are believed to function as protective antioxidants in the macular region of the human retina. Carotenoids have also shown protection against cataract formation, coronary heart diseases and stroke [47-49]. *β*–carotene has shown other health benefits, that may be related to their antioxidant potential, such as enhancement of the immune system function [50], protection from sunburn [51], and inhibition of the development of certain types of cancers [52].

The main carotenoids found in broccoli are lutein and β–carotene with ranges of 707–3,300 and 291–1,750 µg 100 g^{-1} fw, respectively [53-55]. Lutein is also the major carotenoid found in kailan-hybrid broccoli with 1,480 µg 100 g^{-1} fw lutein content [37].

1.2.9. Antioxidant Compounds and Their Classification

The reactive oxygen species (ROS) are chemically reactive molecules containing oxygen. The ROS include oxygen ions (i.e., $^1O_2$), free radicals (O_2^-, ·OH, NO·, etc.) and peroxides (H_2O_2, ONOO$^-$, etc.). ROS are highly reactive due to the presence of unpaired valence shell electrons. ROS are natural by–products of the normal metabolism of O_2 and have important functions in cell signalling and homeostasis (see Chapter 5). However, under exogenous (heat exposure, ultraviolet light, O_3, contaminants, additives, tobacco, drugs, etc.) or endogenous (monoelectronic O_2 reduction, auto–oxidation of carbon compounds, catalytic activation of several enzymes, etc.) stresses, ROS levels can increase dramatically. This may result in damage to cell structures. Cumulatively, this is known as oxidative stress. In this way, the antioxidants are compounds that at low concentrations, compared to the substrate, delay or prevent the oxidation of that substrate during an oxidative stress [56]. According to its nature, these compounds may be classified as enzymatic or non–enzymatic antioxidants. The total antioxidant capacity (TAC) of a sample is determined by the synergistic interactions between different antioxidant compounds and for the specific reaction mechanism of each of them. The TAC can be influenced by physiological (i.e., ripening, senescence) and technological factors, such as storage and processing conditions [7].

Several epidemiological studies have shown that fruit and vegetable–rich diets reduce the incidence of cardiovascular and other chronic and degenerative diseases related to the oxidative damage [57, 58]. Thus, the protective effects of the fruit and vegetables consumption have been associated to the presence of antioxidant compounds, mainly polyphenols and vitamin C [59]. Kailan-hybrid broccoli showed about 1.6-fold higher TAC than the conventional Parthenon broccoli [6].

2. FIFTH RANGE VEGETABLES

In developed countries, due to socio-economic development, including consumer protection, technology, cultural and information access, among others, the consumer is being more exigent in food selection and more receptive to the newest food innovations. The new culinary trends search for traditional regional cuisine with local products, grown ecologically friendly or organic and/or handmade with a different relatively cheap nutrition, but more balanced, nutritive, healthy and sustainable in contrast with the usual fast food. The increasing audience for gastronomy television programs of, both traditional and innovative, is a clear example of these new consumer trends. Accordingly, in the last few years the ready–to–eat vegetable industry has developed new products in order to diversify the production and enlarge the offer for a consumer who demands new natural healthy products with high quality and reduced preparation time. The Fifth Range industry has found in the cooked vegetables sector a good market opportunity. Some of this demand also comes from the catering services and fast food chains that require larger volumes of these products.

The application of heat treatments is the most widespread food preservation technique. The sterilization treatment has allowed the appearance of canned ready–to–eat meals from traditional recipes and with a long commercial life without refrigeration. However, this treatment is commonly very aggressive against the nutritional and sensory properties of food, and especially with vegetables, causing some rejection by consumers. In order to solve these technological limitations, mild cooking techniques with a subsequent refrigerated storage have appeared to configure the Fifth Range industry of vegetables [5]. The technology used to preserve the Fifth Range vegetables includes hermetic packaging, heat treatment and cooling and can be described by the following characteristics:

- Heat–treated products, ready–to–eat and marketed under refrigeration.
- Heated prior to consumption, usually in microwave or conventional oven.
- Usually packaged in plastic materials.
- Keeping the cold chain until consumption (processing, packaging, storage and distribution).

The name of Fifth Range vegetables has been attributed primarily to vacuum–packaged boiled ready–to–heat vegetables. Lately, the Fifth Range vegetables have been described as plant based products partially vacuum packaged and heat treated (usually cooked), ready to heat and eat, ensuring a minimal conservation of six weeks [60]. As an Anglo–Saxon term, the Fifth Range products are sometimes referred [61] as 'Refrigerated Pasteurized Foods of Extended Durability' (REPFEDs). This Fifth Range vegetable definition could be completed as vegetables ready-to-heat which have been heat treated (65-95°C) and packaged with plastic polymers under vacuum or modified or normal atmospheres, prior or after heat treatment. The process is followed by rapid cooling (quenching) and marketed under refrigeration or, less frequently, at ambient temperature. The shelf life (usually 2-3 months) has to be indicated on the label. The most intense heat treatments of Fifth Range vegetables are used to inhibit the growth of pathogenic and spoilage microorganisms in their vegetative and spore forms, particularly when they contain meat products, and also to reduce the stringiness of certain vegetables.

The Fifth Range products sector has considerably grown in recent years. Europe is by large the most active market in this sector, with a 50% of worldwide share, followed by USA with a 23% [62]. The UK leads the top–five list of countries with the highest turnover of Fifth Range products. Their increase of consumption is related to the fact that it perfectly meets the following consumer expectations:

- High sensory and nutritional quality.
- Adequate to the new habits and lifestyle.
- Natural products.
- Healthy properties.
- Microbiologically safe.

The recent technological advances have allowed one to obtain new products with better nutritional and sensory quality, which has also favored the increase of their consumption. As an example, the sautéed (stir–frying) vegetables dishes represent a 30.1% over the total turnover [63].

3. CONVENTIONAL AND INNOVATIVE COOKING METHODS: POTENTIAL USE IN THE FIFTH RANGE VEGETABLES INDUSTRY

The actual increasing demand of low and easy–preparation foods has attached a considerably long expiration date (usually more than six weeks), expected by the consumers. Along the recent and emerging trajectory of the Fifth Range vegetable industry, conventional cooking techniques, such as boiling, steaming, deep–frying and grilling have been applied. Together with these latter cooking methods, new techniques like vacuum cooking (*cook vide*), *sous vide* ('under vacuum' from French) and microwave (MW) are being adapted to the Fifth Range vegetable industry in order to:

- Diversify the product offer.
- Minimize the nutritional losses during thermal treatments.
- Maximize the sensory properties of the product.
- Reduce the production costs (versatile and effective equipment, less energetic cost, etc.).

These new techniques allow cooking at lower temperature and reduced time in order to obtain products with the aforementioned characteristics.

3.1. General Processing Operations Prior to Cooking

The current manufacturing technology of Fifth Range products is based on the 'cook and chill' concept. Furthermore, when this kind of food is destined to catering services, it is also necessary to implement effective packaging techniques that guarantee its safety and long distance commercial distribution and extended retail sale periods. The 'cook and chill' is a system where food is prepared and subjected to enough heat treatment, packaging (prior or after cooking), fast cooling (blast chilling) and chilling storage until consumption. The rapid decrease in temperature inhibits the growth of spoilage and pathogenic microorganisms in their both vegetative and spores forms [64]. The steps of the 'cook and chill' technology are summarized in the Figure 3.

3.1.1. Raw Material Reception and Storage
The first step once the raw plant material arrives at the factory is a quality control that ensures the right quality attributes necessary for the subsequent Fifth Range processing. If the required quality standards are met, it will go for further processing or will be stored (0–4°C; 90–95% RH), depending of the factory supply requirements.

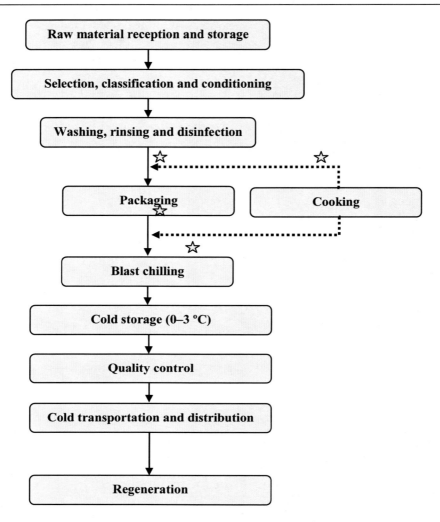

Figure 3. Flow chart of the 'cook and chill' technology in the Fifth Range industry. Critical factors affecting the commercial life of the Fifth Range products.

3.1.2. Selection, Classification and conditioning

The selection, classification and conditioning step for the Fifth Range processing (Figure 3) of vegetables is detailed in Figure 4.

3.1.3. Cooking

3.1.3.1. Boiling

Usually, the most common cooking method for vegetables (although it can be applied for all kinds of food) has been boiling. The advantages and disadvantages of boiling are detailed in Table 5.

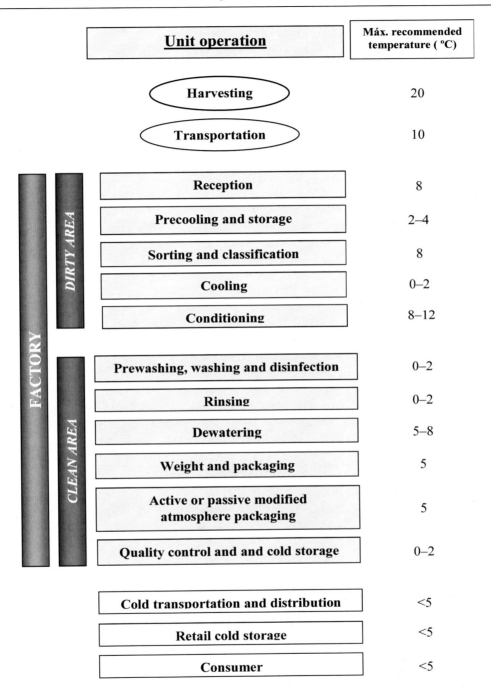

Figure 4. General flow chart of vegetable processing (elaborated from [65]).

Table 5. Advantages and disadvantages of boiling

Advantages	Disadvantages
• Safe and simple method. • Appropriate for large–scale cookery. • Boiling makes digestible older and tougher meat and poultry. • Nutritious, well flavored stock is produced. • Maximum color is retained when cooking green vegetables.	• Loss of nutritional value of the product (if the water is discarded), such as water soluble vitamins. • Some boiled foods can look unattractive. • Can be a slow method of cooking.

In the Fifth Range industry, boiling treatment can be performed by using big pots (discontinuous system) or by conveyor belts, carrying the product, submerging it in boiling water (continuous system).

3.1.3.2. Steaming

Steaming has its origin in China back about 3,000 years with rudimentary stoneware steamers. This cooking method can be employed for almost all kind of food. In Western cooking, steaming is most often used to cook vegetables (it is rarely used to cook meats), while this cooking method is commonly used for seafood and meat dishes in the Oriental cuisine. Steaming is widely considered as a healthy cooking technique, especially for vegetables, since it allows obtaining a high nutritive, light and easy–to–digest product. Furthermore, steaming is an excellent technique to retain the color and flavor of vegetables.

Steaming technique cooks food by moist heat (steam) under varying degrees of pressure. Depending on the pressure used, there are two methods of steaming: atmospheric or low pressure (LP) combined with high pressure (HP, about 0.1 MPa) steaming.

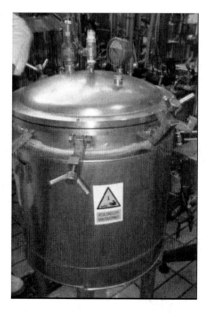

Figure 5. Discontinuous steamer (pilot plant scale).

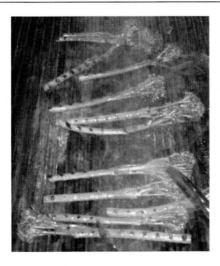

Figure 6. Grilling of kailan–hybrid broccoli,

In the Fifth Range industry, the continuous LP steaming method consists of special tunnels where the product, which circulates over a conveyor belt, is cooked by the vapor injected by an external generator. The discontinuous steaming (LP and HP) method is made in industrial steamers similar to an autoclave (Figure 5). Usually, the discontinuous equipments have a pressure valve that allows steaming the product at LP (opened) or HP (closed).

3.1.3.3. Deep–Frying

The deep–frying is an ancient and popular cooking method that originated in the Mediterranean area due to the olive oil influence [66]. The frying temperatures range from 130 to 190°C, although the most common is the range 170–190°C [67]. The frying equipment used in the industries consists of a long recipient with oil (at the desired frying temperature) that can be used combined with a conveyor belt inside that transports the product during the frying process (continuous system).

3.1.3.4. Grilling

Grilling is a cooking method that involves dry heat applied to the surface of the food product, commonly from above or below. Heat transfer to the food can be made via thermal radiation or by direct conduction, depending upon whether the product is or is not in contact, respectively, with the grilling source. Direct heat grilling can expose food to temperatures over 260°C. Grilled products acquire distinctive roast color marks (Figure 6) and aroma from the Maillard reactions, which take place at temperatures over 155°C [68].

Grilling is often presented as a healthy alternative to cooking with oil (deep–frying), although the fat and juices lost by grilling may render a dry product. However, grilling (together with frying) can lead to the formation of the carcinogenic heterocyclic amines, benzopyrenes and polycyclic aromatic hydrocarbon [69]. However, it has been found that meat marinating (with red wine or beer) may reduce the formation of these compounds [70]. Industrial grills (continuous or discontinuous) are coupled with a sear marker device in order to obtain the characteristic grilling marks on the final product.

3.1.3.5. Vacuum Cooking ('cook vide'): Frying and Boiling

Vacuum cooking, or *cook vide*, is defined as the cooking process that is carried out under pressures well below atmospheric pressure. Owing to the low temperature and oxygen content during the process, vacuum cooking presents some advantages for the Fifth Range product, including better preservation of natural color, flavors and nutritional value [71]. Vacuum frying is used for value–added products such as fruit and vegetables (i.e., potato, banana and mango chips). Kailan–hybrid broccoli is an excellent vegetable suitable for the vacuum cooking.

Over the last decade, chefs have introduced these innovative cooking techniques into their kitchens creating the binomial 'scientific–kitchen.' In this way, they have developed equipment such as the Gastrovac® (ICC Company) that allows frying or boiling under controlled vacuum–pressure conditions (Figure 7).

3.1.3.6. Sous Vide and Its Variant Sous Vide–Microwaving

The *sous vide* is a technique developed by the French cook George Pralus in 1967. It is derived from the traditional cooking method known as *papillote*. The *sous vide* technology is widely used in France (present in around 10–15% of French kitchens) and Belgium. This cooking method is being used by well-known chefs (Ferran Adriá and Joan Roca I Fontané), who recently developed *sous vide* equipments such as Roner® [72].

The most complete definition for *sous vide* was the proposed by the *Sous Vide* Advisory Committee (SVAC) as follows: Catering discontinuous system in which a food, raw or precooked, is vacuum packed in bags or containers of laminate plastic, subjected to a heat treatment under controlled conditions, cooled rapidly, chilled stored and reheated prior to consumption [73]. The *sous vide* technique is usually applied to vegetables since they do not require a pre–cooking step, as do meat or fish.

The increasing interest of the Fifth Range industries in the *sous vide* technique has led to a wide commercial offering of *sous vide* equipments. Among these equipments are those based on: air–steam combination, heating/cooling with water (Thermix and Afrem® systems from the company Armor Inox), streaming water (Steriflow® from the company Barriquand steriflow) and microwave heating (*sous vide*–MW).

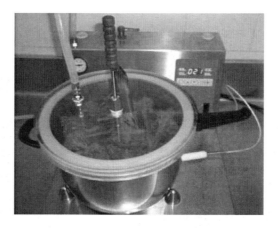

Figure 7. Vacuum boiling of kailan–hybrid broccoli in a Gastrovac® device.

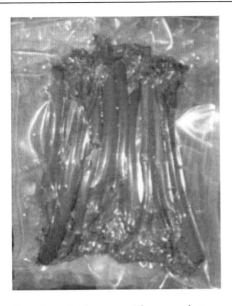

Figure 8. Kailan–hybrid broccoli packaged prior *sous vide* processing.

The *sous vide*–MW uses a magnetron as a heating source. This technique usually uses the Darfresh® and Cryovac® (Figure 8) packaging systems (Cryovac Inc. Company) before exposure to heat.

The election of the temperature/time binomial is very important during the cooking procedures to achieve a good sensory quality and safety. Depending on the product, the shelf–life of the *sous vide* plant food may vary from 7 to 45 days. In particular, that binomial acquires a crucial connotation in the *sous vide* method since the relatively low cooking temperatures used may jeopardize the product safety. Regarding other products, such as meat and fish, vegetables need higher processing temperatures (90–100°C, depending of the product) for acceptable texture [74]. According to our recent studies in pilot plant, the optimum temperature/time for kailan–hybrid broccoli is 90°C/15 min at 900 W. This recommendation accomplishes the minimum heat treatment requirement for pasteurization [75].

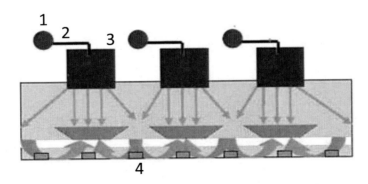

Figure 9. Schematic diagrams of microwave systems.

Table 6. Advantages and disadvantages of microwaving

Advantages	Disadvantages
• Allow in–pack or out–pack cooking. • Minimal damage to the structure and nutritional value of the product. • Quick heat penetration and maximum heating rate. • Low energy consumption. • Allow continuous processing.	• Integration in the processing lines. • Limited heating penetration in some products. • Uniformity of heating: need of computerized design methods for controlling the heating on edges and corners. • Validation and process control: variability of heating times and final temperature controls.

The advantages and disadvantages of microwave cooking are shown in Table 6.

3.1.3.7. Microwaving

Microwaves have a determined frequency of 2,450 MHz, which sometimes, may be 896 MHz in Europe and 915 MHz in USA [76]. Figure 9 shows a diagram of a MW system with the four common parts (1, Magnetron; 2, Waveguide; 3, Applicator; 4, Strips).

The advantages and disadvantages of microwave cooking are shown in Table 6. The most used in–pack MW cooking systems by the Fifth Range industries are MicVac® (Figure 10) and MES® technologies (MicVac Company).

3.1.4. Packaging

The packaging step is crucial due to its importance for inhibiting the chemical and microbiological deterioration during the processing, storage and distribution periods [77]. The container may prevent the exit of water and volatile compounds, as own aromas and flavors from food. Apart from these characteristics, the container must satisfy some technical, commercial and legal conditions.

The following main types of packaging technologies are used in the Fifth Range industry [77]:

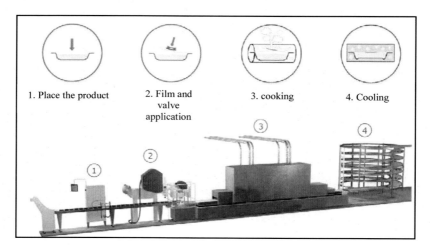

Figure 10. MicVac® system (MicVac Company).

1. Vacuum: the air from the container is completely evacuated.
2. Controlled atmosphere: a single gas or mixture of gases is injected into the container after removing the air. It is subjected to a constant control during the storage period. The most used gases are CO_2 and N_2.
3. Active modified atmosphere: similar to the latter technology but there is no control during the storage period.

The vacuum packaging has an inhibitory effect on the aerobic microorganisms (spoilage and pathogens) growth and on fat oxidation. The low O_2 partial pressures achieved within the container inhibit the growth of mesophilic aerobics. The applied partial vacuum (total vacuum is avoided to prevent the tray collapse) is usually compensated with N_2 and CO_2 residual partial pressures with the purpose of preventing oxidation and microbiological alterations [64]. This packaging method allows the obtaining of products with a long commercial life compared to other conventional cook–chill methods [78].

The heat–sealed bags and plastic trays are the preferred presentations for the Fifth Range products. Vacuum chambers for bags (Figure 11) and tray sealers (Figure 12) are the most used packaging equipments for these products. These devices allow packaging under vacuum or by injecting the desired gas.

3.1.5. Blast Chilling

The temperature and RH conditions reached after the cooking step might favor a rapid microbial growth in the Fifth Range products. The 12–50°C range presents the highest growth risk of the spore–forming bacteria resistant to thermal treatment [79]. With the aim of avoiding the undesired microbial growth, the maximum time to start the blast chilling must be 30 min, and an internal product temperature of 0 to 3°C must be reached in a maximum time of 90 min [80]. Air, water and plates blast chillers, and cold rooms are the most used devices to decrease the temperature of the cooked product [81]. However, new technologies for blast chilling, such as vacuum cooling, have shown excellent results in cooked broccoli [82].

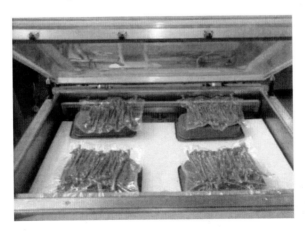

Figure 11. Vacuum chamber during kailan–hybrid broccoli packaging.

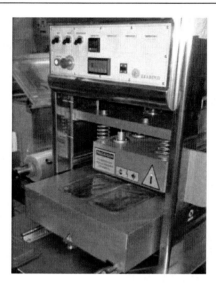

Figure 12. Tray sealer during kailan–hybrid broccoli packaging.

3.1.6. Cold Storage, Transportation and Distribution

Refrigeration is very often crucial for the storage conditions of Fifth Range products. The main hazard associated with the chilled storage is the possible germination and growth of spores that have survived to the thermal treatment. The storage temperatures of these products must be within the range of 1–4°C; it is important that the accuracy on the control of the cold room temperature is within ±0.5°C [64]. The cold room should be close to the blast chiller to avoid excessive temperature fluctuations. In this way, the refrigerated transport and distribution will retard the microbial growth and, depending on the commodity and on the cooking method, a relatively long shelf–life of 7–42 days.

3.1.7. Regeneration

The regeneration is the warming–up of the Fifth Range product prior to consumption. The purpose of this process is to reach a temperature over 65°C. The maximum time for consumption after regeneration is about 1 h (at room temperature) or 2 h (at refrigerated storage). After consumption of regenerated commodity, the remaining product must be discarded. The most used regeneration systems are MW, convection and infrared ovens, water baths (bain–Marie) for soups and sauces and regeneration cars.

4. EFFECTS OF CONVENTIONAL COOKING ON NUTRITIONAL AND BIOACTIVE COMPOUNDS OF BROCCOLI

The cooking methods, when improperly selected, can produce the greatest nutritional quality losses of products both in the food industry and domestic consumption. Therefore, the intrinsic properties of the product should condition the recommended method of cooking to obtain a final Fifth Range food that satisfies consumer expectations related to sensory and nutritional characteristics, and safety. Several scientific-technical works have reported the effects of different cooking methods on the nutritional quality of horticultural products.

One of the first works referring the effect of cooking methods on the nutritional quality of vegetable–based products is on broccoli [83]. This study showed vitamin C retentions of 86, 9.4 and 7.3% for *sous vide*, boiled or HP steamed broccoli, respectively, after 5 days of chilled storage. Table 7 also shows the nutritional components changes of some vegetables after *sous vide* cooking. Vitamin C is among the vitamins that attain the highest losses during cooking owing to its high thermolabile and hydrosoluble nature.

Petersen [84] studied the effect of *sous vide*, steaming and boiling on the L–AA, vitamin B_6 and folacin retention in broccoli (Shogun cv). Generally, L–AA, carotenoids and phenolics in broccoli all decreased significantly with time during boiling or MW cooking [85]. Among the different cooking methods studied to date, boiling is considered as the one that produces the highest nutritive and bioactive compounds losses (phenolics, glucosinolates, carotenoids, vitamins, minerals, etc.) due to lixiviation processes. Steaming, on the other hand, has been widely reported to achieve good retention of those compounds owing to the short cooking time and limited cooking liquids used [84-87].

The aliphatic glucosinolates are generally more stable than indole glucosinolates during postharvest and cooking treatments of *Brassica* vegetables [89, 90]. Vacuum pressure of 97% is recommended for *sous vide* processing of broccoli since the L–AA retention (100°C for 40 min) was significantly enhanced compared to a low vacuum level (92%), meanwhile vitamin B_6 was unaffected [84].

Some mild cooking treatments achieve better bioactive content retention than more aggressive cooking methods. Matusheski et al. [91] showed that heating broccoli at 60°C for 5 min, or more, inactivated the epithio specifier protein (which favors nitrile production over ITC in broccoli under certain conditions), resulting in a higher sulforaphane conversion from glucosinolates. This occurred while myrosinase was not inactivated; myrosinase inactivation requires a thermal treatment of 100°C for 5–15 min. Other studies have reported apparent increased TAC, total phenolics and lutein content in a range of 1.2–1.3–fold after boiling, steaming and MW of broccoli [85, 92, 93]. However, the latter increases were attributed to a cellular tissue disruption, which would release the bioactive compounds from the insoluble portion of the plant tissue.

The achieved good phytochemical retention with less aggressive industrial cooking methods may, however, be greatly reduced if processes after thermal treatment such as quenching, conservation, refrigerated distribution and regeneration prior to consumption are not correctly conducted [74].

5. CASE STUDY: EFFECTS OF INNOVATIVE VACUUM COOKING METHODS ON THE HEALTH-PROMOTING COMPOUNDS OF KALIAN-HYBRID BROCCOLI

Our Research Group studied the effects of vacuum-based cooking techniques on several health-promoting compounds of kalian-hybrid broccoli relative to conventional cooking methods and their changes throughout a shelf life of 45 days at 4-5°C [5, 37, 94]. The processing flowchart is summarized in Figure 13. The sensory quality attributes, microbiological quality and food safety of the products were also studied. A Gastrovac® device was used for some of these vacuum-based cooking techniques.

Table 7. Vitamin retention in *sous vide* processed vegetables after 21 days of chilled storage and subsequent regeneration [88]

Compound	Retention (%)			
	Carrots	Green beans	Cauliflower	Potatoes
β–carotene	–	89	100	–
Vitamin E	–	100	100	–
Vitamin C	63	86	40	69
Vitamin B_1	86	67	86	56
Vitamin B_2	100	100	71	86
Vitamin B_5	84	63	90	37
Vitamin B_3	48	62	65	61
Vitamin B_6	80	100	79	63
Vitamin B_9	100	100	85	100

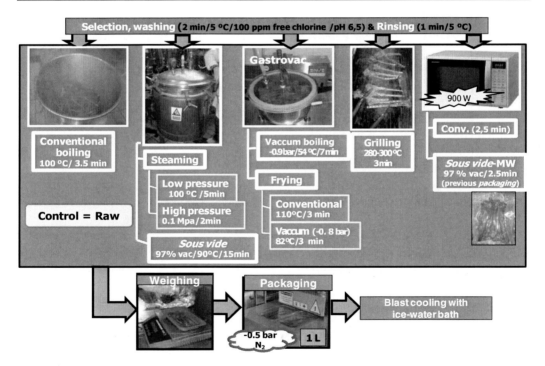

Figure 13. Processing flowchart of Fifth Range kalian-hybrid broccoli cooked with conventional and vacuum-based techniques.

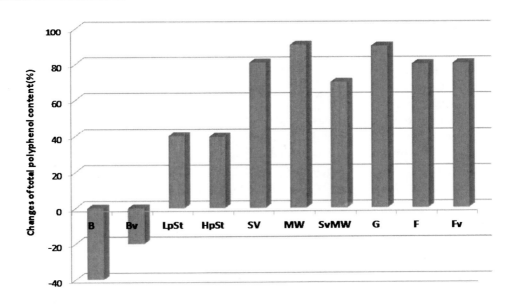

Figure 14. Effects of different conventional and innovative vacuum-based cooking methods on total polyphenols content of kalian-hybrid broccoli (elaborated from [5]). B: conventional boiling; Bv: vacuum boiling; LpSt: low pressure steaming; HpSt: high pressure steaming; Sv: *sous vide*; MW: microwave; SvMW: *sous vide*-microwave; G: grilling; F: frying; Fv: vacuum frying.

The total polyphenol content (TPC), carotenoids and total antioxidant activity of kalian-hybrid broccoli was increased up to 250% after cooking as observed in Figure 15 [5]. The order of TPC increments was MW>G>Sv>F-Fv > SvMW > LpSt > HpSt (see abbreviations in Figure 14). Similar increments in those phytochemicals have been reported in other studies with conventional broccoli cvs [92, 93]. The increase in TPC could be due to the cellular tissue disruption after heat treatment, releasing phytochemicals more accessible for the TPC extraction procedure. This cellular tissue disruption may be higher as the temperature and cooking time increase [95]. On the other side, TPC decreased 40% after conventional boiling due to lixiviation processes. However, vacuum boiling did not show significant TPC decreases.

As above commented, vitamin C is very thermolabile and any heat treatment induces it loss. Accordingly, the initial total vitamin C content decreased after all cooking methods, except for frying (Figure 15). The observed AA retention after stir-frying with extra virgin olive oil may be found in the oil quality and composition. These findings prompt future studies on the effects of different stir-frying treatments (different oil temperatures compared with oil quality and composition) on vitamin C composition. Conventional and vacuum boiling samples registered the highest and the lowest vitamin C losses by 0.6- and 0.3-fold respectively regarding the uncooked control, registering conventional and vacuum boiling waters 0.1- and 0.2-fold of raw broccoli vitamin C content. However, in terms of AA content, conventional boiling showed 3.7-fold higher amount than vacuum boiling. A high DHA content in vacuum-boiled samples was due to the high AA to DHA enzymatic conversion allowed by the low temperature (54°C) of this treatment and also by the great DHA instability (especially at low acid conditions of broccoli). Meanwhile, the absence of DHA in conventional boiling may be due to two main reasons: the inactivation of the AA- to DHA catalyzing enzymes produced by the high temperature of conventional boiling, and the easy and rapidly undergoing of DHA hydrolytic cleavage to form 2,3-DKG, a compound without antiscorbutic activity [5]. Grilled broccoli registered a 47% total vitamin C decrease compared to raw broccoli. The short grilling time probably does not allow broccoli to reach very high temperatures at the center of the stems, thereby allowing the enzymatic conversion of AA to DHA by ascorbate oxidase as well as allowing non-enzymatic conversions. The remaining treatments registered reductions from 33 to 40% regarding initial values, in agreement with previous data for conventional broccoli [84, 12, 85-87].

Conventional boiling induced the largest (80%) total glucosinolates losses in kailan-hybrid broccoli (Table 8) as reported in conventional broccoli after domestic boiling [96, 97]. LP steaming, *sous vide*-MW and microwaving appeared to minimize total glucosinolate losses, reaching the lowest decreases (56–60% over raw values). This low glucosinolate decrease after LP steaming is due to their slower migration to the cooking water because of the lack of direct contact of the vegetable with water, and therefore a lower disruption of their structure. Kailan-hybrid samples that were submerged in water for boiling registered a higher boiling water glucosinolate content than found in the condensed water from LP steaming, with 33.5 and 22.5 mg total glucosinolates, respectively, leached into the cooking liquid per 100 g fw vegetable cooked [37]. The glucosinolate degradation in the grilled samples may be due to the high cooking temperature, since glucosinolates are degraded above 100°C. The total glucosinolate content decline after HP steaming could be due to a high plant cell disruption after treatment, which released more glucosinolates for thermal degradation, as well as the enhanced myrosinase activity by high pressures, since myrosinase activity did not increase at normal atmospheric pressure. The aliphatic glucosinolate glucoraphanin recorded a higher thermostability after cooking (Table 8) with lower decreases (40–67% over raw content) than indole glucosinolates (glucobrassicanapin, glucobrassicin, 4-methoxyglucobrassicin, neoglucobrassicin). Among the latter, glucobrassicanapin and neoglucobrassicin were the most thermolabile with decreases of 80–98% and 85–92%, respectively, compared to raw samples. The best glucoraphanin retention of 60–46% was reached by *sous vide*-MW, LP steaming, microwaving and HP steaming. Grilling, *sous vide* and boiling induced the greatest glucoraphanin reductions, with 82% over the raw kailan-hybrid. *Sous vide*-MW LP steaming and MW showed the highest glucobrassicin retentions (around 54%), while boiling and grilling induced the greatest decrements (78–77%) compared to raw samples. After cooking, glucobrassicanapin and 4-methoxyglucobrassicin showed decreases of 79–98% and 68–95%, respectively, compared to raw samples. On the other hand, neoglucobrassicin did not record any noticeable degradation after cooking [37].

Lutein is the main carotenoid of broccoli and kailan-hybrid broccoli. Cooking of kailan-hybrid broccoli increased the lutein content owing to a better carotenoid extraction. Among treatments, *sous vide*-MW apparently increased 7.1-fold the lutein content [37].

Nutritional and bioactive compounds of Fifth Range kailan-hybrid broccoli decreased progressively throughout shelf life (45 days at 5°C), especially vitamin C. However, *sous vide*-MW induced the lowest vitamin C losses (8%), while conventional microwave induced vitamin C losses of 80% [37].

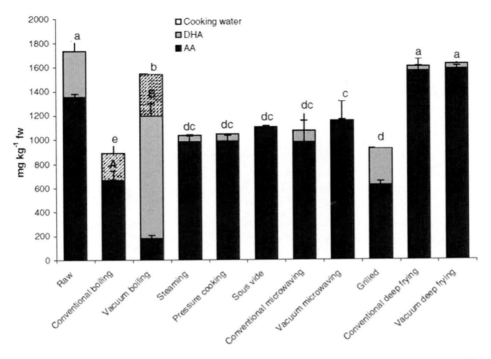

Figure 15. Effects of different conventional and vacuum-based cooking methods on ascorbic acid (black areas) and dehydroascorbic acid (grey areas) contents of kalian-hybrid broccoli and leached total vitamin C (sum of ascorbic and dehydroascorbic acids) to cooking water (lined bars) [5].

Table 8. Effects of different conventional and vacuum-based cooking methods on glucosinolate contents of kalian-hybrid broccoli (elaborated from [37]). B: conventional boiling; LpSt: low pressure steaming; HpSt: high pressure steaming; Sv: *sous vide*; MW: microwave; SvMW: *sous vide*-microwave; G: grilling

Cooking treatments	Glucobrassicin	Glucoraphanin	Glucobrassicanapin	4-methoxyglucobrassicin	Neoglucobrassicin
Raw	4.76	3.47	1.45	1.74	0.60
B	1.06	1.15	0.03	0.07	0.05
LpSt	2.59	2.07	0.13	0.25	0.08
HpSt	1.52	1.59	0.09	0.17	0.07
Sv	1.37	1.21	0.12	0.21	0.07
MW	2.07	1.86	0.27	0.48	0.09
SvMW	2.28	1.85	0.29	0.53	0.06
G	1.11	0.61	0.31	0.55	0.07

6. OVERALL QUALITY OF FIFTH RANGE BROCCOLI

Cooking is a culinary procedure that may attain good sensory characteristics of the food due to certain physical–chemical processes (matrix softening, pH changes, undesirable compounds elimination, etc.) obtaining a product with milder flavor. However, it is difficult to draw general conclusions regarding the sensory quality of cooked products for the following reasons [98]:

1. The experiments are designed to assess changes in specific sensory attributes (caused by different storage temperatures and different cooking times) or to make comparisons between the innovative and traditional cooking for the same food or other processing systems.
2. Some studies applied different treatment conditions for the same cooking method, which does not allow a proper comparison with other studies.
3. Scales, attributes, procedures and statistical tests used in the studies are not the same, which sometimes makes it quite difficult to compare results.
4. Some experiments have reproducibility problems when making comparisons. For example, when a freshly prepared sample with many ingredients is compared with another sample that is stored.

Sous vide emerged as a great cooking method that allows one to better keep the sensory properties of the food products after cooking. For this reason, many of the relevant studies, refers to the effect on the sensory properties of food products of any cooking method compared to the *sous vide*. The following general conclusions about the *sous vide* culinary technique may be stated:

- In terms of texture, aroma, flavor and appearance, significant differences between chilled *sous vide* and frozen *sous vide* products are found.
- When comparing traditional cooking methods with *sous vide*, flavor is further enhanced by *sous vide* treatment, although this sensory parameter may undergo undesirable changes during storage.
- High processing temperatures are needed for vegetables to ensure an acceptable texture for consumers.
- The shelf–life of *sous vide* products is very long compared to other more aggressive methods that induce excessive matrix disruption of the product with more nutrients available for the spoilage microorganisms.

Petersen [84] studied the effects of boiling, LP steaming and *sous vide* on the sensory quality of broccoli (Shogun cv), reporting that the LP steamed and *sous vide* samples showed better acceptability than the boiled samples. Furthermore, the *sous vide* treatment had a better effect on the flavor. However, the *sous vide* treatment enhanced the bitter taste, which was not the case for the boiled samples. Varoquaux et al. [99] established that a *sous vide* treatment not exceeding 90°C for 2 h was enough to reach the best sensory quality for lentils. Thus, any heat treatment above 90°C, or processing time exceeding 2 min, caused excessive lentils softening. Goto et al. [100] compared the *sous vide* method with different traditional Japanese dishes like *takikomigohan* (steamed rice with other ingredients), *saba–nituke* (boiled mackerel with soy sauce) and cabbage rolls. The appearance, color, taste, smell, smoothness and overall preference of the latter dishes did not show significant differences compared to the *sous vide* samples. When comparing *sous vide* with other dishes, such as *nikujaga* (cooked meat and potatoes with soy sauce) and boiled chicken with fig cream, the *sous vide* treatment was preferred [100]. That research also studied the effect of the cooking on some fruit–based products, such as the kiwi sauce, reporting the *sous vide* samples had better color than the traditional methods. In the same study field, Goto et al. [100] found that the aroma and flavor of the *sous vide*–processed (100°C for 1.5 min) mitsuba (*Cryptotaenia japonica*), an aromatic plant Japanese used in the preparation of soups, were better than the boiled samples (1 min). Werlein [101] reported that the *sous vide* carrots (98°C for 20 min) were also preferred, even at the end of storage (21 days at 2°C), than boiled samples (12 min).

FINAL REMARKS AND CONCLUSION

There are some practices that should be taken into account to achieve Fifth Range products with excellent quality, safety and commercial shelf life. They include raw materials with first rate quality, always meeting the food safety aspects; production under strict hygienic conditions and with trained personnel and with well designed and maintained processing plants and installations; use of Good Agricultural Practices and Good Manufacturing Practices during production and elaboration; use of non-aggressive cooking methods, in particular those vacuum-based methods; use of appropriate packages and atmospheres (if any); maintain the cold chain between 0 and 5°C until consumption; and finally regenerate the product for assembly or direct consumption in optimal conditions.

Innovative vacuum-based cooking methods are considered as excellent alternatives to conventional ones to prepare Fifth Range vegetables as it has been shown for kailan-hybrid broccoli. Fifth Range products with similar or better sensory properties, nutritional and microbiological quality, and food safety can be achieved with these vacuum-based cooking techniques regarding conventional methods. *Sous vide* showed greater sensory quality than conventional cooking methods. Furthermore, microbiological quality and food safety of the vegetable after *sous vide* was similar or even higher compared to conventional methods. Vacuum boiling reduced phenolic losses compared to conventional boiling. Vacuum frying achieved the same enhancement of health-promoting compounds than conventional frying while reaching better sensory quality.

Multidisciplinary actions are needed to stimulate the fruit and vegetables consumption, while overcoming the major challenges of the industrial-commercial sector of Fifth Range vegetables. Related protagonists should cooperate in integrated programs to accomplish that what the consumer requires: diversity, safety, quality, availability and reasonable cost. For achievement of these objectives it will be essential interacting with consumers.

REFERENCES

[1] Martínez-Hernández, GB; Gómez, P; Artés, F; et al. New broccoli varieties with improved health benefits and suitability for the fresh-cut and fifth range industries: An opportunity to increase its consumption. In: Lang M, editor. Brassica: characterization, functional genomics and health benefits. New York, USA: Nova Science Publishers, 2013, 67-91.

[2] Tomás–Barberán, FA; Gil, MI. Improving the health–promoting properties of fruit and vegetable products. Boca Raton FL, USA: CRC Press, 2008, 9-13.

[3] Gonçalves, EM; Alegria, C; Abreu, M. Benefits of Brassica Nutraceutical compounds on human health. In: Lang M, editor. Brassicaceae, characterization, functional genomics and health benefits. New York, USA: Nova Science Publishers, 2013, 19-66.

[4] Souci, W; Fachmann, W; Kraut, H. Food composition and nutrition tables. 6th edition. London, UK: Medpharm Scientific Publishers CRC Press, 2000, 697.

[5] Martínez–Hernández, GB; Artés–Hernández, F; Colares–Souza, F; et al. Innovative cooking techniques for improving the overall quality of a kailan–hybrid broccoli. *Food Bioproc Tech*, 2013, 6, 2135-2149.

[6] Martínez-Hernández, GB; Gómez, PA; Artés, F; et al. Nutritional quality changes throughout shelf-life of fresh-cut kailan-hybrid and 'Parthenon' broccoli as affected by temperature and atmosphere composition. *Food Sci Technol Int*, 2015, 21, 14-23.

[7] Tarazona–Díaz, MP. Aprovechamiento de subproductos procedentes de la industria de procesado en fresco: Obtención de un zumo funcional de sandía. Cartagena, Spain: Ph.D. Thesis. *Universidad Politécnica de Cartagena*, 2011, 1–50.

[8] Zhuang, H; Hildebrand, DF; Barth, MM. Temperature influenced lipid peroxidation and deterioration in broccoli buds during postharvest storage. *Postharvest Biol Technol*, 1997, 10, 49–58.

[9] Rosa, EAS; Haneklaus, SH; Schnug, E. Mineral content of primary and secondary inflorescences of eleven broccoli cultivars grown in early and late seasons. *J Plant Nutr*, 2002, 25, 1741–1751.

[10] Davey, MW; Montagu, MV; Inzé, D; et al. Plant L–ascorbic acid: Chemistry, function, metabolism, bioavailability and effects of processing. *J Sci Food Agr*, 2000, 80, 825–860.

[11] Padayatty, SJ; Levine, M. New insights into the physiology and pharmacology of vitamin C. *CMAJ*, 2001, 164, 353–355.

[12] Vallejo, F; Tomás–Barberán, FA; García–Viguera, C. Potential bioactive compounds in health promotion from broccoli cultivars grown in Spain. *J Sci Food Agric*, 2002, 82, 1293–1297.

[13] Gogus, U; Smith, C. n–3 Omega fatty acids: A review of current knowledge. *Int J Food Sci Technol*, 2010, 45, 417–436.

[14] Simopoulos, AP. Essential fatty acids in health and chronic disease. *Am J Clin Nutr*, 1999, 70, 560–569.

[15] Page, T; Griffiths, G; Buchanan–Wollaston, B. Molecular and biochemical characterization of postharvest senescence in broccoli. *Plant Physiol*, 2001, 125, 718–727.

[16] Martínez-Hernández, GB; Artés-Hernández, F; Gómez, P; et al. Combination of electrolysed water, UV-C and superatmospheric O2 packaging for improving fresh-cut broccoli quality. *Postharvest Biol Technol*, 2013, 76, 125-134.

[17] Lule, SU; Xia, W. Food phenolics, pros and cons: A review. *Food Rev Int*, 2005, 21, 367–388.

[18] Redovniković, IR; Repajić, M; Fabek, S; et al. Comparison of selected bioactive compounds and antioxidative capacity in different broccoli cultivars. *Acta Alimentaria*, 2012, 41, 221–232.

[19] De–Kleijn, MJ; Van–der–Schouw, YT; Wilson, PW; et al. Intake of dietary phytoestrogensis low in postmenopausal women in the United States: The Framingham study (1–4). *J Nutr*, 2001, 131, 1826–1832.

[20] Lin, L; Harnly, JM. Identification of the phenolic components of collard greens, kale, and Chinese Broccoli. *J Agric Food Chem*, 2009, 57, 7401–7408.

[21] Cartea, ME; Francisco, M; Soengas, P; et al. Phenolic compounds in *Brassica* vegetables. *Molecules*, 2011, 16, 251–280.

[22] Martínez-Hernández, GB; Gómez, P; Pradas, I; et al. Moderate UV-C pretreatment as a quality enhancement tool in fresh-cut Bimi® broccoli. *Postharvest Biol Technol*, 2011, 62, 327-337.

[23] Wallsgrove, RM; Bennett, RN. The biosynthesis of glucosinolatos in *Brassicas*. In: Wallsgrove RM, editor. Amino Acids and their derivatives in higher plants. Cambridge, UK: Cambridge University Press, 1995, 243–259.

[24] Fahey, JW; Talalay, P. Antioxidant functions of sulforaphane: A potent inducer of phase 2 detoxication enzymes. *Food Chem Toxicol*, 1999, 37, 973–979.

[25] Fahey, JW; Zhang, Y; Talalay, P. Broccoli sprouts: An exceptionally rich source of inducers of enzymes that protect against chemical carcinogens. *P Natl Acad Sci U S A*, 1997, 94, 10367–10372.

[26] Jeffery, EH; Brown, AF; Kurilich, AS; et al. Variation in content of bioactive components in broccoli. *J Food Compost Anal*, 2003, 16, 323–330.

[27] Jones, RB; Faragher, JD; Winkler, S. A review of the influence of postharvest treatments on quality and glucosinolate content in broccoli (*Brassica oleracea* var. Italica) heads. *Postharvest Biol Technol*, 2006, 41, 1–8.

[28] Rosa, EAS; Heaney, RK; Fenwick, et al. Glucosinolates in crop plants. In: Janick J, editor. Horticultural Reviews, Volume 19. Oxford, UK: *John Wiley & Sons, Inc*, 1996, 99–215.

[29] Zhang, Y; Talalay, P; Cho, CG; et al. A major inducer of anti–carcinogenic protective enzymes from broccoli: Isolation and elucidation of structure. *Proc Natl Acad Sci U S A*, 1992, 89, 2399–2403.

[30] Talalay, P; Fahey, JW; Holtzclaw, WD; et al. Chemoprotection against cancer by Phase II enzyme induction. *Toxicol Lett*, 1995, 82, 173–179.

[31] Munday, R; Munday, CM. Induction of Phase II detoxification enzymes in rats by plant–derived isothiocyanates: comparison of allyl isothiocyanate with sulforaphane and related compounds. *J Agric Food Chem*, 2004, 52, 1867–1871.

[32] Huang, C; Ma, WY; Li, J; et al. Essential role of p53 in phenethyl isothiocyanate induced apoptosis. *Cancer Res*, 1998, 58, 4102–4106.

[33] Musk, SR; Smith, TK; Johnson, IT. On the cytotoxicity and genotoxicity of allyl and phenethyl isothiocyanates and their parent glucosinolates sinigrin and gluconasturtiin. *Mut Res*, 1995, 34, 19–23.

[34] Smith, TK; Lund, EK; Musk, SRR; et al. Inhibition of DMH–induced aberrant crypt foci, and induction of apoptosis in rat colon, following oral administration of a naturally occurring glucosinolate. *Carcinogenesis*, 1998, 19, 267–273.

[35] Fahey, JW; Haristoy, X; Dolan, PM; et al. Sulforaphane inhibits extracellular, intracellular, and antibiotic–resistant strains of *Helicobacter pylori* and prevents benzo[a]pyrene–induced stomach tumours. *P Natl Acad Sci U S A*, 2002, 99, 7610–7615.

[36] Wu, L; Ashraf, MHN; Facci, M; et al. Dietary approach to attenuate oxidative stress, hypertension, and inflammation in the cardiovascular system. *Proc Natl Acad Sci U S A*, 2004, 101, 7094–7099.

[37] Martínez–Hernández, GB; Artés–Hernández, F; Gómez, P; et al. Induced changes in bioactive compounds of kailan–hybrid broccoli after innovative processing and storage. *J Funct Foods*, 2013, 5, 133-143.

[38] Schonhof, I; Krumbein, A; Brückner, B. Genotypic effects on glucosinolates and sensory properties of broccoli and cauliflower. *Mol Nutr Food Res*, 2004, 48, 25–33.

[39] Funamoto, Y; Yamauchi, N; Shigenaga, T; et al. Effects of heat treatment on chlorophyll degrading enzymes in stored broccoli (*Brassica oleracea* L.). *Postharvest Biol Technol*, 2002, 24, 163–170.

[40] Lemoine, ML; Civello, PM; Chaves, AR; et al. Effect of combined treatment with hot air and UV–C on senescence and quality parameters of minimally processed broccoli (*Brassica oleracea* L. var. Italica). *Postharvest Biol Technol*, 2008, 48, 15–21.

[41] Dashwood, R; Negishi, T; Hayatsu, H; et al. Chemopreventive properties of chlorophylls towards aflatoxin B1: A review of the antimutagenicity and anticarcinogenicity data in rainbow trout. *Mutat Res*, 1998, 399, 245–253.

[42] Egner, PA; Muñoz, A; Kensler, TW. Chemoprevention with chlorophyllin in individuals exposed to dietary aflatoxin. *Mut Res*, 2003, 523, 209–216.

[43] Lanfer–Marquez, UM; Barros, RMC; Sinnecker, P. Antioxidant activity of chlorophylls and their derivatives. *Food Res Int*, 2005, 38, 885–891.

[44] Tawashi, R; Cousineau, M; Denis, G. Crystallisation of calcium oxalate dihydrate in normal urine in presence of sodium copper chlorophyllin. *Urol Res*, 1982, 10, 173–176.

[45] Artés, F; Mínguez, MI; Hornero, D. Analysing changes in fruit pigments. In: MacDougall DB, editor. Colour in food. Improving quality. Cambridge, UK: CRC Press and Woodhead Publishing Ltd, 2002, 248–282.

[46] Maiani, G; Periago–Castón, MJ; Catasta, G; et al. Carotenoids: Actual knowledge on food sources, intakes, stability and bioavailability and their protective role in humans. *Mol Nutr Food Res*, 2009, 53, 194–218.

[47] Chrong, EWI; Wong, TY; Kreis, AJ; et al. Dietary antioxidants and primary prevention of age related macular degeneration: Systemic review and meta–analysis. *BMJ*, 2007, 335, 755–759.

[48] Ribaya–Mercado, JD; Blumberg, JB. Lutein and zeaxanthin and their potential roles in disease prevention. *The Journal of the American College of Nutrition*, 2004, 23, 567–587.

[49] Snodderly, DM. Evidence for protection against age–related macular degeneration by carotenoids and antioxidant vitamins. *Am J Clin Nutr*, 1995, 62, 1448–1461.
[50] Bendich, A. Carotenoids and the immune response. *J Nutr*, 1989, 119, 112–115.
[51] Mathews–Roth, MM. Plasma concentrations of carotenoids after large doses of beta–carotene. *Am J Clin Nutr*, 1990, 52, 500–501.
[52] Nishino, H. Cancer prevention by carotenoids. *Mut Res*, 1998, 402, 159–163.
[53] Larsen, E; Christensen, LP. Simple saponification method for the quantitative determination of carotenoids in green vegetables. *J Agric Food Chem*, 2005, 53, 6598–6602.
[54] Leth, T; Jakobsen, J; Andersen, NL. The intake of carotenoids in Denmark. *Eur J Lipid Sci Technol*, 2000, 102, 128–132.
[55] Murkovic, M; Gams, K; Draxl, S; et al. Development of an Austrian carotenoid database. *J Food Compost Anal*, 2000, 13, 435–440.
[56] Devasagayam, TPA; Tilak, JC; Boloor, KK; et al. Free radicals and antioxidants in human health: Current status and future prospects. *J Assoc Physicians I*, 2004, 52, 796–804.
[57] Balasundram, N; Sundram, K; Samman, S. Phenolic compounds and agri–industrial by–products: Antioxidant activity, occurrence, and potential uses. *Food Chem*, 2006, 99, 191–203.
[58] Dragsted, LO. Antioxidant actions of polyphenols in humans. *Int J Vitam Nutr Res*, 2003, 73, 112–119.
[59] Scalbert, A; Manach, A; Morand, C; et al. Dietary polyphenols and the prevention of diseases. *Crit Rev Food Sci Nutr*, 2005, 45, 287–306.
[60] Tirilly, Y; Bourgeois, CM. Tecnología de las hortalizas. *Zaragoza, Spain: Editorial Acribia*, 2002, 187–206.
[61] Mossel, DAA; Struijk, CB. Public health implication of refrigerated pasteurised (*sous vide*) foods. *Int J Food Microbiol*, 1991, 13, 187–206.
[62] Mintel. Prepared meals. London, UK: Mintel Reports, 2010.
[63] Sainz, H; Fálder, A; Vera, D; et al. Platos precocinados y preparados. In: Alimentación en España. Producción, industria, distribución y consumo. *Madrid, Spain: Empresa Nacional Mercasa*, 2008, 336–338.
[64] Díaz–Molins, P. Calidad y deterioro de platos *sous vide* preparados a base de carne y pescado y almacenados en refrigeración. Murcia, Spain: PhD. Thesis. *Universidad de Murcia*, 2009, 23–120.
[65] Artés–Hernández, F. Fresh–cut unit operations. In: Colelli G, Kader AA, editors. 5th European short course on quality and safety of fresh–cut produce. CD–Rom. *Berlín, Germany*, 2012.
[66] Varela, G. Current facts about frying of food. In: Varela G, Bender AE, Morton ID, editors. Frying of foods: Principles, changes, new approaches. *Chichester, UK: Ellis Horwood*, 1988, 20–25.
[67] Bouchon, P. Fritura. In: Brenan JG, editor. Manual del procesado de los alimentos. *Zaragoza, Spain: Editorial Acribia*, 2006, 237–290.
[68] Schröder, MJA. Food Quality and consumer value. Delivering food that satisfies. *Berlin, Germany: Springer*, 2003, 330.

[69] Sugimura, T; Wakabayashi, K; Nakagama, H; et al. Heterocyclic amines: Mutagens/carcinogens produced during cooking of meat and fish. *Cancer Sci*, 2004, 95, 290–299.

[70] Melo, A; Viegas, O; Petisca, C; et al. Effect of beer/red wine marinades on the formation of heterocyclic aromatic amines in pan–fried beef. *J Agric Food Chem*, 2008, 56, 10625–10632.

[71] Andrés–Bello, A; García–Segovia, P; Martínez–Monzó, J. Effects of vacuum cooking (*cook–vide*) on the physical–chemical properties of sea bream fillets (*Sparus aurata*). *J Aquat Food Prod T*, 2009, 18, 79–89.

[72] Villarino–Rodríguez, A. Efecto del almacenamiento sobre el valor nutritivo, la calidad higiénico–sanitaria y sensorial de la trucha arco–iris (*Oncorhynchus mykiss*) procesada mediante la tecnología *sous vide*. León, Spain: Ph.D. Thesis. *Universidad de León*, 2009, 56–60.

[73] Sous Vide Advisory Committee (SVAC). Codes of practice for *sous vide* catering systems. Tetbury, Gloucestershire, UK.

[74] Ghazala, S. *Sous vide* and cook–chill processing for the food industry. Gaithersburg MD, USA: Aspen Publishers, 1998, 25–51.

[75] Sheard, MA; Rodger, C. Optimum heat treatments for *sous vide* cook–chill products. *Food Control*, 1995, 6, 53–56.

[76] Fellows, P. Tecnología del procesado de los alimentos. Principios y prácticas. *Zaragoza, Spain: Editorial Acribia*, 1994, 355–364.

[77] Rodgers, S. Innovation in food service technology and its strategic role. *Int J Hosp Manag*, 2007, 26, 899–912.

[78] Church, IJ; Parsons, AL. The sensory quality of chicken and potato products prepared using cook–chill and *sous vide* methods. *Int J Food Sci Tech*, 2000, 35, 155–162.

[79] Gaze, JE; Shaw, R; Archer, J. Identification and prevention of hazards associated with slow cooling of hams and other large cooked meats and meat products. Chipping Campden, UK: *Editorial Campden and chorleywood food research association group*, 1998, 1–12.

[80] Anonymous. Chilled and frozen, guidelines on cook–chill and cook–freeze systems. *London, UK: Department of Health–HMSIO*, 1989, 4–8.

[81] Zhang, Z; Sun, DW. Effects of cooling methods on the cooling efficiency and quality of cooked rice. *J Food Eng*, 2006, 77, 269–274.

[82] Sun, DW; Wang, L. Vacuum cooling. In: Sun DW, editor. Advances in food refrigeration. Surrey, UK: Leatherhead Publishing, 2001, 264–304.

[83] Buckley, C. The vitamin C content of cooked broccoli. Hotel Catering Research. *Centre Laboratory Reports of the Huddersfield Polytechnic University*, 1987, 240, 2–3.

[84] Petersen, MA. Influence of *sous vide* processing, steaming and boiling on vitamin retention and sensory quality in broccoli florets. *Eur Food Res Technol*, 1993, 197, 375–380.

[85] Zhang, D; Hamauzu, Y. Phenolics, ascorbic acid, carotenoids and antioxidant activity of broccoli and their changes during conventional and microwave cooking. *Food Chem*, 2004, 88, 503–509.

[86] Galgano, F; Favati, F; Caruso, M; et al. The influence of processing and preservation on the retention of health–promoting compounds in broccoli. *J Food Sci*, 2007, 72, 130–135.

[87] López–Berenguer, C; Carvajal, M; Moreno, DA; et al. Effects of microwave cooking conditions on bioactive compounds present in broccoli inflorescences. *J Agric Food Chem*, 2007, 55, 10001–10007.

[88] Watier, B; Belliot, JP. Vitamines et technologie industrielle récente. *Cahiers de Nutrition et de Diététique*, 1990, 26, 23–26.

[89] Cieslik, E; Leszczynska, T; Filipiak–Florkiewicz, A; et al. Effects of some technological processes on glucosinolate contents in cruciferous vegetables. *Food Chemistry*, 2007, 105, 976–981.

[90] Rungapamestry, V; Duncan, AJ; Fuller, Z; et al. Changes in glucosinolate concentrations, myrosinase activity and production of metabolites of glucosinolates in cabbage (*Brassica oleracea* var. Capitata) cooked for different durations. *J Agric Food Chem*, 2007, 54, 7628–7634.

[91] Matusheski, NV; Wallig, MA; Juvik, JA; et al. Preparative HPLC method for the purification of sulforaphane and sulforaphane nitrile from *Brassica oleracea*. *J Agric Food Chem*, 2001, 49, 1867–1872.

[92] Turkmen, N; Ferda, S; Velioglu, YS. The effect of cooking methods on total phenolics and antioxidant activity of selected green vegetables. *Food Chem*, 2005, 93, 713–718.

[93] Yamaguchi, T; Mizobuchi, T; Kajikawa, R; et al. Radical scavenging activity of vegetables and the effect of cooking on their activity. *Food Sci Technol Res*, 2001, 7, 250–257.

[94] Martínez-Hernández, GB; Artés-Hernández, F; Gómez, P; et al. Quality changes after vacuum-based and conventional industrial cooking of kailan-hybrid broccoli throughout retail cold storage. *Lebenson Wiss Technol*, 2013, 50, 707-714.

[95] Young, CT; Schadel, WE. A comparison of the effects of oven roasting and oil cooking on the microstructure of peanut (*Arachis hypogaea* L. cv. Florigiant) cotyledon. *Food Struct*, 1993, 12, 59–66.

[96] Jones, RB; Frisina, CL; Winkler, S; et al. Cooking method significantly effects glucosinolate content and sulforaphane production in broccoli florets. *Food Chem*, 2010, 123, 237–242.

[97] Pellegrini, N; Chiavaro, E; Gardana, C; et al. Effect of different cooking methods on color, phytochemical concentration, and antioxidant capacity of raw and frozen brassica vegetables. *J Agric Food Chem*, 2010, 58, 4310–4321.

[98] Creed, PG. The sensory and nutritional quality of *sous vide* foods. *Food Control*, 1995, 6, 45–52.

[99] Varoquaux, P; Offant, P; Varoquaux, F. Firmness, seed wholeness and water uptake during the cooking of lentils (*Lens culinaris* cv. Anicia) for *sous vide* and catering preparations. *Int J Food Sci Technol*, 1995, 30, 215–220.

[100] Goto, M; Hashimoto, K; Yamada, K. Difference of ascorbic acid content among some vegetables, texture in chicken and pork, and sensory evaluation store in some dishes between vacuum and ordinary cooking. *J Jpn Soc Food Sci*, 1995, 42, 50–54.

[101] Werlein, H. Comparison of the quality of *sous vide* and conventionally processed carrots. *Eur Food Res Technol*, 1998, 207, 311–315.

INDEX

#

1-methylcyclopropene, 290, 291, 295, 297
26S proteasomal, 199
4-hydroxyglucobrassicin, 39, 46, 277
4-methoxy-glucobrassicin, 36, 39, 43, 269
6-phosphogluconate dehydrogenase, 113
8-hydroxydeoxyguanosine, 242
8-isoprostane, 228, 242
8-oxo-deoxyguanosine, 230
9-cis-retinoic acid receptor, 72

A

aconitase, 220
acrolein, 193, 243
activator protein-1, 128, 199, 205, 207
acyl-CoA-cholesterol acyltransferase, 230
adipocytokines, 228
adrenal cortical zona glomerulosa cells, 212
advanced glycation end products, 227
Aflatoxin B_1, 113
age, 102, 103, 104, 165, 166, 178, 180, 184
aging, x, 1, 70, 87, 88, 90, 91, 92, 93, 94, 100, 101, 102, 103, 104, 105, 106, 109, 113, 183, 223, 224, 246, 247, 286, 287, 290, 292
air pollution, 6, 243
Albena Dinkova-Kostova, 5
aldehyde dehydrogenases, 56
aldo-keto reductase, 113
aldose reductase, 227
allyl isothiocyanate, 31, 307, 329
amino-terminal jun kinase, 92
AMP-activated protein kinase, 226
androgen receptor, 245, 249
androstane receptor, 72, 78, 85
Angiotensin converting enzyme, 213, 214
angiotensin I, 212, 213, 214
angiotensin receptor-1, 212, 213
angiotensinogen, 213, 214
anthocyanins, 284, 304
anticarcinogenic activity, 4, 34, 275
anti-inflammatory, 94, 104, 105, 109, 126, 127, 128, 129, 130, 131, 133, 134, 137, 140, 141, 145, 167, 186, 188, 197, 198, 199, 203, 207, 226, 228, 229, 233, 235, 283, 287
anti-inflammatory pathways, 126, 226
antimicrobial activity, 288
antioxidant capacity, 188, 192, 193, 225, 228, 234, 267, 284, 285, 286, 289, 290, 292, 293, 309, 333
antioxidant response, 5, 73, 85, 116, 118, 119, 131, 137, 139, 189, 191, 196, 202, 205, 206, 225, 226, 227, 230
anti-oxidant response, 94, 99, 111, 115, 131, 211, 220
anti-oxidant response element(s), 99, 111, 131
apolipoprotein B, 221, 230, 236
arachidonic acid, 127, 220
ARS, 33
aryl hydrocarbon receptor, 85
ascorbic acid, 286
asthma, 130, 132, 139, 239, 248
asthmatics, 243
atherogenic index, 230, 242
atherosclerosis, 209, 210, 222, 224, 237
ATP Binding Cassette (ABC) Transporter, 47, 57, 68, 124
ATP-Binding Cassette C Multidrug Resistance Proteins, 112
autism, 239, 244, 249
Autism spectrum disorder, 244

B

Beneforte, 41, 46
bifunctional, 3, 4

bile salt excretory protein, 68
bioavailability, 8, 123, 203, 272, 278
biofortification, 285
Blast Chilling, 319
blood pressure, 209, 211, 286
boron nutrition, 40, 45
Brassica villosa L, 41
Brassicaceae, 10, 11, 12, 20, 23, 35, 122, 134, 251, 264, 266, 269, 300, 301, 306, 328
Brassicales, 9, 10, 11, 25, 264, 266
Brazil, 283
breast cancer resistance protein, 69, 80, 82, 83, 124, 136
broccoli diet, 217, 287
broccoli seeds, 42, 279
broccoli sprout(s), x, 5, 6, 8, 42, 46, 100, 161, 162, 165, 167, 168, 169, 175, 182, 183, 186, 189, 193, 195, 199, 202, 203, 205, 209, 215, 216, 217, 218, 219, 220, 221, 224, 225, 226, 227, 228, 229, 230, 231, 232, 233, 234, 235, 236, 237, 238, 240, 241, 242, 243, 245, 246, 247, 248, 249, 271, 275, 277, 278, 279, 284, 286, 292, 293, 307, 329
butylated hydroxyanisole, 2, 100

C

Ca^{2+}-calmodulin, 212, 213
calcineurin, 95, 107
calmodulin, 212, 213
caloric restriction, 109
cAMP response element-binding protein, 127
cancer(s), 2, 6, 7, 8, 44, 45, 75, 82, 83, 109, 117, 118, 127, 132, 133, 136, 137, 139, 140, 141, 142, 146, 147, 159, 160, 183, 185, 186, 188, 191, 192, 199, 200, 201, 202, 203, 204, 205, 206, 207, 225, 237, 239, 240, 243, 245, 246, 247, 248, 249, 252, 278, 279, 280, 281, 285, 293, 294, 303, 309, 329, 331, 332
caper, 13
carbonyl reductase, 113
carcinogenesis, 44, 84, 117, 119, 186, 203, 207, 247, 248, 249, 330
Carotenoids, 145, 146, 188, 201, 202, 226, 287, 288, 290, 293, 294, 299, 301, 308, 309, 321, 323, 330, 331, 332
casein kinase, 115, 118, 133
casein kinase-2, 115
caspase 3, 220
caspase-1, 228
caspase-3, 129
catalase, 88, 125, 128, 129, 188, 189, 196, 226, 227
cdc25 phosphatases, 95
cell adhesion molecules, 210, 221

cell-cycle progression, 4
cerebral palsy, 162, 163
chaperone proteins, 199
chloramine, 125
cholesterol, 230
chronic disease, x, 1, 5, 6, 100, 101, 102, 105, 226, 284, 303, 328
c-Jun N-terminal Kinase, 115
clinical trial(s), x, 1, 3, 5, 6, 8, 102, 115, 121, 129, 130, 134, 167, 181, 203, 210, 218, 221, 229, 230, 232, 233, 235, 236, 238, 239, 241, 242, 244, 245, 246, 248
colitis, 294
concentrative nucleoside transporters, 67
C-reactive protein, 128, 130, 138, 228
crotonaldehyde, 243
Cullin 3, 131
cultivars, 33, 35, 46, 253, 258, 259, 277
Cultural Practices, 39, 302
cyclic guanosine monophosphate (cGMP) synthase, 212
cyclin-dependent kinases, 143, 147
cyclooxygenase-2, 137, 187, 228
cyclooxygenases, 126, 127
CYP1, 57, 58, 59, 77
CYP2, 58, 59, 60
CYP3, 57, 58, 60
cysteine, 87, 94
cysteine residues, 73, 87, 94, 95, 96, 101, 106, 113, 114, 189, 197, 198, 199, 227, 242, 276
Cysteine-based phosphatases, 95, 107
cystine, 179
cystine-glutamate antiporter, 112
cytochrome P450, 4, 47, 56, 57, 58, 76, 77, 78, 83, 220, 226, 241, 247
cytochrome P450 enzymes, 47, 58, 77, 241
cytochrome P450s, 4, 56, 57
cytokines, 128, 138
cytosine methylation, 209, 220, 245
cytosine-guanosine repeats, 220

D

developmental disabilities, 162, 163, 177, 184
diacylglycerol acyltransferases, 230
Diesel exhaust particles, 243, 248
diet, 87, 99, 137, 169, 170, 248
dietary Nrf2 activators, 100, 101, 216, 222
dimethyl fumarate, 115, 118
dithiocarbamate(s), 191, 224, 246, 272
dry season, 251, 252, 256, 257, 259, 260
dual specificity phosphatases, 95

E

E3-ubiquitin ligase, 113
Edible coatings, 290, 296
eicosanoids, 220
electrophile response element, 112, 116
endocrine, 225
endothelial dysfunction, 223
endothelial function, 216, 217, 218, 232, 236, 245, 249
endothelin-1, 213, 214
endothelium function, 218
epicatechin-3-gallate, 188, 201
epigallocatechin gallate, 129, 205
epigenetic regulation, 70
epigenetics, 83, 145, 209, 218, 224, 245
Epiprogoitrin, 29, 39
epoxide hydrolases, 56, 60
ERK, 91, 92, 93, 106, 132, 133, 142
E-Selectin, 221
ethoxyquin, 2, 7
exercise, 222
extracellular receptor kinase, 92
extracellular signal-regulated kinase, 105, 133

F

FAD-containing monooxygenases, 58
farnesoid X receptor, 72
fatty acid oxidation, 119, 242
fatty acid synthase, 230
fatty acids, 267
Fe^{2+}-based phosphatases, 95
fetal determinants of adult health, 109, 182, 209, 218, 219, 220, 221, 224
fetal inflammation, 162, 166, 167, 172
Fifth Range industry, 300, 309, 310, 312, 314, 315, 318
Fifth Range products, 299, 310, 311, 312, 319, 320, 327
Fifth Range Vegetables, 309, 311
flavin mono-oxygenases, 60
flavonoids, 135, 295
flavonols, 122, 125, 128, 131, 135, 136, 138, 139, 229, 278, 290, 304
foam cells, 210, 211
folic acid, 302
food, 283
free radical, 88, 102, 125, 153, 154, 156, 158, 165, 173, 179, 211, 213, 227, 276, 286, 294, 309, 331

G

G2/M arrest, 158
gastric cancer, 6, 241, 247
gender, 59, 70, 78, 84, 223
genotoxicity, 147, 158, 159, 330
Genotype versus Environment, 40
glucoalyssin, 39, 269
glucobrassicin, 26, 33, 36, 37, 38, 39, 41, 43, 146, 236, 269, 271, 278, 307, 308, 324, 325
glucoerucin, 39
glucoiberin, 33, 36, 38, 41, 42, 43, 215, 269, 271, 308
gluconapin, 39, 269, 307, 308
gluconapoleiferin, 21, 39
gluconasturtiin, 39, 215, 269, 308, 330
glucoraphanin, ix, x, 4, 5, 33, 34, 36, 37, 38, 39, 40, 41, 42, 43, 45, 46, 145, 146, 147, 167, 190, 191, 195, 197, 199, 203, 205, 209, 215, 216, 217, 218, 219, 221, 226, 239, 240, 242, 243, 245, 246, 248, 263, 264, 269, 270, 271, 272, 273, 274, 277, 279, 280, 289, 290, 293, 295, 307, 308, 324, 325
glucose-6-phosphate dehydrogenase, 101, 113
glucosinolate(s), ix, x, 1, 4, 8, 9, 10, 13, 19, 20, 24, 25, 26, 27, 28, 29, 30, 33, 34, 35, 37, 36, 38, 39, 40, 41, 42, 43, 44, 45, 46, 100, 145, 146, 147, 159, 182, 183, 190, 191, 202, 203, 215, 216, 217, 218, 226, 230, 240, 241, 245, 246, 263, 264, 265, 268, 269, 270, 271, 277, 278, 279, 283, 284, 285, 287, 288, 289, 290, 291, 292, 293, 294, 297, 299, 301, 306, 307, 308, 321, 324, 325, 329, 330, 333
glucuronosyltransferases, 3, 57, 76, 77, 79, 189
glutamate-cystine antiporter, 101
glutathione, 57, 76, 79, 80, 87, 101, 102, 103, 117
glutathione peroxidase, 88, 89, 94, 101, 102, 106, 112, 125, 165, 189, 193, 215, 216, 226, 227, 231
glutathione peroxidases, 88, 101, 112
glutathione reductase, 89, 94, 101, 106, 113, 189, 216, 226, 227
glutathione S-transferase(s), 2, 3, 7, 62, 79, 80, 112, 116, 159, 226, 227, 231
glutathione transferase(s), 7, 34, 76, 80, 118, 189
glutathione-S-transferase(s), 57
glycogen synthase kinase (GSK) 3β, 133
glycogen synthase kinase 3beta, 230
glyoxalase system, 112
goiter, 22
goitrogenicity, 22
grapefruit juice interaction, 71
green chemoprevention, 6, 8
GSH, 88, 89, 90, 96, 99, 101, 112, 165, 188, 189, 191, 193, 215, 216, 220, 227, 272

H

HDL/LDL ratio, 228
HDL-cholesterol, 242
heat shock elements, 199
heat shock factor-1, 199
Helicobacter, 6, 8, 225, 226, 227, 234, 237, 238, 239, 241, 247, 275, 281, 307, 330
Helicobacter pylori, 237
heme oxygenase, 119, 205
heme oxygenase-1, 113, 119, 131, 140, 142, 205
hepatocyte nuclear factor, 72, 83, 85
Hippocrates, ix, 239
Histone Acetylation, 138, 146, 154
histone deacetylases, 4, 94, 107, 155
histones, 149
hormone-sensitive lipase activity, 242
hydroxyl radical, 88, 89, 284
hypertension, 24, 30, 93, 105, 109, 175, 182, 183, 209, 210, 211, 212, 214, 215, 218, 222, 223, 230, 234, 236, 248, 249, 330
hypochlorous acid, 125

I

IKK kinase, 197
IL-1β-, 127, 133, 142
increased intercellular adhesion molecule-1, 217
India, 145
indole-3-carbinol, 38, 45, 145, 146, 159, 236, 271
inducible nitric oxide synthase, 127, 187, 217, 218, 219, 228
inflamm-aging, 92
inflammation, 83, 87, 101, 121, 126, 137, 142, 172, 235
inflammation markers, 130, 147, 235
inflammatory response, 108, 122, 128, 133, 134, 138, 166, 180, 187, 192, 197, 243, 287
insulin, 141, 229
insulin homeostasis, 229
insulin receptor, 97
insulin receptor substrate, 97
insulin substrate protein, 98
insulin-like growth factor receptor, 132
intercellular adhesion molecule-1, 221
interleukin 6, 181, 228
interleukin-1β, 228, 232
interleukins, 128
IP$_3$, 211, 213
ischemia-reperfusion, 99, 109, 159, 224
isothiocyanate(s), ix, 1, 3, 4, 5, 8, 9, 14, 20, 23, 25, 26, 27, 28, 31, 33, 34, 37, 38, 43, 44, 46, 131,145, 146, 147, 159, 182, 183, 186, 190, 191, 202, 203, 206, 207, 224, 226, 230, 233, 234, 237, 240, 241, 242, 245, 246, 264, 267, 268, 269, 270, 271, 272, 273, 275, 280, 284, 292, 293, 294, 299, 306, 307, 329, 330
IκB kinase(s), 126, 134

J

Janus kinase, 130
Jed Fahey, x, 5, 6, 8
JNK, 92, 93, 98, 105, 108, 115, 119, 127, 131, 132, 133, 140, 142
JNK phosphatases, 99

K

kaempferol, 121, 122, 127, 130, 133, 134, 137, 138, 139, 140, 141, 142, 305
kailan, 300, 301, 302, 303, 304, 305, 306, 307, 308, 309, 315, 316, 317, 319, 320, 324, 327, 328, 330, 333
Kailan-Hybrid, 300, 301
Keap1, 5, 8, 73, 85, 94, 111, 113, 114, 115, 116, 117, 118, 119, 131, 134, 139, 140, 186, 189, 190, 191, 192, 194, 195, 196, 201, 202, 206, 227, 234, 247, 276
Keap1-knockdown, 192, 194, 195, 196
Keap1–Nrf2–ARE pathway, 5
Kensler, Tom, 5, 8
keratinocyte chemokine, 221
kidney(s), 47, 49, 51, 53, 56, 57, 58, 59, 60, 61, 64, 65, 67, 68, 69, 72, 73, 92, 104, 107, 130, 134, 147, 160, 193, 201, 209, 214, 216, 217, 220, 223, 224, 230, 249, 308
kinase signalling, 73, 87, 96, 101
kinases, 91, 93, 134

L

LDL-cholesterol, 236, 242, 248
Lewis B. and Dorothy Cullman Chemoprotection Center, 4
lifespan, 90, 100, 102, 242
linoleic, 303
lipid hydroperoxides, 88, 89
lipid phosphatase(s), 87, 95, 97
lipid synthesis, 116, 242
lipogenesis, 226
lipopolysaccharide, 127, 138, 141, 160, 181, 228, 235, 294
lipoprotein lipase, 230

low density lipoprotein receptor-1, 210
Lutein, 284, 308, 309, 321, 324, 330
luteolin, 129, 138

M

macrophage, 127, 129, 141, 186, 198, 199, 206, 207, 216, 217, 228
Maf, 73, 112, 113, 114, 115, 116, 189, 190, 205
malic enzyme, 113, 193
malondialdehyde, 90, 103, 220, 228
MAP kinase phosphatase-1, 98
MAP kinase phosphatases, 98, 108
MAP kinase signals, 98
MAP kinases, 91, 92, 93, 96, 97, 133, 141
MAP/ERK kinases, 92
MAPK, 73, 97, 105, 121, 126, 127, 132, 133, 134, 141, 142, 197
Masayuki Yamamoto, 5
matrix metalloproteinases, 127, 210
MEK kinases, 92
mercapturic acid(s), 3, 146, 191, 243, 272, 273
metallothioneins, 113
methyl jasmonate, 40, 46
Methyltransferases, 57
Michael reaction acceptors, 3
microflora, 62, 124, 146, 190, 195
microwave cooking, 294, 318, 332, 333
migration inhibitory factor, 186, 198, 199, 206, 207
Mitochondria, 58, 192, 193, 204, 242, 276
mitochondrial biogenesis, 116, 119, 139, 193, 205
mitochondrial dysfunction, 141, 192, 204, 227, 244, 249
mitochondrial permeability transition pore, 193
mitogen-activated protein kinases, 105, 106, 126, 132, 138
monoamine oxidase, 58
monocarboxylate transporters, 66
monocyte(s), 129, 133, 142, 160, 209, 210, 211, 221, 224, 228, 235
monocyte chemoattractant protein-1, 129
monocyte chemotactic protein-1, 221
monofunctional inducers, ix, 3, 241
monooxygenases, 56, 77, 78
multidrug and toxin extrusion proteins, 67
multidrug resistance protein 1, 68, 83, 124
multidrug resistance-associated proteins, 69
muscarinic, 211, 212, 213
muscarinic receptors, 213
myosin light chain, 212, 213
myosin light chain kinase, 212

myrosinase(s), 4, 9, 11, 14, 16, 17, 18, 19, 20, 21, 22, 23, 24, 25, 27, 28, 29, 46, 146, 190, 191, 226, 240, 270, 273, 280, 284, 306, 307, 321, 324, 333

N

N-acetyltransferases, 57, 62, 76
NAD(P)H
 quinone oxidoreductase 1, 189
 quinone oxireductase, 112
NAD(P)H oxidase, 96, 97, 98, 210, 213, 214
NADPH, 3, 58, 60, 77, 101, 113, 204, 226, 228
 quinone oxidoreductase 1, 228
neo-glucobrassicin, 33, 36, 37, 38, 41, 43
nephropathy, 230, 231, 236, 237
Nf-κb, 121, 126, 127, 128, 129, 133, 140, 142, 197, 198, 226, 228, 229
niacin, 266
nitric oxide, 223, 237
Nitriles, 20
nitrogen nutrition, 40
NRF2, 121, 126, 131, 132, 134, 142
Nrf2 activation, 119, 160, 193, 217, 230, 231, 234, 242
Nrf2 activators, x, 87, 99, 100, 101, 197, 210, 214, 216, 221, 222, 240, 242, 246
Nrf2 polymorphisms, 101
Nrf2 signalling, ix, x, 90, 100, 101, 111, 115, 116, 118, 119, 219, 239, 244, 247, 276
Nrf2-dependent, 100, 138, 159, 189, 191, 192, 193, 195, 197, 199, 200, 206, 230, 280
Nrf2-independent, 186, 197, 199, 235
Nrf2-knockout, 191, 192, 194, 195, 196, 197
nuclear factor kappa B, 92, 93, 104, 108, 203, 210, 217
nuclear receptors, 85
nuclear respiratory factor-1, 116, 119, 193, 205
nutrigenomics, ix, 113, 239

O

obstructive pulmonary disease, 6, 130
offspring, 168, 181, 216, 218, 219
oligopeptide transporters, 65
organic anion transporters, 66
Organic Anion Transporting Polypeptide 2B1, 112
organic cation transporters, 66, 81
Ornish diet, 101
oxazolidinethiones, 14, 21, 22
oxidative stress, x, 1, 3, 58, 62, 73, 78, 87, 88, 90, 91, 93, 94, 95, 96, 98, 99, 100, 101, 102, 103, 104, 106, 107, 108, 109, 110, 113, 115, 116, 117,

122, 124, 125, 126, 128, 129, 130, 131, 138, 139, 140, 145, 147, 155, 158, 159, 162, 167, 168, 179, 182, 183, 186, 188, 191, 192, 200, 201, 204, 206, 209, 210, 214, 217, 218, 219, 220, 222, 223, 225, 227, 228, 229, 230, 231, 232, 233, 234, 235, 236, 237, 241, 242, 243, 244, 245, 248, 249, 284, 287, 290, 292, 293, 309, 330
oxidized-glutathione, 113, 168, 215

P

p38 MAP kinase, 91, 92, 93, 98
p38 MAPK, 105, 127, 133
p38 mitogen-activated protein kinases, 231
p42/p44 MAP kinases, 92
packaging, 271, 279, 289, 290, 295, 296, 300, 301, 310, 311, 317, 318, 319, 320, 329
PAPOLG, 242
peptic ulcers, 6, 239, 241
perinatal asphyxia, 162, 173, 181
peroxidases, 88, 101, 188
peroxides, 3, 88, 125, 227, 309
peroxiredoxin(s), 89, 96, 106, 108, 113, 132, 140
peroxisome proliferator activated receptors, 226, 229
peroxisome proliferator-activated receptor alpha, 72
peroxisome proliferator-activated receptor γ coactivator-1α, 193
peroxyl radicals, 88, 89
peroxynitrite, 95
p-glycoprotein, 68, 75, 82, 124, 272
P-glycoprotein 1, 124
phase 1 enzymes, x, 3, 5, 112, 191, 241
phase 2 enzymes, ix, x, 1, 3, 4, 8, 111, 112, 116, 131, 167, 202, 203, 204, 225, 233, 240, 243
phase 2 protein inducers, 99, 109, 183, 247
phase I metabolism, 47
phase II enzymes, 51, 56, 57, 61, 62, 63, 70, 71, 73, 124, 147, 227, 228, 237, 275, 276, 281
phase II metabolism, 47, 55, 57
phenolics, 27, 294, 299, 301, 321, 329, 332, 333
phosphatase and tensin homolog, 95, 108, 132
phosphatidylcholine hydroperoxide, 228, 242
phosphatidylinosital-3 kinase, 97
phosphatidylinositol-4,5-phosphate, 97
phospholipase C, 211, 212
photodamage, 186, 196, 197
photoprotective effects, 192
planting dates, 251, 254, 255, 259, 260
plasminogen activator-1 protein, 98
platelet-derived growth factor, 97, 108, 231
polyphenol, 323
postharvest stability, 271, 273
post-harvest technique, 283, 288

pregnane X receptor, 72, 85
Prochaska, Hans, 4
proigoitrin, 307, 308
proinflammatory cytokines, 104, 105, 141, 155
pro-inflammatory cytokines, 128, 129, 130, 133, 134, 187, 188, 192, 210, 228
pro-inflammatory genes, 92, 93, 210
pro-inflammatory processes, 187, 191, 228
prostaglandin D2, 228
prostaglandin-E2, 187
prostaglandins, 127
prostate-specific antigen, 245
protein carbonyls, 90
protein kinase B, 93, 97, 98, 132, 138
protein kinase C, 115, 118, 119, 147, 227, 237
protein phosphatases, 93, 94, 95, 96, 97, 106, 107

Q

Quercetin, x, 101, 121, 122, 123, 124, 125, 126, 127, 128, 129, 130, 131, 132, 133, 134, 135, 136, 137, 138, 139, 140, 141, 142, 143, 241, 247, 289, 304
quinone oxidoreductase, 3, 7, 117, 131, 139, 226, 228
quinone reductase, 7, 34, 118, 275, 276, 279

R

radiation exposure, 145, 147, 155, 158
radiation-induced DNA damage, 145, 155, 158
reactive oxygen species, 73, 96, 106, 108, 125, 127, 129, 130, 140, 145, 147, 149, 159, 179, 186, 187, 188, 198, 210, 211, 226, 227, 235, 249, 292, 309
redox, 78, 87, 90, 92, 94, 99, 101, 103, 104, 106, 107, 108, 110, 111, 113, 114, 115, 116, 117, 118, 125, 126, 131, 136, 140, 142, 165, 188, 202, 204, 210, 211, 216, 222, 223, 233, 239, 242, 244, 245, 247, 249
redox homeostasis, 111, 116, 210
redox sensor, 94, 113
refrigeration, 299, 310, 320, 332
renal disease, 211, 220, 223
renal fibrosis, 231
reperfusion, 117, 209, 220, 234
retinoic acid receptor, 72
Rho kinase, 93, 94, 105, 106

S

schizophrenia, 6, 166, 180, 239, 244, 245, 249
selenium, 44
selenocysteine residue, 101

selenocysteines, 94
serine/threonine phosphatases, 95, 107
signal transducer and activator of transcription 1, 127
sinigrin, 39, 46, 215, 269, 271, 307, 308, 330
skin cancer, 193
skin tumors, 193, 205
Solute Carrier Organic Anion Transporter, 57, 65
Solute Carrier Transporter, 47, 57, 65
solute carrier transporters, 47, 57
sous vide, 311, 316, 317, 321, 322, 323, 324, 325, 326, 327, 331, 332, 333
spontaneously hypertensive stroke-prone rats, 215
Sprague Dawley rats, 215, 216, 217, 219, 220
Src kinase, 130, 137
sterol regulatory element-binding protein-1, 116
stress-associated protein kinases, 92
sulfenic, 96, 99, 106
sulfenic acid, 96, 106
sulfinic, 96, 99, 108
sulfonic acid, 96
sulfonic residues, 99
sulforaphane, ix, x, 1, 4, 5, 6, 8, 33, 34, 37, 38, 39, 42, 44, 45, 90, 99, 101, 102, 107, 109, 115, 117, 131, 139, 145, 146, 147, 148, 151, 153, 154, 155, 157, 158, 159, 160, 161, 167, 173, 175, 182, 183, 185, 186, 187, 189, 191, 197, 198, 199, 203, 204, 205, 206, 207, 209, 210, 211, 214, 215, 217, 219, 220, 221, 224, 225, 228, 231, 233, 234, 235, 236, 237, 238, 239, 240, 241, 242, 243, 244, 245, 246, 247, 248, 249, 261, 263, 264, 269, 270, 271, 272, 273, 274, 275, 276, 277, 278, 279, 280, 281, 284, 286, 289, 291, 293, 307, 321, 329, 330, 333
sulforaphane content, 45, 263, 273, 274, 280, 289
sulfotransferases, 57, 61, 76, 79, 112
sulfur fertilization, 39, 40, 45, 271
superoxidase dismutase, 189
superoxide, 58, 60, 88, 89, 90, 96, 97, 107, 125, 129, 188, 192, 193, 212, 226, 227, 231, 284, 285
superoxide anion(s), 58, 90, 96, 97, 125, 212, 284
superoxide dismutase, 88, 89, 125, 129, 188, 226, 227, 231
superoxide radical, 60, 88, 285
systemic exposure, 47, 48, 49, 50, 54, 56, 68, 69, 70, 71, 72, 74

T

Talalay, Paul, ix, 1, 2, 7, 34, 99, 185
tertiary-butylated hydroxyanisole, 100
tetranor-PGEM, 228
thiamine, 286
thiocyanate(s), 14, 15, 16, 21, 22, 23, 26, 29, 30, 191, 270, 306
thiocyanate ion, 14, 15, 16, 22, 23
thioglucosidase, 24, 240
thiolate ion, 95
thioredoxin, 94, 101, 106, 113, 125, 129, 131, 189, 193, 224, 226, 231, 233
thioredoxin reductase(s), 94, 101, 106, 113, 125, 189, 224, 231
thrombi, 210
toll-like receptor, 93, 127, 129
transforming growth factor-β1, 230
Transporter Associated with Antigen Processing-1B, 112
tropical climate, 251, 253, 254, 259
tubule-glomerular feedback, 214
tumor necrosis factor α, 228
Type 2 diabetes, 100, 105, 109, 122, 183, 221, 222, 224, 225, 226, 227, 228, 229, 230, 232, 233, 234, 235, 240
tyrosine phosphatase, 93, 95, 97, 105, 106, 107
tyrosine-specific phosphatases, 95

U

UDP Glucuronosyltransferases, 57
uercetin, 122, 128, 129
Ultraviolet radiation, 185, 186, 200
urease, 232, 237
uridine diphosphate glucuronosyltransferases, 61
USA, 33
USDA, 33

V

vacuum cooking, 311, 316, 332
vacuum packaging, 319
vascular cell adhesion molecule 1, 231, 287
vascular cell adhesion molecule-1, 221
vascular cell adhesion protein-1, 231
vascular disease, 159, 227, 228, 231, 233, 237
vasorelaxant, 217, 218, 220
vasorelaxation, 211, 212, 213, 214, 217
vitamin A, 267, 302
vitamin B6, 302, 322
vitamin C, 266, 286, 295, 302, 322
vitamin E, 267, 302, 322
vitamin K, 267, 302

W

Wattenberg, Lee, ix, 2
Western-style diet, 100
whey protein, 101, 110

WNT, 121, 133, 134, 142
WNT signaling pathway, 133

X

xenobiotic elimination, 47, 48, 49, 50, 51, 53, 54, 55, 58, 61, 63, 69, 70, 71, 72, 73
xenobiotic elimination system, 47, 48, 50, 51, 53, 73
xenobiotic interactions, 65, 67, 70, 71, 72
xenobiotic metabolism, ix, x, 47, 53, 54, 58, 59, 60, 61, 62, 72, 77, 85, 112
xenobiotic transporters, 56
xenobiotics, 47, 48, 49, 50, 53, 54, 55, 56, 57, 58, 59, 60, 61, 62, 63, 65, 66, 67, 68, 69, 70, 71, 72, 73, 74, 76, 79, 81, 83, 84, 206

Y

yield(s), x, 56, 252, 253, 254, 255, 256, 257, 258, 259, 260, 261

Z

zinc, 107
zinc finger motifs, 94
zona glomerulosa cells, 214

α

α–linolenic, 303
α-lipoic acid, 229
α-tocopherol, 286

β

β cell dysfunction, 228, 229
β–carotene, 308, 309, 322
β-catenin, 121, 133, 134, 142
β-thioglucosidase, 4

γ

γ-glutamylcysteine synthetase, 189